HEALTH CARE SYSTEM AND HOSPITAL ADMINISTRATION

6

SECONDARY AND TERTIARY HEALTH CARE

HEALTH CARE SYSTEM AND HOSPITAL ADMINISTRATION

6

SECONDARY AND TERTIARY HEALTH CARE

DR. S.L. GOEL

Professor of Public Administration (Retd.),
Panjab University, Chandigarh
Editor, Indian Journal of Public Administration, IIPA, New Delhi
Former Member, UGC, Former Member Distance Education Council
Former Member All India Board of Management, AICTE
Member, Executive Council, IIPA, New Delhi.
Former Vice-President, IIPA, New Delhi.
Emeritus Fellow, University Grants Commission
Former Director, State Bank of India (Local Board) Chandigarh
Former Director, National Horticulture Board, Ministry of Agriculture,
Government of India, New Delhi.

DEEP & DEEP PUBLICATIONS PVT. LTD.

F-159, Rajouri Garden, New Delhi-110027

HEALTH CARE SYSTEM AND HOSPITAL ADMINISTRATION
Vol. 6—Secondary and Tertiary Health Care

ISBN 978-81-8450-196-4 (Vol. 6)
ISBN 978-81-8450-198-8 (Set)

Typeset by S.S. COMPOSERS
3190, Mohindra Park, Shakur Basti, Delhi-110034.

Printed in India at MAYUR ENTERPRISES
WZ Plot No. 3, Gujjar Market, Tihar Village, New Delhi-110018.

Published by DEEP & DEEP PUBLICATIONS PVT. LTD.
F-159, Rajouri Garden, New Delhi-110027.
Phones: 25435369, 25440916
E-mail: ddpbooks@yahoo.co.in • ddpubs@gmail.com
Showroom:
2/13, Ansari Road, Daryaganj, New Delhi-110002 • Telefax: 23245122

Contents

Preface

The Health Services are usually organized at three levels, each level supported by a higher level to which the patient is referred. These levels are:

(a) Primary Health Care

This is the first level of contact between the individual and the health system where essential health care (Primary Health Care) is provided. A majority of prevailing health complaints and problems can be satisfactorily dealt with at this level. This level of care is closest to the people. In the Indian context, this care is provided by the Primary Health Centres, Mini-Primary Health Centres, Subsidiary Health Centres; and with community participation along with lot of health providers engaged in the various national programmes.

(b) Secondary Health Care

At this level, more complex problems are dealt with. This care comprises essentially curative services and is provided by the District Hospitals, Sub-Divisional Hospitals, Area Hospitals, Rural Hospitals, and Community Health Centres. This level of services are the first referral level in the health system as the patients are referred to such medical institutes from the periphery health places.

(c) Tertiary Health Care

This level offers super-specialty care. This care is provided by the regional/central hospitals, teaching hospitals and super-specialty hospitals. These institutions provide not only highly specialized care, but also planning and managerial skills and teaching for specialized staff/general staff.

Linkages of Primary, Secondary and Tertiary Level

Hospitals provide a wide variety of services, from basic care to highly specialized diagnosis and treatment, depending on the technological capacity of a specific hospital. There is considerable duplication of services provided at different levels. Tertiary hospitals though equipped with highly sophisticated equipment with advanced technical capacity has to divert considerable 3 Ms to deliver basic secondary and even primary health care.

As either there is a lack of system for secondary and primary health care or the people don't have confidence in them. These hospitals, however, are designed to treat only complicated cases and because of their composition of skilled staff and medical equipment, the cost of treating a patient is much higher than the cost would be for the same type of patient in lower level or specialized alternative facilities in addition the inconvenience to both the patients and their attendants, including the relatives and other well-wishers. This undesirable use of the capacity of tertiary hospitals affects adversely outpatient and inpatient services.

The outpatient departments of large tertiary care hospitals often suffer from overcrowding; this situation is exacerbated by the presence of a large number of patients who require only basic curative care that could be provided in a lower-cost setting such as a district hospital or health centre like sub-divisional hospitals, CHCs or other lower rung medical Centres. If patients requiring basic care could be shifted to medially appropriate lower-level or alternative treatment facilities, health system costs would be reduced and economic efficiency improved as the per capita cost of both outdoor and indoor patients is too high in these hospitals.

Analysis of discharge information by cause and severity of the illness or condition is needed to assess the potential for reallocation of the case load within different hospital systems. In large tertiary facilities perhaps 75% of outpatient care and 30% to 50% of inpatient care could be easily and effectively delivered in district hospitals or at lower levels. A comparison of the cost per outpatient visit or inpatient day between varying levels of hospitals suggests that the savings could be of the order of 50% of current costs per patient.

WHO has advanced the following principles to describe the role of secondary health care institutions:

1. A health care system based on Primary Health Care cannot exist without a network of hospitals with responsibilities for supporting primary care and hospital care. Both are essential parts of a well integrated health care system.
2. An effective primary health care system can only be achieved within the framework of a comprehensive district-based health care system serving a defined population, and the district itself must be a part of regional and national health care system.

We mention here some of the basic problems which need serious attention of policy-makers and Health Experts:

(i) dilapidated conditions of buildings and infrastructure,
(ii) top manpower lacks latest clinical, managerial and technical skills;
(iii) nursing personnel not having job satisfaction and thus have poor rapport with patients and not good relations with doctors;

(iv) lack of reliable Management Information System to regulate patient admissions and registration, medical records management, patient accounting, inventory control;

(v) dis-satisfaction of patients and their relatives to the services of the hospitals;

(vi) lack of linkages among various levels of care—primary, secondary and tertiary; and

(vii) deteriorating quality of Secondary Health Care has led to unnecessary rush at Tertiary Level and mushroom growth of private Nursing Homes, which unnecessarily fleece the people sometimes.

Secondary Level Curative Care

Under secondary level health care services, all types of curative treatment for various diseases are provided. All types of surgeries and other interventions are being carried apart from by-pass and transplantations, which are being carried in the tertiary level institutions (Medical Colleges). In these institutions, all the preventive health care services and other disease control programmes are being taken care of. Let us illustrate in the context of Punjab. Presently, there are 164 secondary level hospitals in Punjab as per following details.

There are 16 District Hospitals having bed range of 50-400 beds. These hospitals are situated in all the districts except in Patiala.

There are 2 Special Hospitals, i.e. Special Gyane Hospital, Mata Kaushyla Hospital at Patiala having 200-beds and Special Children Hospital at Bathinda having 100-beds.

There is one Special Mental Hospital at Amritsar having 400-beds, which has been reconstructed recently and is functioning under the name and style of "Institute of Mental Health", Amritsar, 39 Sub-Divisional Hospitals are there having bed range of 50-60 beds.

Out of 130 above-mentioned CHCs, 107 CHCs are managed by the Punjab Health Systems Corporation (98 CHCs have been recently revamped under World Bank project along with all Districts, Special and Sub-Divisional Hospitals). In these CHCs, apart from preventive health care services mentioned above, curative health services are being provided.

Hospital Services at the Secondary level play a vital and complementary role to the tertiary and primary health care system together form a comprehensive district-based health care system. After prevention, the cure is the only remedy. The Government sector was mainly taking care of preventive measures and insignificant sum of the total was being spent on curative part. It was noticed that District Hospitals, Sub-Divisional Hospitals and Community Health Centres were having critical gaps in buildings, equipment, manpower, and skills and were unable to provide required basic health care services. With an objective to improve efficiency and quality of the health care provided at first referral level hospitals, the State Government took an initiative to prepare a proposal for seeking aid from the World Bank. With the World Bank support, in the year 1996, the Government of Punjab embarked on an ambitious program to improve the state's secondary health services.

Health System Corporations were set-up in different states to improve secondary health services with the help of World Bank assistance. The project aimed at (i) Improve efficiency in the allocation and use of health resources through policy and institutional development; and (ii) Improve the performance of the health care system through improvements in the quality, effectiveness and coverage of health services at the first referral level and selective coverage at the primary level to better serve the neediest sections of society. The achievements of objectives were to be evaluated on the basis of timely implementation of Health Sector Development Programme (HSDP).

Let us discuss in the context of Punjab.

Achievement

The project upgraded 156 secondary level hospitals (including Community Health Centers, Sub-Divisional and District Hospitals) and two Training Institutes. This added approximately 2,100 additional beds in the public sector and provided much needed equipment and medicines. With the help of the project, many studies and activities have been undertaken to revamp secondary health care.

Strengthening the capacity of the Department of Health and Family Welfare for strategic thinking, a Strategic Planning Cell has been established which is functioning under the overall supervision of Managing Director-PHSC-*cum*-Secretary Health. Several studies/activities were undertaken by this Cell which mainly includes:

(i) Equipment Status and Requirement;
(ii) Training need Assessment;
(iii) Size of Private Health Care and Infrastructure in the state;
(iv) Burden of Disease;
(v) Preparation of Draft Nursing Home Registration Act;
(vi) Manpower Study comprising of analysis of staffing position and requirements;
(vii) Analysis on utilization of hospital services and financial analysis on exemptions;
(viii) Assessment of drugs availability in the hospitals;
(ix) Rational usage of drugs;
(x) Mapping pattern of major communicable diseases (GIS);
(xi) A draft policy on public-private partnership;
(xii) Prescribing practices;
(xiii) Study on Health Care Waste Management;
(xiv) Continuous patient's satisfaction surveys;
(xv) Study on Female Foeticide;
(xvi) Maternal Death Audit;

(xvii) Evaluation of training programmes;
(xviii) External validation of HMIS data;
(xix) Preparation and analysis of monthly, six monthly and yearly hospital efficiency report;
(xx) Implementation of IEC strategy;
(xxi) Community perception on utilization of health care services in PHSC *versus* Private;
(xxii) Health Insurance Scheme;
(xxiii) Documentation of processes; and
(xxiv) Revamping/Restructuring of Primary Health Care.

Outcome of the Reform Program

The outcome of the reform program has been impressive, by any standards. Table below indicates the tremendous increase in key performance indicators during the first seven years of the reform program. The number of patients attending secondary care facilities has increased significantly during the last few years. The secondary health care facilities run by the corporation are now dealing with almost 8.5 million outpatients each year, from a total population of approximately 24-million. The table also illustrated that the number of lab tests and diagnostic tests has also short up dramatically.

PHSC Key Performance Indicators: 1996-2004

(Calendar Year)

Performance Indicators	*1996*	*2000*	*2001*	*2002*	*2003*	*2004*	*Increase 2004 over 1996 (%)*
OPD	5197689	5136057	6883072	8347549	8420636	8710854	67.59
No. of Surgeries	39916	118027	143053	152862	229403	319229	699.75
No. of X-rays	80439	196429	307749	460642	551118	633409	687.44
No. of Lab. Tests	278092	1403864	1675987	2283039	3008819	3661952	1180.85
No. of Deliveries	18026	21171	19914	22242	27001	31117	72.62
Diagnostic Tests	358531	1600293	2291485	3204323	3559937	4195361	1070.15

Source: Punjab Health System Corporation.

Let us now discuss about Tertiary Hospitals.

FEATURES OF TERTIARY HOSPITAL

Tertiary Hospitals are of two categories, one set-up by State Governments to cater to the needs of the states. For example in Haryana, it has been set-up in Rohtak. In Punjab, these have been set-up at Patiala, Amritsar, Faridkot. Since, the funds at the disposal of the State Government are limited, therefore, the Government of India, has set-up regional Apex institutions which are highly sophisticated both in infrastructure and quality like All India Institute of Medical Sciences, New Delhi, Post-Graduate Institute of Medical Education and Research, Chandigarh. In addition, the Government of India has set-up apex institutions in specialized areas like eyes, communicable diseases, lung, cancer, chest, etc.

Features of Tertiary Hospitals are:

1. Highly sophisticated having latest diagnostic tools produced by researches in Science and Technology

Tertiary Hospitals occupying top positions in health and medical care system are equipped with latest diagnostic and laboratory instruments which hospitals at lower level cannot afford. These diagnostic tools are used to carry out investigations of diseases of persons who could not be treated at lower level hospitals. In developing countries even tertiary hospitals cannot afford costly equipments. These costly equipments need highly qualified experts to handle them. Such experts are either not available or their cost is so high that tertiary hospital cannot afford.

2. Highly qualified and experienced medical experts are appointed in these tertiary hospitals

Tertiary hospitals are meant for examining and treating exceptional medical cases to ensure expert advice. The best brains within the country and even NRIs are encouraged to join such tertiary hospitals. In India, we do not find such eminent experts resulting into low status of these institutions. Eminent experts are also attracted by private tertiary hospitals as they can compensate them with high perks.

3. Preparing super-specialists in different medical fields

The tertiary hospitals are created to prepare medical specialists in different disciplines through various courses. They are extensively trained in theory and practice of different disciplines. Manpower is the most important requirement for teaching and research.

4. Conduct research in rare areas

Medical experts in tertiary hospitals are supposed to conduct research on rare areas based on theory and case studies. Tertiary hospitals are supposed to carry out research and make available their findings for lower level hospitals. In developing countries like India, medical experts do not find time from their daily routine, to conduct extensive and intensive research. In addition, referral system is not in vogue causing great rush in tertiary hospitals.

5. Make the medical personnel in secondary hospitals aware of the latest development

Medical experts in tertiary hospitals are supposed to provide continuous medical education to medical personnel at lower levels to keep them upto date in medical knowledge.

6. Patients are examined thoroughly as through them experts are exposed to live situations

Patients in tertiary hospitals are examined thoroughly. First of all Medical doctors pursing MS, MD and other high level courses take history and do preliminary examinations thoroughly and prescribe laboratory diagnostic (if needed). After thorough examination, they suggest some remedies. Later on, the Doctor student and the patient approach the Professor and specialist in the areas with all details. The professor goes through the case and discusses with Doctor student in detail. In this way, they reach the diagnosis and prescribe treatment. In this way doctors pursuing higher courses get practical training besides the theoretical classes. That is why only critical patients should approach these tertiary hospitals to make the best use of the resources and expertise.

7. Exchange of information among tertiary hospitals in the country and abroad

The tertiary hospitals are repository of information so that collective wisdom may be pooled for the benefit of critical patients.

8. Tertiary Hospitals in the Private Sector

Recently a large number of tertiary hospitals are coming up in private sector as an industry and not merely for the welfare of the patients. They are very costly and poor patients cannot afford their services. Even, these tertiary hospitals lack moral values as they are engaged in making money. There is a need for some legislation to regulate maximum charges as well some free treatment to poor people. These tertiary hospitals should be asked to adhere to their social responsibility.

9. Division of Labour

Since the tertiary hospitals are complex institutions, personnel working in these institutions are given specific duties to promote specialization and competence.

Role Analysis

There are many conflicts among experts. It is the duty of the Director of Tertiary institute to promote role analysis so that experts work in the tertiary hospitals with full devotions and dedications. Role is the point where the organisation and the individual meet. Role analysis aims to decode the actions expectation from the individual and the individual's expectations from his action with the organisation; and brings into focus where these can meet so as to ensure performance and effectiveness. When expectations of role are materially different or opposite, a person tends to be in role-conflict. This generates psychological reactions—low self-actualisation, low self-esteem, job tensions, job disenchantment/alienation, job dissatisfaction. Role analysis may be used to define a role more clearly to pave the way for effectiveness. The purpose of role analysis exercise is to help the role occupant to clarify his role to reduce role ambiguity, so that he may become more effective.

10. Technical and Administrative Reforms in Tertiary Health Organisations

Just as doctors advise us to get our health system examined during normal times to locate problems, similarly, we must examine the tertiary health organisations to weed out unwanted activities and promote good activities which have been developed recently.

11. Effective Leadership

Directors of these tertiary health institutes need be appointed on merit and not political considerations since the Director is to set the standards of such tertiary health institutes. To quote Gita, Sloka 21, Chapter III: For whatever a great man does, that very thing other men also do; whatever standard he sets-up generally of men follow the same. The common run of men begin to follow whatever the great men establishes by his precept and practices as the standard of morality, and perform their duties exactly on the lines laid down by the great man. This is meant by the statement that "whatever standard is set-up by the great men, is followed by the generality of men." Therefore, the great and noble man of knowledge, holding a position of honour in society, should in the interest of the world order very carefully perform his own duties and thus teach men to perform their duties.

Gita in Sloka 7, Chapter XII and in Slokas 2, 3, and 4 mentions the qualities of true leader. Absence of pride, freedom from hyprocrisy, non-violence, forbearance, straightness of body, speech and mind, devout service of the preceptor, internal and external purity, steadiness of mind and control of body, mind and the senses. Non-violence in thought, word and deed truthfulness and softness of speech, absence of anger even on provocation, disclaiming doership in respect of actions, quietude or composure of mind, abstaining from malicious gossip compassion towards all creatures, absence of attachment to the objects of senses even during their contact with the senses, mildness, a sense of shame in transgressing against the scriptures of usage, and abstaining from frivolous pursuits.

There is a need to understand Organisational Behaviour which is deep understanding prediction and management of human behaviour in organisations. Chief executives must work with a good understanding of his colleagues (team work) coupled with the art of motivating them and ultimately lead to excellence. Development is concerned with dynamic changes to achieve results. The process of change calls for administrators to bring about social, economic, administrative and political changes through the knowledge and practice of Modern Management Techniques.

12. Support Secondary Health Care in the Region

The main function of a tertiary hospital is to provide leadership in all discipline and help the experts in secondary health care with latest developments. The experts at tertiary health care remain too busy in routine activities, they hardly find time to keep in touch with secondary health care and that is why rush in tertiary health care is increasing beyond proportion.

13. All Technical and Non-technical people must follow and respect code of Ethics

The document prepared by Deptt. of Administrative Reforms and public grievances has chalked out a Code of Ethics which need implementation. The objective of Code is to prescribe standards of integrity and conduct that are to apply in the public services. The principles stated below underlie and supplement the rules and laws to regulate the public and private conduct of various public services.

Selflessness

Holders of public office should take decisions solely in terms of the Public interest. They should not do so in order to gain financial or other material benefits for themselves, their family, or their friends.

Integrity

Holders of public office should not place themselves under any financial or other obligation to outside individuals or organisations that might influence them in the performance of their official duties.

Objective

In carrying out public business, including making public appointments, awarding contracts, or recommending individuals for rewards and benefits, holders of public office should make choice on merit.

Accountability

Holders of public office are accountable for their decisions and actions to the public and must submit themselves to whatever scrutiny is appropriate to their office.

Openness

Holders of public office should be as open as possible about all the decisions and actions that they take. They should give reasons for their decisions and restrict information only when the wider public interest clearly demands.

Honesty

Holders of public office have a duty to declare any private interest relating to their public duties and to take steps to resolve any conflicts arising in a way that protects the public interest.

14. Tertiary health care

Tertiary health care in India is not functioning well at present, it is no more than advanced secondary health care system. Tertiary health care must bring out creativity and innovation in health care system in the Region/State through making the health institutions at secondary level aware of the new developments. Such institutions must be provided with sufficient/resources, in terms of experts, material and money so that they can discharge their obligations faithfully. Such tertiary health care institutions must be governed efficiently to optimize the use of resources.

Thus, tertiary hospitals are supposed to keep the medical and health care system of a high quality. However, in practice, tertiary hospitals in India, have degenerated into secondary hospitals. We advance the following problems:

1. Funds allocated to tertiary hospitals are limited;
2. Medical experts are in short supply;
3. Referral system non-existent;
4. Political interference;
5. Great rush of patients;
6. No time for research;
7. No relationships with secondary health care;
8. Corruption;
9. Too many legal cases;
10. Lack of team work; and
11. Lack of job satisfaction.

The Government of India and State governments must provide all facilities to maintain their tertiary health institutions perfect. Merit should be the sole criteria in all appointments. In addition, these tertiary health care institutions must promote the development of health institutions in their areas.

The organisational theoreticians and management experts unanimously agree that a sound climate is extremely important for the ultimate achievement of organisational objectives. Organisational climate refers to the general attitude of members of an organisation to life and work in that organisation. Donald Hellriegael and John W. Solcum Jr. have defined the concept of Organisation's climate as a set of properties of the work environment perceived by the employees who work in the environment and is a major force in influencing their job behaviour. The properties include structure, challenge and responsibility, warmth and support reward and punishment systems, performance standards, production orientation and supportiveness.

The organisation of the 21st century must be built around the concept of flexibility, that is, it is committed to moving, adapting, adjusting and changing as required by changes in its environment. The environment (both external and internal) is constantly changing. Organisation being a part of the environment, must adjust itself in order to remain in equilibrium *vis-a-vis* the ever changing environment. Dynamic executives do not wait for the future they make the future by managing change. In order to manage the change, the organisation must control both the external and internal factors. Let us discuss briefly about them.

To overcome resistance is no mean task. Probably because of this reason, Niccolo Machiavelli rightly contended: " . . . it must be considered that there is nothing more difficult to carry out, nor more doubtful of success, nor more dangerous to handle, than to initiate a new order of things."

We mention here only the names of methods and the details can be found in other chapters—

1. Education and Training
2. Participation and Involvement
3. Incentive
4. Explicit or implicit coercion
5. Visionary leadership
6. Re-engineering
7. Strategic Management
8. MBO
9. OD
10. Just in Time (JIT)
11. Computer Integrated Manufacturing System (CIMS)

Charles Handy is in favour of radical changes in the organisation's climate in the new millennium. To quote him, "One thing is sure. The organisation of the next century are going to be very different from the ones which we knew. Most of the past analysis and writing on the subject will be, frankly wrong or at the best irrelevant. That leaves us with a huge challenge. We have to rethink what an organisation is, conceptually, why it exists, for what and for whom."

Eleventh Five Year Plan, 2007-2012, Vol. II observes that:

Administration of the secondary and tertiary care hospitals will be professionalized and trained professionals posted as Medical Superintendents. Hospitals will be allowed to recruit various staff including junior doctors on ad hoc and contract basis. Drugs purchase should be made through centralized rate contract and decentralized distribution with zero stock at headquarter level. Emergency and disaster stock should be located at each hospital. Drugs at all levels with minimum of one year shelf life should be supplied.

District hospitals, which play a key role in providing health services to the poor, need substantial improvement in infrastructure and other facilities to perform their role more effectively. This would also be a key intermediate step in the health strategy, till the vision of health care through PHCs and community health centres is fully realized. The Plan will also complete setting up of 6 AIIMS-like institutions, upgrading 13 existing medical institutes under the Pradhan Mantri Swasthya Suraksha Yojana (PMSSY) and strengthening the Central Government hospitals. Adoption of PPP mode will be explored for these activities.

It is often observed that Government Medical Colleges and Hospitals are on the verge of derecognition mainly because they fail to adhere to the infrastructure, equipment, and staff norms, as laid down by Medical Council of India. This is thought to be due to lack of funding. The Centre and States will have to make provisions for strengthening these institutions.

In this volume 6, "Secondary and Tertiary Health Care", we have divided the volume into 16 chapters. Chapter 1 discusses the Challenges of Health and Hospital Administration in New Millennium. Chapter 2 examines issues and problems of Secondary and Tertiary Hospitals through the analysis of some hospitals. Chapters 3 and 4 concentrate on two case studies of a Regional level sophisticated hospital that All India Institute of Medical Science followed by Chapter 4 a state level tertiary hospital—Rajendra Hospital, Patiala. Chapters 5, 6 and 7 examine the secondary level hospital at District level and Taluka level. Chapter 8 examines the working of secondary hospital in Thailand. Chapters 9, 10 and 11 examine the role of Chief Executive, role of Professionals and Doctor-Patient relationship in Secondary and Tertiary hospitals. Chapter 12 discusses Referral System to link primary, secondary and tertiary health care. Chapter 13 deals with the role of Nursing services administration in Secondary and Tertiary hospitals. Chapter 14 suggests the need, methods and role of quality health care in Secondary and Tertiary hospitals. Chapter 15 examine the role of Medical Education in preparing, personnel for secondary and tertiary health care. Chapter 16 discusses the role of MBO in improving the secondary and tertiary health care system.

What is needed is to lay emphasis on emerging and thrust areas to keep the medical science knowledge and delivery of health services as per the needs of the people. It is hoped that this book on "Health Care System and Hospital Administration—Secondary and Tertiary Health Care" would make a modest contribution to the knowledge and existing literature on this expanding field. Besides, this would help the academicians, national health officials, public health administrations, medical research workers and the policy-makers and planners in the proper understanding of health care delivery system. I will consider my labour well rewarded if the findings of the study are translated to provide decent health care to the millions of people living in rural areas, urban slums and tribal areas. Comments and suggestions from the readers would always be welcome.

Chandigarh S.L. GOEL

1

CHAPTER

Challenge of Health and Hospital Administration in New Millennium

PART I

CHALLENGES OF HEALTH CARE ADMINISTRATION IN NEW MILLENNIUM

Current problems faced by the health care services include:

1. Persistent gaps in manpower and infrastructure especially at the primary health care level.
2. Sub-optimal functioning of the infrastructure; poor referral services.
3. Plethora of hospitals not having appropriate manpower, diagnostic and therapeutic services and drugs, in Government, voluntary and private sector.
4. Massive inter-state/inter-district differences in performance as assessed by health and demographic indices; availability and utilisation of services are poorest in the most needy states/ districts.
5. Sub-optimal inter-sectoral coordination.
6. Increasing dual disease burden of communicable and non-communicable diseases because of ongoing demographic, lift, Style and environmental transitions.
7. Technological advances which widen the spectrum of possible interventions.
8. Increasing awareness and expectations of the population regarding health care services.
9. Escalating costs of health care, ever widening gaps between what is possible and what the individual or the country can afford.

CHART 1.1

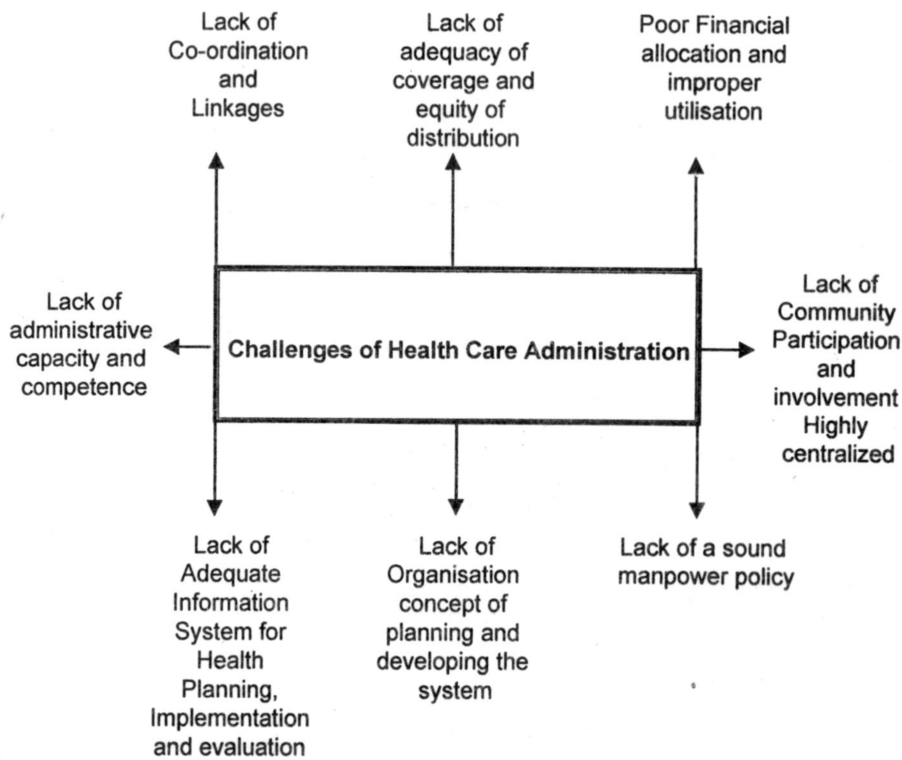

CHALLENGES OF HEALTH CARE ADMINISTRATION

We have examined the present health situation in the developing countries which is quite discouraging though hope-inspiring. There is a great potential in the developing countries to solve all the present and emerging health problems. This needs resolute determination to solve health problems based on proper planning. Health services have become more complex as the result of technological, social and economic advances. In order to reap the benefits of modernisation, a recent UN report has indicated that in both developed and developing countries, "a growing awareness has emerged for the need of a more efficient administration and management delivery of health care services, which will have to be more adapted to local conditions."[1]

We shall discuss the challenges of health administration which need the attention of policy-makers, planners and health administrators, to provide adequate and effective health care to all at the earliest. This calls for strengthening the administration and management of the national health services.

"Effective administration and management all for more intensive preparation and training of senior medical and non-medical administrative personnel, whose functions must be considered in the wider context of the national public administration and not just in the mere limited sphere of public health administration. The major share of national budgets in the future will most certainly go to the departments that develop and use the best systems of planning, performance and programmes accountability ."[2]

Let us now review some of the inadequacies of health administration which need immediate attention to provide decent health care to all. The health care administration has been functioning with the following shortcomings:

(a) The inability of the health care system to make available services required to meet the demands of those most in need, who are usually too poor or too geographically or socially remote to benefit from such facilities.
(b) Wide differences in resources distribution and service and a multiplicity of institutions which are unrelated and not functioning as a system.
(c) The placing of emphasis on medical rather than overall health care. The curative aspect of care has been stressed with insufficient priority to promotive, preventive and rehabilitative care. This has resulted in a fragmentation of the care provided to the individual.
(d) Training of health personnel directed primarily towards medical and institutional care, and largely irrelevant to the tasks and functions required outside institutional settings.
(e) The education and training of health professionals in such a manner as to accentuate the social distance between health professionals and the population, resulting in an inability on the part of the providers of health services to identify with the consumers.
(f) A lack of recognition as well as a rejection of useful, traditional healing practices.
(g) An inadequate assessment of other community resources, imposing unnecessary limitations on the scope of action of health services and often preventing them from approaching major community needs in an effective manner.
(h) The people have rarely been given the opportunity to play an active role in deciding the types of activities they want and have not participated in the actual services they receive. Community interest and resources have too often been Inadequately expressed and activated because there has been a failure to recognise that people will be most interested in and responsive to activities related to their own priority concerns.

We have discussed in detail some of these problems in the various chapters that would follow. We shall concentrate here only on some of the challenges of health care administration.

Lack of Coordination and Linkages

Coordination means bringing about consistent and harmonious action of persons and programmes with each other towards a common goal. The coordination is lacking in the field of health care administration resulting in poor delivery of health services. Professor Mofide (Iran) has rightly indicated the prevailing atmosphere when he states: "In the majority of countries with some or all of these problem (environmental) pollution, uncontrolled population growth; nutritional deficiencies; the high risk of disease; shortages and mal-distribution of trained staff; and insufficient financial, material and physical resources, there exists also a fragmentation of responsibilities for the delivery of health care, with overlapping, conflicting, and competing organisations within the health system and widely scattered funding mechanisms with little control over costs. Health services authorities give only token recognition to those segments of the services that are not under their direct executive or financial control, and often plan only for that part of the national budget that is said to be their responsibility. The state of affairs is unjustified and harmful."[3]

Resources for the health care delivery are limited' in the developing world. An effective health approach and strategy requires the coordinated efforts of sectors and agencies that can contribute directly or indirectly to the promotion of health care. Such coordinated efforts would promote health services that will be more efficiently and effective from both the standpoint of the providers and that of the beneficiaries. The need of coordination is so great that according to Findlay, "It expresses the principles of organisation in toto; nothing less."[4]

The first essential requisite to achieve coordination is to develop—meaningful linkages with sectors of social and economic development which can influence the promotion of health care, e.g., agriculture, public works, housing, communication, education, etc.

The second step is to pool the efforts of all health agencies at all levels in a system to achieve maximum output—public and private; national and international; curative and promotive; peripheral, intermediate and central; western medicine and traditional medicine. This would avoid the dangers of dysfunctional attitudes.

Third, there is the need of welding different aspects of health services into a total health package, e.g., integration of maternal and child care, family planning, prevention of communicable diseases, health education, environmental sanitation.

Coordination and linkages on a systematic, rather than on *ad hoc* basis will definitely reduce costly duplications of effort and lead to increased health coverage of the needy population and neglected area, while making the optimum use of the resources. Most of the countries in their reply to the WHO admitted that the lack of coordination in health care delivery system is a serious challenge. To quote WHO:

> The consensus of opinion is that the most important managerial problems are foreseen in the continued reduction of the imbalance of the system and the lack of integration in the distribution of care with the existence of parallel systems with different objectives. Fragmentation and division of responsibility between the different levels of care have led to a lack of effective communication between the health and social welfare agencies. . . . As there are several agencies providing medical care there is over-lapping and duplication of activities. . . . The major managerial problems. . . .is to recognise the various components of this system in a way that reflects complementarily, eliminates duplication, and minimizes waste of resources."[5]

This problem becomes more acute in a federal country like India where health is a State subject. It becomes important to coordinate the health programmes at the national level. The dilution of health standards in one State may affect adversely the whole country. There is a need therefore, to give more powers to the central authority by making health a concurrent subject. One of the health experts; went on to say: "The present health situation in developing countries, especially India, is in a chaotic condition as no scientific and realistic attempt is visible to coordinate the available inputs to produce maximum output. We can locate a large area without any health care facilities while in some areas, every third shop or house is providing medical care."[6]

How can we achieve effective coordination? According to Dr. White, its achievement may require: "The most delicate insights, the most mature wisdom, and perception of a truly artistic quality."[7]

It has to be achieved through formal as well as informal methods. The effective co-ordination and linkages would automatically result from effective planning, policy-making, manpower planning.[8] After planning and policy-making, the effective instrument to achieve: coordination is to design a sound organisation. Dr. White says:[9]

> "An organisation characterised by clear lines of authority, adequate powers, well-understood allocation of functions, absence of overlapping[8] and duplication of effort and proper delegation of work in itself reduce the necessities of coordination."[9] Besides, if the organisational boundaries are properly demarcated, there would be little scope of confusion and misunderstanding and coordination would naturally flow from this inherent structure.

The coordination among different agencies, however, can be obtained through mutual consultation or information. This mutual. consultation should be encouraged through setting up of inter-departmental agency/ committees for joint planning, joint decision-making and joint action in areas concerning more than one agency. While achieving coordination, we may keep the cost factor in mind. Such inter or intra-agencies can serve a useful purpose when the members come duly prepared with a sense of urgency and commitment. According to Key, "a session of an inter-departmental committee tends to be a place where departmental representatives come well prepared to defend their positions and leave more convinced than before of the correctness of their attitudes."[10]

We are to take care that the benefits achieved though coordination should surpass the expenditure incurred to obtain coordination. Besides formal methods, we should adopt informal methods which are as effective as the formal ones, e.g., the Central Council of Health and the Central Council of Family Welfare (India) uses the informal method to achieve coordination among the different States and between the Union Government and the State Governments. It is the most powerful cement in the whole executive structure.[11]

We must encourage such informal methods at all levels of Government. We must try to achieve coordination to obtain coherency in all the agencies dealing directly or indirectly with health care, all the systems of medicines, all the persons responsible for health care team work and at all the levels through well designed formal and informal organisation with minimum costs to fulfil the goal—the betterment of the health of mankind irrespective of the status and location and to obtain optimum benefit from available and potential resources.

Lack of Equity of Distribution and Adequacy of Coverage in Relationship to Need

According to David Morley:

"Three quarters of our population are rural, yet three quarters of our medical resources are spent in the towns where three quarters of our doctors live. Three quarters of the people die from diseases which could be prevented at low cost and yet three quarters of medical budgets are spent on curative services."

The large population of the people living in rural areas are not being provided even rudimentary health care in this age of modern medicine. The benefits of modern medicine are available only to the chosen few living in metropolitan cities, e.g., 10-20 per cent of the people are consuming 70 per cent of the resources invested in health care in India. What has happened during the last three decades is not in tune with the spirits of the Constitution of India. The Government must serve the millions of people who suffer from chronic poverty, ignorance, disease and inequality of opportunity. The Government must fulfil the aspirations of the people enshrined in the Constitution. Austin summed up the Constitution of India in the following words:

"The Indian Constitution is first and foremost a social document. The majority of its provisions are either directly aimed at furthering the goals of the social revolution or attempt to foster this revolution by establishing the conditions necessary for its achievement. Yet despite the permeation of the entire constitution by the aim of national renaissance the core of commitment to the social revolution lies in Parts III and IV, in the Fundamental Rights and in the Directive Principles of State Policy. They are the conscience of the Constitution."[12]

Have we lived up to the expectations and aspirations of the people? The answer is plain and simple: certainly not. What can we do in future? We can devise technology and organisation objectives and structure that would benefit the largest number of the people and if possible to the last person as desired by Mahatma Gandhi. What is required is change of ideology, philosophy and priorities in favour of the poor people, i.e. any device to improve health care should ensure improvement in the health status of the whole population. This may be possible if our planning in future takes care of the following:

(a) We should attend to the needs of the largest groups rather than meet the demands of a particular group or section of society. We can ascertain the need of the target groups through epidemiological studies.
(b) We may provide that health care to the people through the technology that may reach all. We may not invest in highly sophisticated technology only to be used by the few. The dilemma can be best described as an attempt to ride two horses galloping in different directions. On the one hand is maintenance of the high standard of medical excellence taught in the West. The other is the problem of providing health care for the millions of poor who cannot possibly provide an economic support base for our Western-styled health systems. There is no particular merit in promoting the highest level of medical services when the direct result is medical care casted beyond the reach of four-fifths of the population.[13]

The Government of India is presently thinking of reviving short-term LSMF (Licentiate of the State Medical Faculty) to provide health care to the rural population in 580,000 villages. *The Tribune Editorial* has rightly mentioned:

"The Medical Council of India's opposition to the short-term medical course and the dubbing of Licentiate Doctors as half baked seems strange in view of the fact that in six decades we have failed to remove dichotomy of 85 per cent of the health resources being utilised for the benefit of less than 15 per cent of the country's population. On the contrary, the revival of the licentiate cadre may lessen the burden of the MBBS doctors, especially, general practitioners."[14]

Thus, we must train more and more health personnel of lower categories who can serve the people at large and restrict the few, specialities only for referral services. The United Nations in its 1974 Report on the world social situation reported that:

"Despite the generally greater availability of resources, most governments are faced with difficult choices, because of the recognised need to provide the best possible personnel health care to the rapidly growing population, on the one hand, and because of limitation created by the increase in costs, on the other. Even the most affluent countries have started encountering growing financial difficulties in responding to the health demands of their people. Governments are now paying closer attention to the amount they spend on health services and the value they get in return. They are considering new financing arrangements in the health care field with the objective of reducing the rate of cost escalation and enabling health authorities to achieve flexibility in determining priorities and in pursuing the most efficient and effective approaches to health care."[15]

Kenneth Hill is surprised to notice the opposition of the health experts in the use of Auxiliaries. He says, 'Although the use of intermediary personnel is on the increase, resistance to their recognition continues and this is often even stronger in developing countries than it is elsewhere. It is hard to understand the rationale of such opposition. It is true that there is a remote danger of people with less advanced training developing inflated ideas of their own capabilities, but such people can only be relatively few and they will be found at the fringe."

All this would be possible if the principles of socialism are put into practice. This would encourage political, economic and social democracy. Nehru, in his presidential address at the Lucknow session of AICC in April 1936, expressed his deep faith in the success of socialism. "I am convinced", he said, "the only key to the solution of world's problems and that of India's problems lies in socialism and when I use this word, I do so, not in vague humanitarian way but in the scientific-economic sense. Socialism, however, is something more than an economic doctrine, it is a philosophy of life. . . . I see no way of ending poverty, the vast unemployment, the degradation and subjection of Indian people except through socialism."

If socialism is established in the real sense in the developing world, the entrenched disparities would go away benefiting the poor. This would automatically solve the problems in the field of health care administration as well. As per Declaration on Health Development, South East Asia Region in the 21st Century, (WHO, 1997, p. 4) it is clear that Our Foremost Challenges:

- Closing the gaps and inequities in health in our societies.
- Creating conditions that promotes health and self-reliance.
- Ensuring basic health services to all, especially the poor, women and other vulnerable groups.
- Upholding and enforcing health ethics.
- Placing health at the centre of development.

Overcoming these challenges is the responsibility of governments. But the health sector alone cannot do everything. Partnership must be built with other government sectors, as well as with industry, the private sector, voluntary and non-governmental organisations and with people. We must trust our partners in development, catalyze a demand from the people, set out priorities, lay down standards and stimulate growth with incentives and regulations. Until now, the health sector has largely worked in isolation, yet other sectors have an important role in extending a healthy life to our people. We need to acknowledge this and promote partnerships.

Poor Financial Allocation to the Health Care Delivery and Improper Utilisation of Existing Resources

The developing countries give low priority in the allocation of resources to the health care of their people. We can see from the table given earlier that the expenditure has been very low. The health expenditure to the total expenditure has been very low in South-East Asian countries, i.e. 1.6 per cent in Indonesia, 2.1 per cent in India, 3.8 per cent in Bangladesh. Mongolia has been spending 10 per cent for the health care of its people. There is a need to raise the health allocations to improve the quality of life. Dr. White has rightly said that, "Nothing can be done without the expenditure of money. . . . Available financial resources set a maximum limit on administrative activity as a whole and on each of its separate parts."[16]

A sound state of finance is of paramount importance to the political heath of a nation. . . . The soundness of public finance depends both upon the right policy and good organisation, but a great deal upon the latter.[17] The scarcity of resources affect all aspects of the health delivery system. There is a need to step up the health allocations to the minimum of 10 per cent of the total budget.

Secondly, there is maldistribution of health resources. Most of the health budgets (about 80 per cent) are being spent only on a few people (20 per cent). This deprives the people living in rural areas and urban slums. A WHO study group on the Financing of Health Services which met in Geneva from 21 to 25 November 1977, mentioned the following characteristics which reflect the situation in the developing countries:[18]

(a) Disproportionate concentration of expenditure on health services in urban areas compared with expenditure in rural areas.
(b) Heavy concentration of expenditure on secondary and tertiary care services compared with expenditure on primary care services.
(c) Heavy concentration of expenditure on curative services compared with expenditure on preventive services. We can correct this imbalance through the innovative health policies developed in tune with the needs of the country rather than based on any foreign model.[19]

The third serious problem in this area is of inefficient use of expenditure and non-utilisation of actual and potential resources judiciously and properly. In the developing countries, huge resources are being wasted because of the selection of inappropriate technology,[20] inefficient management[21] and unsatisfactory control mechanism.

Sangita Reddy observed (*Economic Times*, 13 Nov. 2007): Every health care system around the world is constantly working to meet with three objectives. Equitable access, high quality and low cost. For care providers, these are often competing objectives, with the tradeoffs among these goals usually ridden with economic, social and political implications.

The inherent challenge in reconciling the three objectives is common to every health care system, and not unique to any particular country. For instance, many countries have learnt that higher spending does not correlate with higher quality or better outcomes, as is usually perceived by consumers. In fact, the first of the measures that we need to adopt to reduce health care costs focuses on reducing higher spends.

Looking at the history of the evolution of health care systems around the world, we can surmise that throughout, it has been our emphasis on the curative approach, rather than adopting a preventive one, that has been responsible for boosting health care costs. Traditionally, for health care systems, health and wellness are personal matters, while access to care and its financing are more political ones. This view has to be modified considerably to help build an infrastructure to support basic levels of hygiene, and to encourage healthy lifestyles among individuals.

> "It is necessary that public revenue should be raised is an equitable manner and spent economically so that the tax-payers may get full value for his money."[22]

The objects of financial control are to ensure—(i) that no wastage if resources occurs; (ii) that public money is not misused; and (iii) that Intended results are obtained with the money spent. We can exploit the potential resources through careful planning and management. The traditional system of medicine can be of immense value to provide health care at a very low cost provided this is properly tapped by the designers of health services. It was reported in a recent UN Survey that, these adverse trends are despite the higher percentage of government expenditure being devoted to health, compared with 1960s and the fact that ratio of population to the number of beds and of medical personnel have moved favourably. Essentially, the continuance of poor health standards is indicative of a less-than-optimal use of resources available. Some aspects of this are the emphasis on curative, as opposed to preventive techniques embodied in the existing hospital systems, the inadequate development of indigenous medicine systems on which there is a continued reliance and the limited coverage of available medical facilities particularly in rural areas.[23]

In a paper presented by M. Siegel, Assistant Director-General, Department of Administration and Finance, WHO, Geneva, to the Advisory Group on Nursing Administration (16 December 1957) rightly remarked: "If the resources for health work, in trained persons and in finances, were unlimited, the need for constant attention to these factors would not be so great. But the limitation in the number of trained personnel and the lack of adequate financial resources are major obstacles to greatly improved health in the world today. We must, therefore, husband our resources carefully to accomplish as much as possible with what we have available."

The fourth serious challenge in this field is the rising cost of health services beyond the reach of most of the people inhabiting the developing societies. It is very difficult to afford the costly urban-based hospitals using highly sophisticated technology. A huge amount is being spent on costly buildings and equipment which the developing countries cannot afford. The only services which can meet the health needs of the people are low-cost services which should be efficient and effective. This is possible if we use methods and equipment appropriate to the socio-economic environment existing in a country, e.g., the people can contribute voluntary labour to maintain health services. This would reduce the cost. We must take decisions and think of alternative solutions to provide health care to the people as financing and decision-making are complementary functions. The health administrator should encourage the low-cut service programmes beneficial to the larger section of the community.

The fifth problem in this connection is the lack of coordination among different agencies financing health care services. This may result in wasteful duplication of efforts. Besides, many health services may not get the desired financial allocation because of this wastage. The situation can be improved through proper co-ordination among such agencies.

The sixth measure we need to adopt to bring down health care costs is to improve finance mechanism. If we need to insure one billion Indians through a sustainable form of health insurance, we would do well to have a segmented approach to the population. Private health insurance could address the needs of all segments of the society other than the poor in both urban and rural areas. The latter segments will need a public-private partnership approach, and some form of support or subsidy from the government.

The fundamental deficiency in the public health system lies in the gross understanding of the system rather than in the infrastructure per se, which in reality, is far more robust than what is available in several other countries. The public health sector in India is unique in that it must take responsibility not only for producing a steady supply of professionals but also for stimulating demand for them. Optimizing costs is largely dependent on the production, acquisition and management of labour resources, and then on the productive delivery of services.

From a private providers perspective, one can say that improving productivity of processes should mean measurable reduction in service times, as in reducing average lengths to stay and emergency room waiting times. It also means increasing capital productivity as in increasing the number of surgical operation per theatre per day, for instance. Over and above this, we need to strive to optimize costs by making better investments in assets and in technology, and then using them optimally, productively and effectively.

On the whole, there must be an effort to convert our piecemeal approach to interventions at reducing health care costs into a more holistic approach that recognizes the interdependent of seemingly autonomous actions. We need a comprehensive perspective lest our remedy for one aspects generates unintended and potentially negative and costly implication for another act.

The key challenge that India must address to make health care affordable and accessible are liberalizing health insurance, digitization of health care, create awareness about early health as a concept amongst the masses, and increasing the level of integration between government, hospitals and equipment manufacturers to improve the health care system. With insurance covering just 3% of the total population, India remains one of the most under-insured countries in the world. A strong effort must be made to communicate who is covered, how to access benefits, and what screening and other preventive care is available under government and private-pay policies. All consumers of health care will benefit form an increasing understanding of what coverage insurance plans can offer.

Public-private partnerships are the way to revolutionize health care system and make it affordable to the masses. We need to develop health care infrastructure to cater to the projected demand for health care services. Private providers have already made substantial inroads and have set-up facilities both in India and overseas. The government can help this through targeted incentives that can reduce the cost of creation of facilities.

Lack of Adequate Information Required for Health Planning, Implementation and Evaluation

Information is the life-blood of an organisation. According to R.R. Duersch, "it is a system which provides management with the information it requires to monitor progress, measure performance, detect trends, evaluate alternatives, make decisions and to take corrective action."[24]

There is no centralised department in the health organisations to collect, analyse, interpret, store and retrieve information. Confusion between 'Statistical data' and 'information' still prevails, with the result that many statistical services fail to provide public health administrators with the information they need for sound decision-making, planning and evaluation. In most of the health organisations, the data collected from the fields is either not of the required type or is not presented in a form or in time to be really useful to health administrators. Beside, the data is collected without a clear understanding about the use that such information will have. The routine collection of data which is neither reliable nor timely serves no purpose. These defects can be weeded out if we can design a scientific Health Information System or Management Information System (MIS). MIS is an analytical tool which facilitates more informal and better decision to be made and it helps to identify problem areas and to take timely remedial measures. It is in no case a substitute for management decisions but it is management's most important tool for decision-making. As Morton puts it:

> "Good management information system is no cure for bad management. Bad information always leads to bad management, but good information does not in itself ensure good management. Information is only a tool of management. The ability to put information to work is what determines a successful manager."[25]

Four basic processes involved in an information system are the collection of data, storing of data, processing of data and transmission of information. The term data is used to denote the input into the information system while information is the output. MIS should be designed to ensure smooth and proper flow of information into the desired channels. The information must be made available to the management at the required time and in right quantity and quality. It is also to be borne in mind that supplying unnecessary or unwanted information is also a sign of inefficiency of the system. To quote a UNICEF Report: "Information Services should be recast according to the priorities of the health system and should be aimed strictly at problem solving."[26]

Lack of Organisation Concept in Planning and Developing the System

The absence of a clear national health policy in most of the countries has created an environment in which fragmented health services have sprung up haphazardly. There is a need of a balanced health policy. Besides, the health planning though picking up, has yet to be adopted in the right earnest. The planning of health services and their expansion requires special skills and knowledge which must be cultivated among the personnel responsible for planning. Proper identification of the health needs and priorities of the general population is essential for the development of a comprehensive national health plan.[27]

Lack of a Sound Health Manpower Policy[28]

A sound health manpower policy is the main requirement for the development of any functionally effective health care system. Most of the countries in the developing world have never formulated or implemented such a policy.

> "The most crucial factor for the improvement of the World Health situation. . . . is undoubtedly the development of health manpower that is properly attuned to the health problems of the people and suitably, trained to respond to health programme and service need."[29]

We must find the method to achieve greater productivity, efficiency and cost-effectiveness in health manpower utilisation. No society, especially the developing, can long justify investing years of education and training in individuals who later on perform rudimentary duties that could be achieved satisfactorily by people trained in half that time. The critical decisions in health manpower planning concern the kinds of personnel required, the type and adequacy of education and training and financial resources necessary to produce them, their relationship to each other in the health team, and where and how they would practise.

Lack of Community Participation and Involvement

Merle Fainsod remarks: "The most favourable setting for progress in development administration exists where a politically influential and dynamic modernizing elite strongly desires development and can successfully project this attitude into both the bureaucracy and the population at large."[30]

Many well-intentioned and technically sound programmes aimed at solving health problems have been frustrated by a lack of popular acceptance and community participation. It has been observed that such programmes are either not actively associated or passively ignored because they do not 'belong' to the population they are desired to help; they are rather seen by the population as imposed external programmes that belong to the government and consequently deserve and require little, if any, of the population's attention, action, or other response."[31] We must be clear that health cannot be imposed; it can only be acquired. This requires participation based on enlightenment of the beneficiaries.[32]

Dr. Madiou Toure, Director, Hygiene and Health Protection, Ministry of Public Health, Republic of Senegal, in his article, "The Health Revolution", in *World Health* (November, 1979) has rightly said: "The medicine of tomorrow will be shaped by the people for the people, because the people themselves will determine their own condition, their own destiny."

Lack of Administrative Capability and Competence

Administrative capability is *sine qua non* for the success of any programme. It is a major and crucial factor in the success or failure of development programmes. It is the scarcest of all resources in the developing world. The general administrator is fit only for the maintenance of law and order and he is not suitably equipped to deal with the problems of development and welfare economics.

> "According to K.N. Rao: "Unlike advanced countries there is no pool of experienced and well informed leaders of thought available as potential leaders for ministerial positions which greatly handicaps their assuming policy-making and decision-making responsibilities in the Government. This results in over-dependence on the Secretaries who are non-technical general administrators."[33]

The technical experts must be given training in public health administration to make them competent in the art of health planning and administration.

Highly Centralized: Need of Decentralization

The national health system, within whose structure the services Required to deliver care to the urban, sub-urban and rural family nucleus must be organized, is a mechanism of such administrative complexity that it cannot possibly be run on a centralized basis. Hence, the need to decetralize the administrative process. This decentralization should include the extensive delegation of functions from the higher to the intermediate and local echelon, so as to produce effective decentralization in staff management, budgetary control, application of laws and regulations and if possible, financing as well. A consequence of this will be the need to provide administrative facilities at the regional level. An important factor supplementing the mechanisms of decentralization should be the participation of the community and of health professionals in the administration of the regional and local services. In most countries there is a marked trend in the opposite direction, i.e. towards centralization of authority, and it is not always easy to convince the powers that be of the need to decentralize the health services. There are nevertheless many reasons that justify decentralization. One that has already been mentioned is the extent of the facilities needed to provide comprehensive preventive, curative and rehabilitative services to the whole population of a country. This requires a large multi-disciplinary staff which must deliver an enormous variety of services involving different technologies to a population composed of millions of individuals of widely differing cultural levels and with different health needs. The administrative machinery required to operate this gigantic service is so complex that its management cannot be centralized—furthermore, if planning and evaluation of these services is to be conducted locally, it is essential that the implementation of the health activities also be directed at the local level, with the effective participation of the suppliers and consumers of health services.

MEETING THE CHALLENGES

On the basis of our discussion and analysis the following suggestions are given in brief to revitalise the health care delivery system, to meet the challenges and fulfil the basic health needs of the people:

(i) Need of will and determination on the part of the political elite, to accept innovative measures to meet the population's health needs and priorities.
(ii) Identification and implementation of a clear and comprehensible National Health Policy.
(iii) Need of decentralised planning involving the participation of the target community
(iv) Mobilisation of existing and untapped resources-community, government (local and national), bilateral, multilateral and non-governmental to provide adequate health care for all.
(v) Establishment of appropriate administrative structures with necessary competence and capability and devolution of authority and responsibility for the implementation and development of the programme in a team spirit and a well-designed information system to help in planning, implementation and evaluation.
(vi) Manpower development for national health needs.
(vii) Strengthening existing rural establishment and graded extension of national administrative structures to provide adequate and accessible referral, supervisory, logistical and other supporting services to ensure the judicious use of health services.
(viii) More allocation of financial resources based on the principles of equitable distribution and maximum utility.
(ix) Encouraging integration and coordination.
(x) Reorientation of Medical Education to suit the needs of the community.
(xi) Designing health technology to suit the environment and making the best use of existing technology of traditional system of medicine.
(xii) Improving research and development capacity to solve health problems.
(xiii) Devising measures to promote the use of simple, standardized equipment and drugs, placing reliance on available local resources whenever possible to foster self-reliance.
(xiv) The preventive health measures are crucial for sustained improvement and must be intensified to attain:
    (a) Total coverage of the entire urban and rural population in

the country with assured potable drinking water supply and sewerage;

(b) The disposal of urban wastes should also be given a high priority to ensure clean environment;

(c) For improving the environmental sanitation and hygiene, high priority must be given to town and country planning, provision of better working and living conditions, removal of congestion through the increased tempo of housing construction, slum clearance and prevention of water and air pollution;

(d) The nutritional status of the population must be raised and total prevention of food adulteration and drugs control should be achieved through rigorous controls; and

(e) Health education should be an integral part of all health programmes.

SUGGESTIONS GIVEN BY NINTH FIVE YEAR PLAN

(a) Creation of a functional, reliable health management information system and training and deployment of health manpower with requisite professional competence.

(b) Multi-professional education to promote team work.

(c) Skill upgradation of all categories of health personnel, as a part of structured continuing education.

(d) Improving operational efficiency through health, Services research.

(e) Increasing awareness of the community through health education.

(f) Increasing accountability and responsiveness to health needs of the people by increasing utilisation of the Panchayati Raj institutions in local planning and monitoring.

(g) Making use of available local and community resources so that operational efficiency and quality of services improve and the services are made more responsive to user's needs.

Other Suggestions

(i) An absolute and total commitment to improve access to, and enhance the quality of primary health care in urban and rural areas by providing an optimally functioning primary health care system as a part of the Basic Minimum Services;

(ii) To improve the efficiency of existing health care infrastructure at primary, secondary and tertiary care settings through appropriate institutional strengthening, improvement of referral linkages and operationalisation of Health Management Information System (HMIS);

(iii) To promote the development of human resources for health, adequate in quantity and appropriate in quality so that access to essential health care services is available to all so that there is improvement in the health status of community, periodically organise programmes for continuing education in health sciences, update knowledge and upgrade skills of all workers and promote cohesive team work;

(iv) To improve the effectiveness of existing programmes for control of communicable diseases to achieve horizontal integration of ongoing vertical programmes at the district and below district level; to strengthen the disease surveillance with the focus on rapid recognition, reporting and response at district level; to promote production and distribution of appropriate vaccines of assured quality at affordable cost; to improve water quality and environmental sanitation; to improve hospital inflation control and waste management;

(v) To develop and implement integrated non-communicable disease prevention and control programme within the existing health care infrastructure;

(vi) To undertake screening for common nutritional deficiencies especially in vulnerable groups and initiate appropriate remedial measures; to evolve and effectively implement programmes for improving nutritional status, including micronutrient status of the population;

(vii) To strengthen programmes for prevention, detection and management of health consequences of the continuing deterioration of the ecosystems; to improve linkage between data from ongoing environmental monitoring and that on health status of the population residing in the area including health in impact assessment as a part of environmental impact assessment in developmental projects;

(viii) To improve the safety of the work environment and worker's health in organised and unorganised industrial and agricultural sectors especially among vulnerable groups of the population;

(ix) To develop capabilities at all levels for emergency and disaster prevention and management; to implement appropriate management systems for emergency, disaster, accident and trauma care at all levels of health care;

(x) To ensure effective implementation of the provisions for food and drug safety; strengthen the food and drug administration both at the Centre and in the States;

(xi) To increase the involvement of ISM&H practitioners in meeting the health care needs of the population;

(xii) To enhance research capability with a view to strengthening basic, clinical and health systems research aimed at improving the quality and outreach of services at various levels of health care;

(xiii) To increase the involvement of voluntary, private organisations and self-help groups in the provision of health care and ensure inter-sectoral coordination in implementation of health programmes and health-related activities; and

(xiv) To involve the Panchayati Raj Institutions (PRIs) in planning and monitoring of health programmes at the local level so that there is greater responsiveness to health needs of the people and greater accountability; to promote inter-sectoral coordination and utilise local and community resources for health care.

Action-oriented Responses from WHO

A series of challenges call for action-oriented responses from WHO:

- Maintaining a commitment to health for all and primary health care, including oversight of related policy and programme responses throughout the state.
- Ensuring commitment to the values underlying health for all, including the universal right to health, and equity-oriented and gender-sensitive policies and strategies.
- Establishing ethical and scientific norms and standards for health and health care, and monitoring progress in advancing health throughout the Region.
- Promoting combined health and development agendas so that health and other sectors function interactively and complementarily.
- Supporting sustainable health system development, including health system responses—both public and private—to health as a human right and equity as essential commitments.
- Establishing and maintaining surveillance systems for threats to health.
- Supporting human resource development, including encouraging population-based and community-oriented educational experiences in the overall context of health system function.
- Building capacities for science and technology, and contributing to health policy development based on reliable, scientific evidence;
- Facilitating technical cooperation and mobilizing resources in support of health development, particularly for the poorest and backward districts.
- Promoting partnership for change, including commitment to overcome obstacles to health and well-being involving public, private as well as local communities.
- Envisioning likely futures for the health and well-being of the populations of the state and suggesting response options for the state.

It is hoped that the implementation of these suggestions would ensure wider and more evenly distributed health care based on social justice, greater involvement and satisfaction of the beneficiaries and more efficient and more economical health services.

Part II

HOSPITAL ADMINISTRATION

Hospital infrastructure has grown in both size and complexity as well as hospitals have grown both in size and direction, making its management a challenging task. With the coming in of polyclinics and big hospitals in private sector, the problems of hospitals administration have compounded. What are the problems that are likely to be encountered by hospitals in new millennium? What can be done to make them serve the cause of health of the community? How can we translate the definition of health given by WHO to make the lives of people healthier. Let us discuss some of the potential problems and their solution that the hospitals are likely to face in the new millennium. We may keep the following words in mind. We cannot continue doing what we have always done. Tomorrow cannot be just more of yesterday. We need flexibility and pragmatism as much as innovation. But the stress must invariably be on action.

In *World Health*, in an article, "Globalization and Public Health, a new challenge for WHO", (51st year No. 2, March-April 1998), it was emphasized that it is important to note, however, that the implications of globalization for public health are not all negative. The diffusion of modern technologies and ideas between countries present promising opportunities for improving global health in the future. Recent advances in telecommunications technology, can be exploited for health purposes, which include: telemedicine, interactive health networks, disease surveillance systems, communication links between health workers, human resources development and continuing education, and distance learning.

In summary, a strong case can be made that the globalization of public health represents an important trend for the 21st century. Although some transnational health problems have historical precedents, many new issues are emerging which are unique to our time. The 1997 Kyoto conference on climate change under-scored the fragility of the world's ecosystem, and showed how interdependent the health of all of humanity has become. Shared global problems transcending state borders call into question conventional paradigms which divide countries into North and South, or developed and developing. Let us discuss important problems and their solutions. (See Chart 1.2)

CHART 1.2

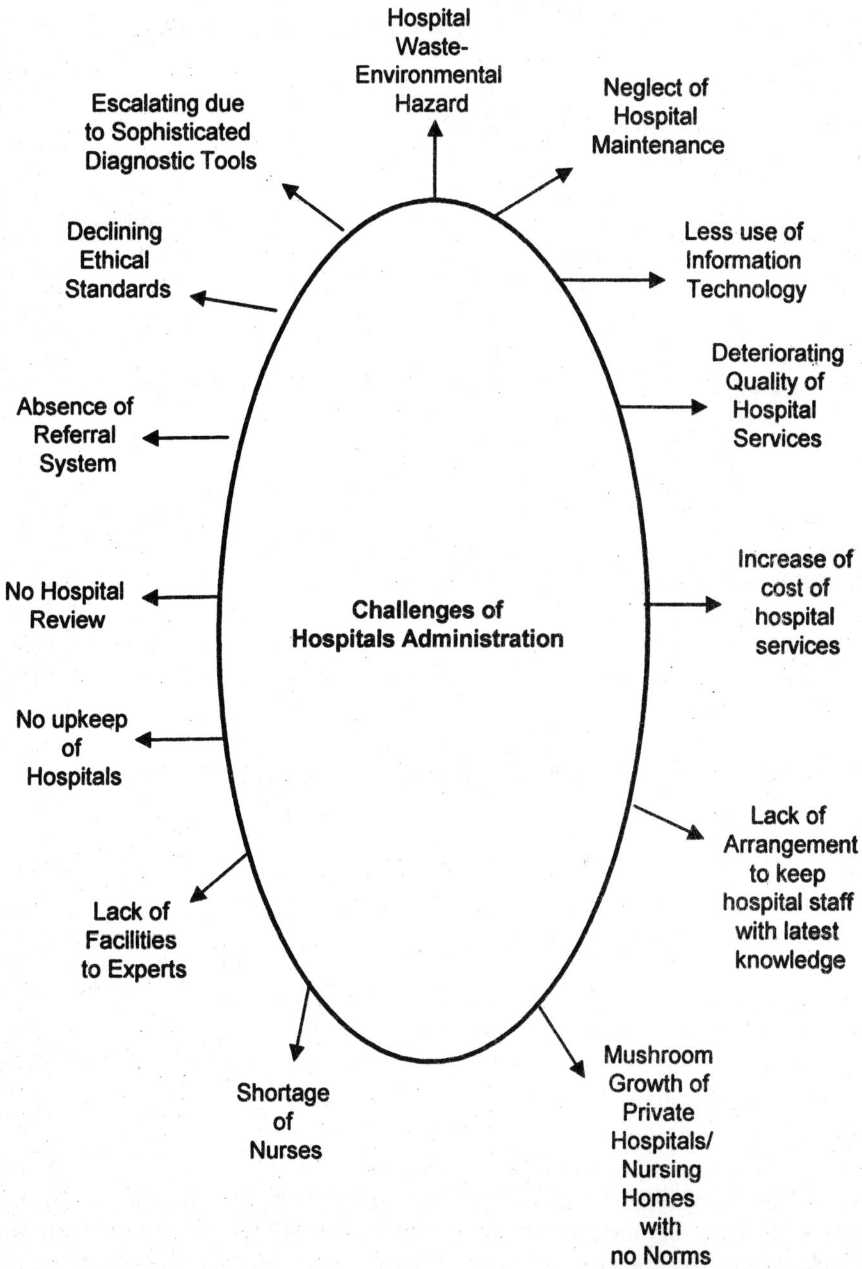
Hospital Waste- Environmental Hazard
Neglect of Hospital Maintenance
Escalating due to Sophisticated Diagnostic Tools
Declining Ethical Standards
Less use of Information Technology
Deteriorating Quality of Hospital Services
Absence of Referral System
Increase of cost of hospital services
No Hospital Review
Challenges of Hospitals Administration
No upkeep of Hospitals
Lack of Arrangement to keep hospital staff with latest knowledge
Lack of Facilities to Experts
Mushroom Growth of Private Hospitals/ Nursing Homes with no Norms
Shortage of Nurses

I. COMPLEXITY OF HOSPITALS CREATED BY EVER INCREASING SOPHISTICATED DIAGNOSTIC TOOLS RESULTING INTO HIGH COSTS BEYOND BUDGETARY ALLOCATION: NEED OF ANALYSIS AND PLANNING

The developments in science and technology has resulted into the designing of complex medical equipments which can help medical experts in easy and accurate diagnosis and treatment. The development is so fast that old instruments become outdated after 3-4 years. All these equipments cost heavily and are mostly beyond the reach of many hospitals. Even if some hospitals acquire them, they have to cut on essential items, thus badly affecting the efficiency of hospital services. It is a paradox as to how to get the best of medical equipments as well as remain within financial constraints. This is a dilemma for many planners of the hospital. Based upon personnel observation, discussion and study, i.e. suggest here some points to come over this serious problem.

(a) Need of Defining the Objective of the Hospitals

First of all, it is necessary to define the objective of the hospital, i.e. what level of health care is to be provided and to meet that care, what instrumentation and medical equipments are required? Upon the answers to this question would depend the purchase and use of equipment. What happens in practice, equipment available is not used, equipment needed is not available. It needs a thorough analysis before equipping the hospital with any new equipment.

(b) Need of Ensuring the Technical Manpower to Handle Costly Equipments

In most of the Government hospitals, equipments are lying idle and becoming junk because of not appointing the required technical personnel to handle the instrument. Even if the personnel are available, these become outdated and thus need be trained to make use of the latest knowledge.

(c) Need of Maintaining the Output to Ensure Benefits

Most of the equipment in Government hospitals either remain non-functional or work at lowest output resulting into highest per unit cost. It is done intentionally so that the patients may be referred to private laboratories to oblige/earn commissions. The technician's salary should be dependent and made conditional to the minimum output. His responsibility should be fixed and he should be held personally responsible for all the lapses. It may be mentioned here that he must be associated with the purchase of the machinery. He should be given necessary authority. Equipment should be used at least in two shifts and even private patients may be encouraged to use the services at some premium.

(d) Essential Use of these Equipments should be Encouraged but not a Routine Affair

It has been seen that it has become a fad with most of the specialists to prescribe unnecessary tests using complex instruments to make their false reputation and prestige resulting into wastage of resources both of the hospitals and the patients. It is suggested that doctors should prescribe only essential tests and move from simple to complex and not jump to complex examination. Doctors should be encouraged to develop more and more of their clinical sense.

Besides, costly equipment either not used or mostly remain non-functional causing losses worth crores of rupees. Let us illustrate with some examples reported by Poonam Bath in Tribune dated July 13, 2000. She stated that Machines worth lakhs of rupees are not being put to any use in the Department of Physiotherapy, PGI. While, some of them are out of order, a few other which are brand new, are yet to be used

The department, which has been recently shifted to the new OPD block, has a daily OPD attendance of 100-150 patients. It offers patients, at least five different forms of the therapy. This includes electro therapy, exercise therapy, heat therapy, hydrotherapy and manual therapy. But the non-functioning machines are causing problems not only for the patients but for the doctors as well, who are forced to recommend an alternate therapy in the absence of the required therapy. Sources reveal that a bio-tech machine worth Rs. 25 lakhs was purchased by the institute in 1997. But till today it is lying locked up in the department. Even a short wave diathermy machine, which is used for heat therapy, is out of order most of the time. Similarly, another machine for heat therapy, which is an essential equipment used to reduce the muscle spasm and various kinds of body pains, is not being put to its optimum use as half of its screen is damaged. One of the regular patients, who comes here for exercises, said earlier this machine was being used to give heat treatment to facilitate exercises, but this is not being used now.

(e) Private Laboratories may be Identified and Contracts Entered to Facilitate Cheap and Efficient Services

Even if the hospitals are overloaded or cannot provide the services, they may enter into contract with private laboratories to provide cheap and efficient services.

(f) Indigenous Equipment of Quality Need be Preferred

It has become a fashion to use imported equipments resulting into loss of foreign exchange and unemployment. Our equipment manufacturers can supply quality equipment provided corrupt practices are strictly dealt with and transparency in purchases is ensured.

2. DECLINING PROFESSIONAL ETHICS AMONG SPECIALISTS AND OTHER HOSPITAL STAFF: NEED OF DEVELOPING ETHICAL STANDARDS

The tendency to make money is on the increase in the profession. Medical professionals attend on priority the wealthy and influential people who can compensate them directly or indirectly while neglecting the common man. This tendency is on the increase and can become a big problem in new millennium.

Bertram M. Gross, an eminent Professor of Urban Affairs, Hunter College, City University of New York, has remarked: "One of the most important characteristic of a genuine profession—in addition to a recognized body of knowledge or skill and some organized provision for training, recruitment or certification—is a code. of ethics. Professional codes of ethics, recognize the special power that may be exercised by someone with expert skill and knowledge. They are desired to protect clients against the abuse of such power by the professional—whether he be a doctor who penetrates bodily secrets of clients or a lawyer who learns the details of their private affairs."[34]

Large scale bureaucratic management, particularly when equipped with the most refined calculational techniques, can develop—to use Erich Fromm's words—a spirit "inhospitable to life, joy, independence, love, compassion, meaningful human relations, real intimacy and sharing between people." If the public administrators, managers and political leaders in developing countries cannot develop non-bureaucratic methods and institutions, "the result will be increasing loneliness, boredom, aggressiveness, competition, consumption—from cars to sex, liquor and drugs-and cruelty as the result of a lack of compassion."[35]

We can thus say that there is a need to develop both human and modern technology to improve efficiency. We must, however, give priority to human development. As stated in a UN Report: "There are two aspects to development technical and human. Organisations had usually been more sensitive to possibilities offered to them by the achievements of modern technology than to the refinements of human behaviour as revealed by the sciences of Sociology and Psychology. On the other hand, lessons drawn from experience showed that technical innovations derived from the engineering sciences encountered considerable resistance unless supported by corresponding changes in human attitudes and behaviour. In an era of rapid change, the improvement of management in its human aspect had become a critical issue. It was important to make full use of the findings of social sciences which endeavoured to be instrumental in giving guidance in behaviour of individuals and groups in varying circumstances. Organisations should, therefore, be conceived as complex, socio-technical systems whose management required both technical skills and insight into the motives of human behaviour."[36]

It is widely agreed that manipulation and lack of integrity produce strong negative side-effects and reduce organisational effectiveness. With this important value commitment the organisation may shift their styles and climate from one of direction, control and surveillance to one of providing help, support and instruction. Mutuality and collaboration between the leaders and the led, self-control and mutual support are essential for creating an organic organisation. Let the newcomers strive to set-up organized society with social democracy and high human values settings up ideal societal or public management institutions and if such timely warnings are not accepted, social upsurges are bound to develop in a mild or a violent form.

J.S. Neki has rightly said that "to help, to heal, to reconstruct, to comfort—and all along the line to act with compassion—all these bear testimony to the moral consciousness of the doctor. Whatever the new strains imposed upon medical ethics this structure will survive and continue to guide doctors in their professional conduct. Level and juridical obligations they have, of necessity to fulfil. But these are not genuine ethics. Genuine ethics has to be integrated into character and does not have to depend upon external controls."[37]

R.S. Pathak, former Chief Justice of India rightly mentions that the vitality of an ethical dimensions in the discharge of public responsibilities is essential to a developing nation. In a developing nation, the release of nascent national energy is a great moment. It provides the power necessary for building of a nation.[38]

We suggest here some points to make ethical standards practicable and feasible:

(i) Top leadership should follow ethical standards to serve as bacon light for the health functionaries at the lower level.
(ii) We should encourage professional standards to inject in the medical team the spirit of service.
(iii) New entrants need be supervised properly so that wrong behaviours may be corrected in the initial stages.
(iv) There should be code of ethics which should be followed by all.
(v) Environment of the hospital should be such which can inspire confidence and loyalty.
(vi) Medical team should be respected and given due status.

3. ABSENCE OF REFERRAL SYSTEM CAUSING MISUSE OF RESOURCES

We may mention here that we cannot afford the scarce resources for health services being wasted in duplication, overlapping and mismanagement. There is at present no proper referral system in place. Once a patient is received at particular institution, the doctor examines the patient and decides whether he/she can be managed there itself, or needs a referral to a higher level facility. There is complete lack of coordination among the peripheral institutions, on the one hand, and between the institutions and district hospitals, on the other. There are no guidelines or procedures that govern the peripheral institutions and the higher-level hospitals in a referral chain. No written or unwritten conventions exist as to what types of conditions are to be treated, from where and when. There is also no prioritization of referred cases, either from private or government institutions. Lower-level facilities lack even basic facilities, equipment and major specialists, leading to a large number of self-referrals and overcrowding in the higher level facilities. In the new millennium, we must promote forward and backward linkages among all levels and institutions of all systems of medicine to provide decent health services in new millennium. At present, our hospitals are working in isolation causing misuse of services. In the new millennium, we must define the clear-cut referral system to provide integrated health services and pooled wisdom of health experts.

Conceptually a multi-tier system which combines preventive, curative and specialized care is efficient when it provides patients access to levels of care that are appropriate to their health needs with a minimum of inconvenience and delay. It works best when the lowest tier is easily accessible to the community and provides the bulk of the preventive care as well as curative care services for common illnesses. Patients with more complex problems are identified in a timely and systematic manner and referred to the appropriate higher level. Each successive level provided services that are more complex and therefore more expensive. In such a system, the higher tier provides technical leadership and support for the lower tiers, and the community has confidence in the quality of care provided at each tier and the patients understand they will be in accordance with patient needs.[39]

4. HOSPITAL WASTE CAUSING ENVIRONMENTAL POLLUTION AND LEADING TO NEGATIVE RECYCLING WITH SERIOUS MEDICAL AND HEALTH CONSEQUENCES—NEED OF SERIOUS THINKING AND ACTION

Hospital waste is causing great health hazards especially in metropolitan and big cities where large number of hospitals are located. Hospital wastes include both infectious and non-infectious substances coming out of different wards, OTS, OPD, Emergency services, etc. Such wastes can create hospital infection as well pose major cause of environmental pollution. Hospital waste will contain injurious items such as: infective tissues, or dressings; radioactive materials; and contaminated syringes and needles. Special care must be exercised in disposing of these items by incineration, burial, or other means. In particular, disposable syringes and needles may be sought by drug abusers, and should be rendered unusable. The channels for disposing of hospital waste will depend on local circumstances and legislation. There is a need for every hospital to set-up hospital waste system. The hospital waste can cause infectious problems to:

(a) Patients and their relatives who come to the hospital.
(b) Personnel providing hospital services from doctors to sweepers.
(c) Impact on environment causing many health problems—Where hospital wastes are dumped, it becomes an ideal breeding ground for rodents, mosquitoes, bacteria, virus, flies, leading to many complex diseases. These can contaminate the water and air and can cause serious health problems for the residents.

The quantity of hospital wastes is on the increases as more and more disposal items are being used. In the new millennium, it may be very high. So, there is a need of scientific management of hospital wastes. It means removal and disposal of waste economically and hygienically on a scientific basis.

Generally two methods of waste treatment are in existence:

(i) Incineration.
(ii) Steam Sterilization.

Incineration is a process which converts solid wastes into harmless gases at 1400 degree Fahrenheit. While steam sterilization uses steam penetration. Hospitals in India both Government and Private are not using scientific methods. They are dumping the wastes nearby or throw them at some distance of the hospital. In this way hospitals are becoming the cause of environmental degradation and causing many health hazards than providing good health care. Even, where incinerators are provided, these are non-functional. In the new millennium, we suggest that hospital waste management must be given top priority, otherwise we would be creating our own health problems. We suggest the following to be done in new millennium:

(a) All hospitals with 30 beds and above should install incinerators.
(b) All health centres must dispose of the wastes carefully,
(c) All health institution should have a manual on waste handling procedure and those made responsible for it should be provided a training for it.
(d) Strict supervision must be done by directors/medical superintendents and local administration over the waste disposal.
(e) No private health establishment should be allowed to function until and unless they have developed proper waste disposal system.
(f) Care should be taken that unscrupulous element may not recycle the waste.

The Tribune, May 19, 2000 nicely reported the situation of waste disposal in Rohtak and Jhajjar districts. The Drug Control Department, Haryana has reportedly taken strict measures to check the sale and storage of medical waste in the state in view of the reports regarding the development of a "nexus" leading to the supply of used disposable syringes and intravenous (IV) sets for recycling and resale in market. According to sources the Drug Control Department has alerted its officials and directed them to conduct raids at clinics and hospitals in rural and urban areas in the state. While the focus area remains the districts lying in proximity of the national capital, 'raids' can be conducted at any clinic anywhere in the state.

Officials of the department have conducted several "raids" in Rohtak and Jhajjar districts. According to reports the authorities had "recovered" used disposable syringes and Intravenous (IV) sets weighing about four kg from a clinic run by a registered medical practitioner (RMP) at Barahi village in Bahadurgarh sub-division, about 40 kms from Jhajjar. However, some of RMP's working in the same village fled before the officials reached their clinics. The "accused" medical practitioner is charged with storing used syringes and intravenous (IV) sets instead of destroying these immediately after use.

The authorities produced the samples of seized material in the court. The officials also recovered some expired medicines from a chemist's shop at Badli village in Jhajjar district. The shop is run by Ramesh Kumar. Meanwhile, according to sources raids had also been conducted in Bahadurgarh and Rohtak towns, but with no major success. A senior official, however, said raids would continue.

The officials reportedly became alert after reports in the media regarding the recovery of two truck loads of medical waste (used syringes and IV sets) from Delhi. The matter became serious when the issue was raised in parliament and the government assured that proper action would be initiated to check the "entry" of recycled medical waste into market. The recycled hospital waste poses a risk of the spread of AIDS and Hepatiti B.

The Drug Controller, Haryana, has issued instructions to the district drug inspectors and officials of the Health Department to step-up the campaign and identify the persons engaged in storing, selling and recycling of medical waste.[40]

However, the shortage of staff and inadequate infrastructure in the department could hamper the campaign against recycling of medical waste. Hospital waste poses a great hazard as it can spread infection, but most hospitals don't follow any standard waste disposal method. Government hospitals as well as the private nursing homes dump their waste just like ordinary garbage. Needless, syringes, dressings, swabs immersed with blood, pus or other body fluids, culture stocks, infected or unused blood are all disposed of in the same way. Only placenta and body parts are buried or burnt. Advent of new technologies has revolutionised the diagnosis and treatment methods, but at the same time it has also added to the quantum of hazardous waste.

The Ministry of Environment and Forests formulated certain rules called the Biomedical Waste (Management and Handling) Rules, 1998, to be followed throughout the country, but these are being flouted everywhere.

For evolving national guidelines on hospital waste management, the All India Institute of Medical Sciences (AIIMS) organised a two-day expert committee meeting in November, 1998, where medical officers and health administrators evolved guidelines, which were published and circulated to all states. But they have hardly been followed. The Ministry of Environment and Forest has categorised and notified two types of medical waste in the bio-medical handling and management rules. Each category needs a separate disposal treatment. But this is not done in most hospitals. The whole lot is dumped with waste from other sources infecting the latter also. Scavengers are the potential carriers of infections.

Rajan Kashyap in his article "Dangers from Medical Wastes—Need for multi-disciplinary approach" in *The Tribune,* dated July 13, 2000 stated that even as hospitals provide solace and relief from disease, the dangerous wastes generated by them have become a serious hazard which threatens public health. Indiscriminate disposal of hospital wastes is indeed" a major source of pollution and infection. Bio-medical wastes from hospitals, nursing homes and clinics include hypodermic needles, scalpel blades, surgical gloves, cotton, bandages, clothes, medicines, blood and body fluid, human tissues and organ, body parts, radio-active substances and chemicals. Some of these contain harmful organisms. Reuse of discarded syringes/needles can transmit lethal disease like AIDS and hepatitis. Similarly, indiscriminate recycling of used cotton, clothes and medicines poses a host of health hazards.

For a solution, it is necessary to appraise both visible and invisible factors. A multi-disciplinary approach would have to be adopted for the management of bio-medical wastes. This must incorporate the following:

Legal Measures

- The Ministry of Environment and Forests, Government of India, has framed Bio-Medical Wastes (Management and Handling) Rules, 1995. The Central Pollution Control Board has formulated guidelines for safe handling of hospital wastes. Compliance must be enforced.
- Allocation of resources of the Central Government and the state government for an integrated programme of bio-medical waste management.
- Closer coordination between the Department of Health of the state government and municipal administration.
- The establishment of a commonly managed and integrated system of final disposal of medical wastes, linked to a fair debiting of costs to the generators of the hazardous wastes.
- Drastic reform measures in municipal administration for raising

adequate financial resources for optimal utilisation for the management of hazardous wastes.

- Involvement of non-governmental agencies which are closely linked to the people who suffer the adverse impact of mishandled hazardous wastes.
- A well-directed public awareness campaign.
- Harnessing technology for achieving clearly developed objectives.
- Structured training programmes for all staff members engaged in the handling of the wastes. These could include the introduction of specific diploma or even degree level courses in medical or engineering institutions, as also some practically-oriented courses for workers.
- A strong monitoring system, which determines accountability of the polluter and of the handler of the hazardous wastes.
- Enforcement of the polluter pays principle.

5. MUSHROOM GROWTH OF PRIVATE HOSPITALS WITH NO NORMS—NEED OF DEFINITIONS

Private hospitals are coming in a big way to make good the inefficiency of Government hospitals but with a heavy price. Ravinder Sood, reporting from Palampur (H.P.) said (*The Tribune*, May 22, 2000) that health services in this remote comer of the state has received a big boost with the setting up of a private hospital in the town. However, he cautioned that it is a sad state of affairs that despite spending crore of rupees every year, still, the government hospitals in the state has failed to meet the medical needs of the people. Every year the state government is spending over Rs. 120 crores on health services in the state but still the common man is deprived of health facilities.

In the new millennium hospitals would become big business exploiting both the doctors and the patients and benefiting the owners. Satya Prakash Singh in his article in *The Tribune*, dated May 30, 2000 rightly observed that given the same environment and budget, hospitals in private sector provides better service, and can see the mushrooming of private nursing homes in a city like Chandigarh, which has the prestigious PGI and a modern government hospital. It would be tantamount to complacency if one thought that the growth of private nursing homes in the city was only due to the increased demand for medical service and that government hospitals were not able to cope up with.

There is a definite shift from government hospitals to the private sector. The future therefore, is that of private sector hospitals. Due to competition the quality of medical services is expected to improve to a satisfactory level for those who can afford to pay. The future of medical service for the teeming millions below the poverty line (and one should not believe that those above the poverty line are not poor) is indeed bleak. Even if the blissful world of perfect competition prevailed, in distant future, where the services would be produced and sold at a level of "prices equal to the marginal revenue equal to the minimum marginal cost", the poor would still not adequately be served. That level of minimum cost too would be too high for them to afford. There is no harm in supplementing health services by private hospitals but with some state laws, norms and controls. State must help in providing various inputs in setting up private hospitals and also exercise its regulatory authority in respect of the following through medical council of India:

(a) Doctors engaged by private hospitals should be paid at least as per the government pay scales.
(b) Security of service must be ensured through service rules.
(c) Fees from patients need be approved by government for various services.
(d) Regular inspections need be done by experts to ensure quality of essential services.
(e) Hospital should not be located away from residential complexes.
(f) Mechanism of redressal of grievances of patients must be devised.
(g) Hospital must report on a pre-designed performa after a regular interval of time.
(h) Parameters for setting up private hospitals/nursing homes need be defined so that they may not become nuisance to people living nearby.
(i) Norms of services should be spelt out.

There is a need to make use of the private initiative in a big way and associate them as an equal partner in the provision of Health Care. As the population is booming, with resultant increase in pressure on medical services, the inadequacies of Government managed hospital facilities are coming into focus. While the Government cannnot wish away its role in providing some basic health and medical services to those, who can't afford it against cost, it is becoming increasingly evident that system failures can no longer be put under the carpet.

Now the time has come, when Government should restrict its role to providing primary health care and promote/support the private sector to establish and provide the remaining medical services. Let the private sector get pre-eminent role in management of health services, with administrative and financial support coupled with some controls of the Government. This will save the public exchequer from unnecessary and wasteful expenditure and available costs of Governance in health and medical sector.

We can thus say that the government should come forward with a legislation defining parameters for setting up private hospitals/nursing, homes, otherwise, the government would have to face greater challenges.

However, there are many health institutions or private practitioners who are doing good work. The Government should encourage them and associate them in the total process of health care.[41]

6. LACK OF ARRANGEMENTS FOR KEEPING THE HOSPITAL STAFF EQUIPPED WITH LATEST KNOWLEDGE IN NEW MILLENNIUM IN CLINICAL, TECHNICAL AND MANAGERIAL COMPETENCE— NEED OF DESIGNING NEW METHODS

There is no doubt that the efficiency of the hospital service depends to a substantial extent on the clinical, technical and managerial competence of the hospital staff. However, it has been seen that doctors technicians, supporting staff, hospital administrators, once appointed, on working in their narrow grooves. New millennium is unfolding man's new skills in every area to make hospital system efficient and effective A lot of research is being undertaken at various places in new method but these do not reach to most of the hospital personnel and thus the benefits of new knowledge are never translated in practice. What can done to overcome this? How can we keep hospital staff in tune with new millennium? How can we make them think tank of the hospitals? We suggest here some points which can keep the hospital staff effective and efficient.[42]

(i) There is a constant need of in-service training both for the government and private practitioners.

(ii) Teaching-cum-research institutions like PGI, AIIMS, etc. should start some evening classes or a fortnight course where doctor can undergo training in latest techniques. Medical associations, speciality associations and alumni associations medical colleges can also play a significant role in this behalf.

(iii) Teaching-*cum*-research institutions can send the speciality in the concerned field to make doctors in the field aware of the latest development as well as distribute literature in the are concerned.

(iv) An Open Medical University may be set-up where courses in all areas are available. This can benefit in a big way. Mode techniques like tele-conferencing, computers may be used to reach the health and medical personnel in the remotest area.

(v) Telemedicine, a new technique can help the doctors to be in touch with the latest developments in the institutions in entire world benefiting both the doctors and the patients.

Health Telematics is defined as a composite term for health-relation activities, services and systems carried out over a distance by means information and communications technologies for the purpose of global health promotion, disease control and health care, as well as education management and research for health.[43]

Dr. Prakron Vuthipongse, permanent Secretary, Ministry of Put

Health, Thailand, in Inter-country Workshop on Tele-Medicine for Health Development in 21st century from 30th March-3 April, 1998 at Bangkok said that as a decision-maker he was aware of the advancement in today's technology, especially in its applications which will help to bring better quality of health care to people in remote and rural areas in a cost-effective manner. He also said that the initiation of Tele-Medicine in the Ministry of Public Health has emerged from the fact that, in remote and rural areas, there has been mal-distribution of medical specialities, resulting in poor health care services. He expected the workshop to come up with fruitful recommendations on regional and national plans of action as well as on inter-country cooperation.[44]

However, this very conference cautioned about the use of Telemedicine: Health Telematics raises certain ethical issues, such as the acceptability of transmitting personal information across cultural boundaries; young doctors getting professionally affected, and the confidentiality of the relationship between the patient and the treating doctor. Full cooperation of the medical and paramedical staff involved, as well as patients is essential. Even in the most advanced form, Health Telematics might not provide a blanket solution for each situation. There would be cases where human intervention is needed. It also raises concern on widening the gap between the poor and the privileged.[45] Thus, in the new millennium the use of tele-medicine offers a potential source of latest knowledge, however, we must use it with great caution and thought.

Dr. R.A. Mashelkar, Director General, Council of Scientific and Industrial Research, delivered the convocation address at the 30th Convocation of Indian Institute of Technology, New Delhi. He said, "Knowledge without innovation is of no value. It is through the process of innovation that knowledge is converted into wealth and social good. Innovative nations lead the world today. When one looks at India, one feels that centuries of subjugation have perhaps undermined our capacity for innovation and creativity, which has got to be revived. We cannot allow the 'I' in India to stand for imitation and inhibition, it must stand for innovation. This requires an all pervasive attitudinal change towards life and work-a shift from a culture of drift to a culture of dynamism, from a culture of idle prattle to a culture of thought and work, from diffidence to confidence, from despair to hope. Revival of creativity and the innovative spirit needs to be made into a national movement today, in the same spirit and on the same scale as marked our freedom struggle.[46]

Dr. R. Chidambaram, Chairman, Atomic Energy Commission and Secretary to the Government of India, Department of Atomic Energy, delivered the Convocation Address at the Third Annual Convocation of Shivaji University, Kolhapur, he said, "For a nation to grow and advance rapidly, it has to strive for excellence in all its spheres of activity. Dr. Shivayogi P. Hiremath, Vice-Chancellor, Kuvempu University, Shimoga (Karnataka) delivered the Convocation Address at the Graduation Day—1999 of JJM Medical College, Davanagere. He said:[47]

"Doctors on the net is a common caption in most of the Western Countries. Why are so many people turning online for medical information? Experts suggest that there is something inherent in the quick turnover medical office visits that it leaves patients wanting more and more connection, more personal interest, more explanation and more help."

A doctor has to be a constant student and should always work hard to keep abreast of the field by regularly attending the Continuing Medical Education (CME) programme.[48]

7. INCREASING COST OF HEALTH SERVICES: NEED OF RESOURCES MOBILISATION AND COST CONSCIOUSNESS

In the new Millennium, the cost of hospital services would increase beyond the capacity of the hospital resources. The expenditures on salary, equipment and drugs would be an ever increasing pressure on the capacity of the hospitals. The result would be either dilution of quality of services or limiting the hospital services. In both situations, hospital services and prestige would be affected. Let us explains with the help of Indira Gandhi Medical College, Shimla—As reported in *The Tribune* (June, 2000) out of even sanctioned strength of 186 posts comprising of 55 Class I, 70 Class II and 70 Class III are lying vacant while the number of OPD patients increased from one lakh in 1993 to 2.30 lakhs in 1999, and indoor patients increased from 11,295 to over 16,000 during the same period. Because of financial shortage, these posts instead of increase, have not been filled. Patient care has deteriorated. Patient care has been far from satisfactory as there are not enough nurses in the 661-bed hospital as against a requirement of 600 only about 200 were in position.

Even all the existing posts have not been filled and at present 186 posts, including 55 Class I, nine Class II and 70 Class III posts were vacant. While CT scan, ultrasound and other facilities were introduced, no new posts were created.

What can be done to keep the hospital services in operation in the new millennium? We suggest here some facts and suggestions:

(i) Hospitals should set-up an economy committee which should scrutinise the current activities, their mode of financing and their utility. An examination would indicate a great scope for curtailment of unwanted expenditure.

(ii) the Director/Medical Superintendent through financial experts apply the modern management techniques like performance budgeting, zero-base budgeting, cost accounting, etc. to ascertain the genuineness for expenditure and its utility, e.g. what is the cost per patient admitted to an emergency? What is the cost per operation? In this way, we can locate where expenditure can be controlled without affecting the delivery of quality health services.

(iii) Hospital staff should be made cost-conscious so that they should use hospital resources judiciously and economically. They should use only those services which are essential.

(iv) Since a large part of the hospital expenditure is on the salary of medical and supporting personnel there is a need to ensure optimisation of their services. It has been seen that a lot of time is wasted by the hospital staff in non-medical activities. By making use of method study, work measurement, activity analysis we can improve upon the utilisation time of hospital staff. Hospital authorities have to be strict on punctuality and availability of hospital staff to justify their salaries. In India, most of the hospital staff remain busy with private practice and work in private hospitals, therefore, they cannot justify their work in hospitals. Strict action is required on this account as doctors are already paid NPA.

(v) For resource mobilisation, there can be users' charges. The appropriateness of adopting cost sharing principles depends on the type of service provided. Hospital services are mostly patient-related curative services. There is a scope to charge on curative services provided, a mechanism exists to adjust fees depending on the patient's ability to pay. However, the additional revenues generated by cost sharing may not be adequate to cover fully the expenditure in improving quality through better facilities in terms of equipment and drugs. The argument for cost sharing is based on efficiency. If no fee is charged there will be an "excess demand" for services especially hospital beds. Government hospitals are crowded and often the resourceful but the undeserving people get free access, whereas the poor have to incur "transaction costs" to get treatment or a hospital bed. Graded cost recovery from the non-poor is expected to restrict demand for beds thereby releasing beds for the poor. Thus, cost sharing may be a step in restoring equity; the poor may benefit proportionately more than the non-poor.

Charging fees for services may only slightly affect the demand negatively for health services because demand for in-patient and out-patient care is highly inelastic. However, consumers will be the responsive to the quality of care, time costs and the relative prices alternative types of care givers. Cost sharing will augment resources for the health sector and should, therefore, lead to improvements in supply both in Qualitative and quantitative terms. Sustainability would also be promoted to a large extent beause the revenue realized would finance a portion of the operational costs thereby, relieving the budgetary constraint. Cost sharing would result in improvements in the quality care if the resources generated internally by a hospital are ploughed back for improving the availability of drugs and equipment in that hospital. Introduction of measures to augment resources will not automatically raise the level of infrastructure unless the concerned institution is in a position to reinvest a substantial portion on the hospital. Ideally, each secondary and tertiary level hospital should establish a "Development Fund" and open a Bank account where the collections from Cost Sharing would be remitted.

All hospitals should also be entitled to receive donations from philanthropic organisations and individuals, undertakings in the private and public sector, etc. and credit to its "Development Fund" which can then be used for undertaking civil works, purchase equipment, drugs, hospital supplies, etc. Mobilisation of resources and injecting economy are the two important areas which can ensure the quality of hospital services in new millennium.

8. DETERIORATING QUALITY OF HOSPITAL SERVICES—NEED OF INTRODUCING HOSPITAL ACCREDITATION—QUALITY OF HEALTH CARE IN HOSPITALS IS DETERIORATING

The hospital system suffers from major handicaps. It was reported in *The Tribune* (June 2, 2000), that Doctors prescribes medicines of sub-standard companies. To quote: "The Government Zonal Hospital has not been supplied stationery for a long time and various things like the OPD slips, in-door patient chart", X-ray prescriptions are being sought through donations. The hospital laboratories too are in a sorry state of affairs. The ambulance service is also reported to be miserable. The three drivers have been posted on shift duties, but usually two of them remain on furlough. The only driver on duty takes his own time for attending emergency calls.

There is no casualty ward service available. The laboratory and X-ray technicians do not attend the emergency duties in protest against the failure of the government to pay them 10 percent house rent emergency allowance. The ECG technician has not been posted for past two years. A Class IV employee has been deputed for taking ECG.

Budgets meant for maintaining equipment and building need to be stepped up. The hospital system in the State suffers from many handicaps. Budgets meant for maintaining equipment and building need to be stepped up. Diagnostic facilities, equipment, ambulance and trained personnel require strengthening. Existing norms for staffing at various levels have to be reviewed, given the heavy pressure on the hospital system which currently results in poor quality of services. Similarly, norms for equipment and the range of clinical services at each level need to be worked out on a rational basis. The infrastructure needs thorough overhauling as well as expansion to meet the needs of the over strained hospital system. Management skills at the hospital level need to be continually upgraded. The overall environment in which the hospitals function need improvement.

Quality of health care is defined as "the degree to which health services for individuals and populations increase the likelihood of desired health outcomes and are consistent with current professional knowledge" (National Academy of Sciences, USA, 1997).

Quality of health care can be assured if the government introduces accreditation of hospitals in 21st century. WHO, South Asia Regional Office organised a workshop in "Hospital Accreditation" at Bangkok, Thailand from 7-11 Dec. 1998. The group found the following advantages of accreditation:[49]

- Stimulates improvement of care.
- Strengthens community confidence.
- Reduces unnecessary costs.
- Increases efficiency.
- Promotes personnel training.
- Provides credentials for education.
- Can protect against lawsuits.
- Provides comparative data.

The Indian government proposed to take the following measures to introduce accreditation:

(1) Initiate the process for setting up a core group in the Ministry of Health.
(2) Sensitization of policy-makers by organizing national-level workshop by January 1999 for generating awareness about the need for hospital accreditation.
(3) Sensitization of professional bodies, service providers, and consumer groups by organizing regional workshops.
(4) Organize discussions on proposed legislation for compulsory registration of hospitals.
(5) Set-up expert groups to suggest minimum conditions for hospital registration.
(6) Set-up expert groups to suggest standards for hospital accreditation.[50]

Accrediation is going to be beneficial to both the providers and receivers of the services. Providers would be clear as to what standards are to be maintained and the receivers would know what to expect from the particular hospital. In this way, there can be a race among hospitals to get accreditation for better marketing of their services. Even in universities and colleges accreditation is being done in a big way National Assessment and Acreditation Council (NAAC), an Inter-University Centre of University Grants Commission. Health Department of the Union and State governments can set-up such accreditation councils for hospitals under the auspices of Medical Council of India. We have to take care that this work should be done in association with professional associations, research institutes, so that there may be resistance at the implementation level

9. NO HOSPITAL REVIEW: NEED OF STUDY AND RESEARCH IN DIFFERENT AREAS OF HOSPITAL ADMINISTRATION

Hospital administration is being run by hit and trial methods without undertaking in-depth studies in various areas of administration affecting hospital services.

In the new millennium, the hospitals should be run on scientific lines. This would require research and in-depth study of various administrative issues impinging on the medical services. Some of the areas may be mentioned here:

- the effective use of hospital services, e,g. X-rays, beds and imaging and other services;
- staff issues such as job satisfaction and the retention of staff members, particularly nurses and other highly trained personnel;
- patient satisfaction;
- a clinical data, such as readmission rate, length of stay for various illnesses, and the effectiveness and efficiency of referral to and from the hospital and health centres;
- cost-benefit analysis of different programmes;
- the incidence, etiology, and prevention of infection; a design of new aids and gadgets for the care and comfort of patients, especially the disabled;
- management of human, financial, and material resources;
- a quality assurance in hospitals;
- cost accounting of various services;
- a utilization time of different categories of persons; and;
- transport efficiency.

10. NEGLECT OF HOSPITAL MAINTENANCE: NEED OF MAINTENANCE AND BEAUTIFICATION

The first impression of the visitors to the hospital depends upon the proper upkeep of buildings, equipment, water-supply, electricity supply, etc. A visit to a number of hospitals revealed the following which should be taken care of in the new millennium:

(i) The surroundings of the hospital are covered with congress grass and is full of dirt. Even in many hospitals there are no boundary walls. It is suggested that green grass and plants should be grown to make the hospitals clean and greener.

(ii) Buildings of the hospitals are in bad shape. Because of the shortage of funds, these are not maintained properly. These become the breeding ground of insects and cause infection. In the hospitals, buildings must be maintained properly at regular intervals of time to avoid deterioration.

(iii) Sweepers and ward boys must be encouraged to keep the hospital clean. They must be told that cleanliness is very important for the recovery of patients.

(iv) Lavotaries are in bad shape and even stinking. Hospital authorities must attend to it seriously otherwise the foul smell make the whole environment of the hospital unpleasant.

11. NEED OF HARNESSING POTENTIALITIES BEING OFFERED BY NEW DEVELOPMENTS IN THE FIELD OF REGENERATIVE MEDICINE AND INFORMATION TECHNOLOGY

At the dawn of 21st century, we find the most important development in medicine is development of the science of Human Genome, involving human genetic engineering which will change the contours and contents of medical science. William Haseltine in his article, "What the genome map means to your health." Enormous potential for both good and bad in *The Tribune*, dated July 2, 2000 clearly says that:

- Molecular medicine leads to improved diagnosis of disease; earlier detection of genetic predispositions to disease, rational drug design; gene therapy and control systems for drugs; and pharmacogenomics "custom drugs."
- Microbial genomics explores new energy sources (biofuels); environment monitoring to detect pollutants; protection from biological and chemical warfare; and safe, efficient toxic-waste clean-up.
- Risk assessment assesses health damage and risks caused by radiation exposure, including low-dose exposures; assess health damage and risks caused by exposure to mutagenic chemicals and cancer-causing toxins; and reduce the likelihood of heritable mutations.

Though less than a decade in the works, it is already clear that the combination of the genetic and information revolution will change medicine within the next 50 years more than in the past several centuries.

12. NEED OF STREAMLINING THE UP-KEEP OF HOSPITALS THROUGH METICULOUS PLANNING OF HOSPITAL SERVICES

It has been seen that specialists and other staff are handicapped because of Non-availability of minor facilities which indicate callousness on the part of hospital authorities. For example, many a times, it has been found, trolleys are either not available or out of order, services of barber, bearers, communication facilities, transport facilities are not available. There is a need of planning in toto and not for some services only, as the absence of small services can lead to the death of a patient. Poonam Bath reporting about the death of a girl in (Chandigarh, *The Tribune*, dated July 2, 2000) mentioned the following factors responsible for it:

- Ambulance not available,
- CT scan machine out of order, and
- No barber to shave patient's head.

Besides the mother of the deceased complained of rude behaviour of the hospital staff, 'The rude and callous behaviour of nurses and security staff also added to our woes. Nurses were busy chatting even as we kept requesting them to suck out blood from her lungs as she was finding it difficult to breathe."

Thus, the medical Superintendent must ensure the availability of these facilities or get these arranged from outside and not leave all these to be arranged by the patient's family as they are in a state of psychological trauma and shock. Director of PGI, Chandigarh, where the death of the girl took place, instituted an enquiry into the incident and confirmed that the CAT Scan remains out of order till today (Chandigarh, *Newsline*, July 4, 2000).

In a government hospital in Cuttak (Orissa), three women died because of the infectious saline water. These cases are a daily occurrence and can be avoided with careful hospital management.

13. CONSTRAINTS WITH WHICH MEDICAL PERSONNEL WORK AND LIMITATION IN SUCCESS OF TREATMENT

While endorsement of inefficiency or sheer neglect on the part of a hospital or its staff is uncalled for, it would be prudent to understand the constraints under which the hospitals and the medical personnel have to serve the ever increasing number of critical patients, some of which may not respond to a well proven treatment or the nature of infection may be incurable or the delays in administration of treatment may occur despite the best efforts of the doctors on duty-due to multifarious pressures and bottlenecks, while judging their performance it is imperative to examine, whether the person was adequately skilled to handle the situation, whether there was intention to help to the best of his capability, whether an all out effort was made to render the service promptly and properly. If the answer to the above questions is 'Yes' no charge of negligence can be made out. It goes without saying that the staff has been accessible, humane, committed sympathetic with patients.

It is to be brought home loud and clear that medical treatment/

hospitalization does not guarantee cure/amelioration in all cases. Things often go wrong, inspite of earnest care, concerted effort, advanced investigation, skillful surgical/medical treatment. The adverse outcome of cases involved in serious injuries, often leads to sudden grief, manhandled of the medical and paramedical personnel and eventual media headlines, showing the medical profession/hospital in bad light. This require education to public on a continuing basis, besides providing security/ insurance against outbursts of violent/anger leading to danger and risk to the life and property at the hospital.

It is suggested that local NGO/Red Cross play an important role in planning of utilization of services available and provide personnel services like transport, wheel chairs, drug, stores, barbers, bearers, etc. This can cut down an un-necessary delays, thus savings vital time between the onset of emergency situation and active intervention. Any undue adverse publicity in the media against premier hospitals, will lead to greater stress on the minds of treating physicians/surgeons and prove counter-productive. However, the hospital administration should take seriously to healthy criticism and effect efficiency and improvement, whenever possible.

14. USE OF INFORMATION TECHNOLOGY

India is the world's IT hub. However, very few hospitals in India have started to digitize their hospital and patient records. IT will enhance efficiency of the hospital and productivity of doctors drastically. It has also resulted in better utilization of real estate as the storage of patient files is now digital. Another area India can do well is tele-technology and tele-cardiology. Given the shortage of skilled health care professionals, experts can provide diagnoses and second opinions remotely. We can overcome the shortage of nurses/manpower and reach more people in the rural areas, potentially saving millions of dollars and inconvenience in the process.[51]

15. SHORTAGE OF NURSES

Hospitals are facing shortage of Nurses: Nurses with higher qualifications are leaving hospitals because of better pay scales in the Private Sector.

Better avenues in the private sector for nurses has left a brunt on the quality of patient care in the PGI, which is facing a shortage of more than 10 per cent of staff in the department of nursing.

The department is run by diploma nurses in a majority of cases as the institute has failed to retain post-graduates and graduates in the department. The death of a newborn on October 26, allegedly due to the negligence of a nurse, is a glaring example of the decline in patient care due to fewer qualified nurses, an official said on condition of anonymity. There are only 1,320 nurses at the institute against 1461 posts. A majority of nurses leaves after acquiring higher qualification in the field.[52]

16. HEALTH SECTOR REFORM

South-East Asia Regional Office in its Declaration suggests the need of Health. Sector Reform to make Implementation on Health Planning a reality:

- Accord highest priority to alleviate the burdens of disease, disability, premature death and suffering afflicting our people, especially the poor: The burden of disease is of greater magnitude in this Region than in any other. We call for urgent policy, budget and programmatic initiatives.
- Ensure universal access to quality health care: We will initiate reforms of the health sector (needed to respond to the broader concept of health and contemporary core values) to ensure the new role of government in relation to health which emphasizes, policy formulation, facilitation, regulation and coordination functions, in addition to the traditional provider role. This includes strengthening the infrastructure, equitable financing, decentralized decision-making and governance, promoting private sector panicipation and improving emergency preparedness and response
- Invest in women's health and development to eliminate gender discrimination and disparities: In this we recognize the inextricable link between women's health and the development process and the vital contribution women make to family and community life. Gender issues will be brought into the mainstream of development.
- Encourage application of scientific knowledge and technology: Science is an essential feature of health development and requires strong links with policy-makers. We will strive to ensure that both the generation and the application of scientific knowledge and technology are relevant and appropriate to the needs of the community.
- Mobilize financial resources for health and promote their effective and efficient use: We will advocate for increased allocation of funds for health development and ensure their optimal utilization. Indeed, voices must rise from society as a whole, insisting that adequate resources are made available for basic health care.
- Involve communities as active partners in health development: We recognize that communities are essential resources for health development. They must be actively involved in planning, implementing and monitoring policies and programmes for health.
- Propagate and preserve medicinal plants: We will ensure that in the conservation of biological diversity, the great wealth of

medicinal plants in our Region is preserved and their extinction or exploitation for mere commercial gain prevented. The scope for inter-country cooperation in this area is great. We urge other countries to transfer technical know-how on favourable terms to the developing countries.

- Promote traditional medicine: Our Region has a rich heritage of indigenous systems of medicine. We will strive to integrate these into the mainstream of health care, promoting traditional systems that provide relief, are scientifically proven to be safe, and are easily available, accessible and affordable.[53]

CONCLUSION

Besides, in the new millennium, the hospitals should attend to maintenance of buildings, equipment, dietry services, security services, registration services, etc. to maintain the prestige and dignity of the hospital as well as ensure quality health care in new millennium. In this great venture, hospital authorities may seek the involvement and co-operation of the people to make the medical services, patient-oriented.

Hospitals in the new millennium should provide an environment of extended family where the patients can get professional and expert medical care and homely environment. Patients should be welcomed in this extended family type hospital services. A spirit of service and dedication must pervade among the providers of the health care as they are considered second God on earth by the receivers of health care. In the new millennium, we must empower the patients for looking after them carefully and making them feel important.

The progress and achievements of the past 50 years are solid foundations for a healthier and better world. Life in the 21st century could and should be better for all. We can pass no greater gift to the next generation than a healthier future. That is our vision. Together, the people of the world can make it a reality.

Notes and References

1. UN, 1974 Report on the World Social Situation, New York, 1975, p. 218.
2. WHO, WHO Office Records, No. 226, 1975, p. 113.
3. WHO, Public Health Paper, 55, p. 83.
4. RM. Findlay, Art of Administration, Edinburgh, Oliver, 1952, p. 48.
5. WHO, Public Health Papers, 55, p. 61.
6. Based on personal discussion.
7. L.D. White, Introduction to the Study of Public Administration, Macmillan, pp. 213-14.
8. For details refer to the respective Chapters.
9. L.D. White, *op. cit.*, p. 214.
10. V.O. Key, Politics and Administration in White (Ed.), The Future of Government in the United States, p. 155.

11. S.E. Finer, Primer in Public Administration, London, 19SO, p. 68.
12. Granville Austin, The Indian Constitution: Cornerstone of a Nation, Clarendon Press, Oxford 1966, p. 50.
13. Christian Medical Comimission: An Exercise in the Development of Health Care Priorities", Geneva, 1974 (unpublished document-CMC/47/6), p. 1.
14. *The Tribune*, Chandigarh, August 1979.
15. UN, 1974 Report on the World Social Situation, New York, 1975, p. 219.
16. L.D. White: Introduction to the Study of Public Administration, Macmillan, N.Y., p. 201.
17. Gyan Chand, The Financial System of India, p. 1.
18. WHO, Technical Report, 925, p. 18.
19. Refer to the Chapter on 'Health Policy'.
20. Refer to J.H. Bryant, Health and the Developing World, Ithaca, N.Y., Cornell University Press, 1969.
21. WHO, Modern Management Methods and the Organisation of Services, Geneva, WHO, 1974 (Public Health Papers, No. 5).
22. P.K. Wattat, Parliamentary Financial Control in India.
23. UN (ESCAP), Economic and Social Survey of Asia and the Pacific, 1976, Bangkok, April 1977, p. 18.
24. Raymond J. Coleman and M.J. Rilley (Ed.), Management Dimensions, Holden-Day, INC, San Francisco, California, p. 5.
25. Morton F. Meltzer, The Information Centre: Management Hidden Asset, American Management Association, New York, 1967, pp. 136-37.
26. UNICEF, Health and Basic Services: Keys to Development, p. 50.
27. For details, refer to the Chapter on 'Health Planning'.
28. For details, see the Chapter on Health Manpower Planning and Development.
29. WHO Chronicle, 31:123-126 (1971), "Health Challenges for 1978-83."
30. Merle Fainsod, "Structure of Development Administration" in Irving Swerdlow (ed.), Developmrnt Administration: Concepts and Problems, (Syracuse, N.Y., Syracuse University Press, 1963, p. 1).
31. WHO Chronicle, 30 (19/6), pp. 177-78.
32. For details, refer to the Chapter on Primary Health Care Administration.
33. R.N. Rao, Home Challenges in Health Administration, Background document to Xth Staff College Course at NIHFW, Mimeographed.
34. U.N.: ST/TAO/M/52/Add. I, p. 53.
35. Erich From: "Thoughts on Bureaucracy" (guest editorial), Management Science (Providence, R.I.), August, 1970.
36. U.N. Inter-Regional Seminar on Administration of Management Improvement Services (Vol. I), Cohagen, Denmark, 28 September-6 October, 1970, pp. 6-7 (ST/TAO/M/56).
37. J.S. Neki, Medical Ethics: A View Point from the Developing World, *World Health*, July 1979, p. 15.
38. R.S. Pathak, Ethics in Public Life, Some Observations, in *IJPA*, July to Sept. 1995, p. 265.
39. Government of Karnataka, Karnataka Health System Development Project, Bangalore, 1996, p.102.
40. *The Daily Tribune*, May 19, 2000.
41. *The Daily Tribune*, May 28, 2IXXJ.
42. *The Daily Tribune*, May 30, 2IXXJ.
43. WHO: SEARO, Health Telematics, Report of a WHO Inter-country Workshop on Tele-medicine for Health Development in the 21st Century, Bangkok, Thailand, 30th March-3rd April, 1998, p. 4.
44. *Ibid.*, p. 2.

45. *Ibid.*, p. 5.
46. AIV, *University News*, Sept. 20, 1999.
47. AJU, *University News*, April 21, 1997.
48. AJU, *University News*, Aug. 19, 1999.
49. WHO: SEARO, Hospital Accreditation Report of an Inter-country meeting, Bangkok, Thailand, 7-11, December, 1998.
50. *Ibid.*, pp. 41-42.
51. Raja, CEO, GE Health Care, "How can health care be made affordable", *The Economic Times*, Chandigarh, 15th Nov., 2007.
52. Chandigarh, *Tribune*, Saturday, Nov. 17, 2007.
53. Health Development in the South-East Asia Region in the 21st Century, WHO, 1997, pp. 5-6.

2

CHAPTER

Administration of Hospital Services

(A Typical Secondary and Tertiary Hospital)

A. NATURE, CLASSIFICATION AND INDICES FOR THE MEASUREMENT OR THE EFFICIENCY OF HOSPITAL

Nature

Since many health problems require a level of medical treatment and personal care that extends beyond the range of services normally available in the patient's home or in the office of the physician, modern society has developed formal institutions for patient care intended to help meet the more complex health needs of its members. The hospital, the major social institution for the delivery of health care in the modern world, offers considerable advantages to both patient and society. From the standpoint of individual, the sick or injured person has access to centralized medical knowledge and technology so as to render treatment much more thorough and efficient. From the standpoint of society, hospitalization both protects the family from many of the disruptive effects of caring for the ill in the home and operates as a means of guiding the sick and injured into medically supervised institutions where their problems are less disruptive for society as a whole.

Functions

(a) Patient Care

The first and foremost function of a hospital is to give care to the sick and injured and restore the health of diseased persons. Ethically, this care should be given to all without discrimination of social, economic or racial nature. However, the hospitals as national investments in people's health and as centres for scientific practice of medicine, must do many more things than 'produce' medical care. The success with which a hospital contributes towards meeting the patient's need can be measured by the illness of the life he is able to lead on leaving it.

(b) Training

The education and training of doctors and nurses have traditionally been carried out in hospitals. It is a workshop wherein the student learns by seeing what his superiors and peers do. Radiology, laboratory, radiotherapy, highly advanced surgical techniques demand a variety of skills and knowledge, all of which cannot be mastered by the doctor specialist. These activities have created the need for a large number of skilled technicians who are today the vital support to the specialist whether he is the surgeon, physician, diagnostician or therapeutist. These people are indispensable for the all-round excellence of all specialist work. To develop these technical skills, a programme should be organized by the hospital under the direction of people who have the required experience, knowledge and aptitude to teach others. The purpose of in-service education and training programme is to develop such knowledge and skills in all categories of para-medical personnel as are required to make them fit for the job they hold and keep them attuned to the growing needs of their jobs.

(c) Medical Research

The third important function of hospital is to give support to medical research. A good hospital, where the quality of professional work is excellent, is an ideal ground for medical research. As a matter of fact, excellent professional care of patients largely results from the fruits of research into new problems. An attitude of enquiry and investigation should permeate through the day-to-day care of patients. The hospital can develop facilities for research with comparative ease and speed if the staff and administration are properly motivated. True, elaborate research is expensive. There, nevertheless, remain clinical investigations of applied nature that call for little capital investment. Responsibility for creation of new knowledge is that of any enlightened profession. It is in a hospital that opportunities exist, if not abound, for organized as well as individual initiative for research.

(d) Health Education

The fourth and final object is to support and assist all activities carried out by various public health and voluntary agencies to prevent disease and promote positive health attitudes in the community through health education. Health education, immunization, social and economic rehabilitation are some of the many activities for which the hospital may provide assistance in terms of physical facilities and advisory services to staff. As a matter of fact, in the western countries, this aspect of the hospital as a community health centre is being emphasized more and more. Many ways are being devised to integrate the hospital with the activities of community health agencies.

The main function of a hospital is to promote the health of the community which it serves. Hospitals in the past were set-up primarily as charity institutions for poor and weaker sections of society. These were considered as alms houses. The only function of such institutions was the care of the sick and the poor. The hospital was considered only a shelter for the socially unfit. Hospitals are being re-oriented from just being the centres for medical care and treatment to hospitals which are supposed to provide comprehensive system of preventive and curative medicine and rehabilitation services. It has been stated in a WHO document that the hospital is an integral part of a social and medical organisation, the function of which is to provide for the population, complete health care, both curative and preventive, and whose out-patient services reach out to the family in its home environment; the hospital is also a centre for the training of health workers and for bio-social research[1] and "an institution that provides in-patient accommodation for medical and nursing care." The hospital has a noble purpose expressed in the phrase "Promotion of health and welfare of the people." Hospitals have now become indispensable to the proper care of the broad spectrum of health problems.

In the dynamic society, the hospital occupies a unique place to accommodate explosion of science into medicine and the whole galaxy of new treatment techniques, new equipment and proliferation of services which have made a profound impact on the provision of care facilities and services. Besides this, the development of socio-politico, cultural and educational systems have made the people conscious of their rights and they demand that modern and best means of medical and health care be made available to them; not only within the four walls of the hospital but at their doorstep or in the vicinity of living places. These impacts had made a hospital a complex organisation.[2]

Administration of such a complex organisation requires blending of technical and administrative competence in the right quantity, at the right time, at the right place, by the right man and in the right way or process. Each hospital is a distinct entity and as such each has to be tailored to the specific aims to be accomplished, the specific tasks to be performed, the volume of Services to be rendered and the type of the community to be served. The basic purpose of the hospital is "better patient care" and return the patient back to the community as a productive unit of that community. Hospital administration is an activity to secure better output through optimum utilisation of inputs.

Classification of Hospitals

Each hospital is distinct in its characteristics as it differs in structure, functions, performance and the community it serves. However, we can classify the hospitals into different types depending upon different criteria.

According to the objectives, hospitals can be classified into categories:

1. Teaching-cum-Research Hospitals

The main objective of these hospitals is teaching based on research and the provision of health care is secondary, e.g., All-India Institute of Medical Sciences, New Delhi, Post-Graduate Medical Education and Research Institute, Chandigarh.

2. General Hospitals

The main objective of these hospitals is to provide medical care to the people while teaching and research is secondary and incidental, e.g., district or taluka hospital, PHCs.

3. Special Hospitals

These hospitals concentrate on a particular aspect or organ of the body and provide medical care in that field e.g Cancer, Dental, Psychiatry Hospitals, T.B. Hospitals, etc. On the basis of ownership, hospitals can be classified into four categories:

1. Government Hospitals
2. Semi-Government Hospitals
3. Voluntary Agencies' Hospitals
4. Private/Charitable Hospitals.

According to the system of medicine we can have the following categories:

1. Allopathic Hospitals
2. Ayurvedic Hospitals
3. Homoeopathic Hospitals
4. Unani Hospitals
5. Hospitals of other systems of medicine.

Classification According to the Size

One of the major recommendations of the Health Survey and Development Committee (Bhore Committee) was the setting up of Peripheral Health Centres catering to a population of 40,000 each, which were to be linked up with secondary health centres and hospitals for purposes of referral services. In 1962, the Mudaliar Committee went further into this problem. The infrastructure for the delivery of health and medical care has closely followed the recommendations of these committees, However, the Government felt it necessary to set-up a study group on hospitals in 1966. This group submitted its report in 1968. The group found that out of 335 districts in the country, only 125 had more than 200-bed hospitals, and out of 3000 taluks, only 2,053 had hospitals. However, out of 5,080 primary health centres planned for the country, 4,973 were found to be established. It also found that there was unequal distribution of hospitals in various areas of the country. It recommended that the following pattern of development for hospitals be adopted:

Teaching Hospitals	500 (to be increased according to the number of students).
District Hospitals	200 (may be raised upto 300 beds depending on population).
Tehsil/Taluk Hospitals	50 (may be raised depending on population).
Primary Health Centres	6 (may be increased to 10 depending on needs).

The bed strength of 125 districts which have at least one 200-beds hospital may be raised to 300 depending on the population served. In the remaining 210 districts, hospitals having less than 200 beds, the strength should be raised to a minimum of 200 beds. Ordinarily, the distribution of these beds should be as under:

Medical	60
Surgical	40
Gynaecology and Obstetrics including Maternity	35
Paediatrics	15
Orthopaedics	5
Eye	10
ENT	10
Skin	5
Emergency	5
Isolation	10
Psychiatry	5
	200

Since the district hospital is to serve as a referral centre it should provide specialist services in Medicine, Surgery, Obstetrics, Gynaecology, Eye, ENT, Paediatrics, Dentistry, Psychiatry, VD, T.B. Clinic, etc. The staff norms as fixed by the Government for the different kinds of hospitals in India are as under:[3]

Sr. No.	*Name of the Post*	*No. of Posts (norms)*
	50 BED HOSPITAL	
1.	Medical Officer PCMS I	1
2.	Medical Officer PCMS II (including one Female)	2
3.	PJMS	—
4.	DENTAL SURGEON	1
5.	Pharmacists	3

6.	Nursing Sister	1
7.	Staff Nurses/ANMS	8
8.	Lab. Technician (Grade I), Lab. Technician (Grade II)	1
9.	Radiographer	1
10.	Clerk-*cum*-Storekeeper	1
11.	Cooks	2
12.	Mali	1
13.	Dhobi	2
14.	Class IV including Sweepers	17

50 BED HOSPITAL

1.	Medical Officer PCMS I	1
2.	Medical Officer PCMS II	3
3.	Dental Surgeon	1
4.	Anaesthetist	1
5.	Radiologist	1
6.	Pathologist	1
7.	Casualty Medical Officers	3
8.	House Surgeons	5
9.	Matron	1
10.	Nursing Sisters	4
11.	Staff Nurses	20
12.	Pharmacists	5
13.	Storekeepers	2
14.	Clerks	4
15.	Accountant	2
16.	Lab. Technician Grade I	7
17.	Lab. Technician Grade II	2
18.	Lab. Attendant	1
19.	Cooks	2
20.	Helper	2
21.	Radiographer	1
22.	Carpenter/Painter	1
23.	Chowkidar	3
24.	Class IV including Sweepers	50
25.	Biochemist	—
26.	Operation Room Asstt.	2
27.	Cashier	1
28.	Head Clerk	1
29.	Electrician	1
30.	Plumber	1

200-BED HOSPITAL

1.	Medical Officer PCMS I	2
2.	Medical Officer PCMS II	4
3.	Anaesthetist	1
4.	Pathologist	1
5.	Radiologist	1
6.	Biochemist	1
7.	Dental Surgeon	1
8.	Casualty Medical Officers	3
9.	House Surgeons	10
10.	Matron	1
11.	Nursing Sisters	10
12.	Staff Nurses	32
13.	Radiographer	1
14.	Pharmacists	5
15.	Lab. Asstt. Grade	I 4
16.	Lab. Asstt. Grade	II
17.	Lab. Attendants	2
18.	Dietician	1
19.	Cooks	4
20.	Head Cook	1
21.	Stenographer	1
22.	Accountant	1
23.	Storekeepers	2
24.	Clerks	2
25.	Dental Mechanic	1
26.	Carpenter/Painter	1
27.	Caretaker/Steward	1
28.	Chowkidar	3
29.	Mali	2
30.	Other Class IV posts including Sweepers	81
31.	Registrar	-
32.	Hawaldar	-
33.	Assistant Matron	1
34.	Cashier	1
35.	Head Clerk	1
36.	Operation Room Assistants	2
37.	Electrician	1
38.	Barber	-
39.	Plumber	1

Indices for Measuring the Efficiency of a Hospital

It is very difficult to measure the efficiency of a hospital because of the complex nature of problems that it entails. There are many indices which can help us in evaluation of its quantitative performance. But, what about quality? It can be ascertained only through specially designed surveys. These surveys may be conducted both by persons inside the organisation and outside the organisation to locate the problems and suggest remedies for its future performance. Very few studies are available which have been conducted in this field. The studies carried out by NIHFW on different aspects of hospital administration throw light on various issues. Besides, the Committees of Parliament have done a useful work in analysing the performance of the All-India Institute of Medical Sciences and the three hospitals of Delhi. Research institutions and the universities should take interest and help the hospital management to their services. We mention below some of the indices which are commonly used to measure the efficiency of hospitals:

1. Bed occupancy ratio $= \dfrac{\text{Number of patient-days' during the year}}{\text{Number of bed-days during the year}} \times 100$

This ratio tells us to how far the available bed capacity has been utilised.

2. Average duration of illness $= \dfrac{\text{The Number of patient-days' during the year}}{\text{Total number of in-patient admissions during the year}}$

The index is complementary to the other index 'average turn-over interval'. This is more useful if computed for individual diseases.

3. Turn-over interval $= \dfrac{\text{The total vacant bed-days during the year}}{\text{The number of in-patients' admission during the year}}$

The index indicates the number of days on an average per patient for which a bed has been remained unused.

4. The average out-patient admission $= \dfrac{\text{The total number of out-patients during the year}}{\text{The total number of out-patients admissions during the year}}$

5. Average daily out-patient admission $= \dfrac{\text{The total number of out-patients during the year}}{\text{The total number of new out-patients admissions during the year}}$

The index tells the average workload on OPD.

6. Cost of daily diet $= \dfrac{\text{Total expenditure on diet during the year}}{\text{Total number of in-patient days}}$

7. Average cost of medicine $= \dfrac{\text{Total cost of medicines for in-patients for the year}}{\text{Total number of in-patients' admissions}}$

8. Fatality rate $= \dfrac{\text{No. of in-patients' deaths during specified period}}{\text{No. of discharges during the same period}} \times 100$

9. Autopsy rate $= \dfrac{\text{No. of autopsies performed}}{\text{No. of in-patients' deaths}} \times 100$

Staff Services and Auxiliary Services

Let us discuss some of these services to understand the mechanics of hospital administration.

B. ASPECTS OF HOSPITAL SERVICES

The services provided in a hospital differ from one hospital to another. It is very difficult to discuss all these services here. We can classify these services into three categories e.g., Line services, Supporting Services and Auxiliary Services.

Line Services

(a) Emergency Services (Casualty Services) (See Chart 2.1)

The casualty department provides round-the-clock, immediate diagnosis and treatment for illness of an urgent nature and injuries from accidents. Simple cases after administering preliminary treatment are discharged with instructions to attend OPD as a follow-up measure. Cases of serious nature are admitted in emergency wards to provide immediate medical care. Such patients are either discharged after 2-3 days or are transferred to permanent in-patient wards. Emergency service is acquiring increasing importance due to modern problems arising out of urbanisation and mechanisation. The best services must be provided to the patients in the Emergency wards as the patients and their relatives are under emotional strain and surcharged with suspense and anxiety about the consequences of the disease or calamity that has come up suddenly. Such an approach would alleviate a large part of sufferings born out of fear and suspicion of the unknown. The Public Accounts Committee (1977-78) suggested that:

In order that the emergencies are attended to quickly at effectively, it is necessary to have an efficient set-up, well-knit with other departments of the hospitals with well laid-out procedure and work distribution.

(b) Out-Patient Services

The out-patient department is one of the most important department. All the patients suffering from diseases of minor, serious, acute and chronic nature are examined. It should be designed to provide services to one per cent of the population of the area. It should be large enough to avoid congestion. The functions of the out-patient services are provision of

CHART 2.1

Procedure in an Emergency Service

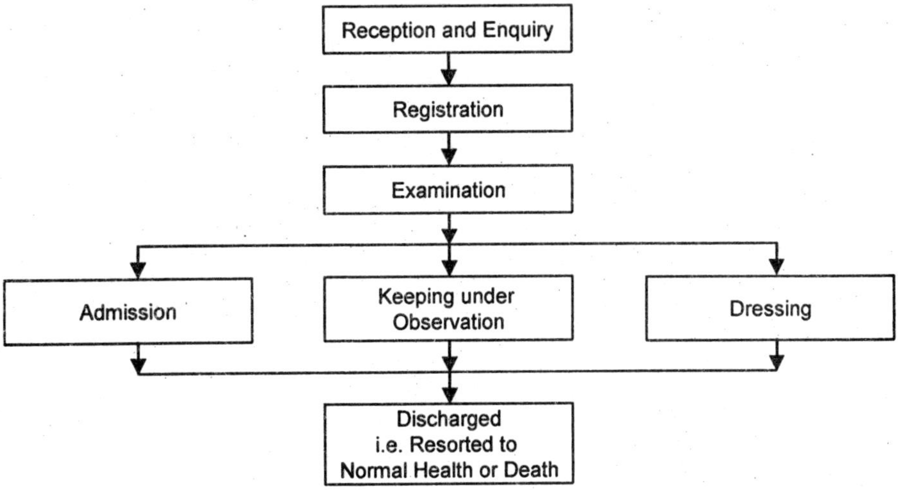

diagnostic, curative, preventive and rehabilitative services on an ambulatory basis. We can explain the whole process with the help of a flow diagram. (See Chart 2.2)

Out-patient department should be so planned that the building is separate from the indoor area. It should be well connected to the laboratories, X-ray department and other supportive services. It should have enough accommodation to avoid congestion. Depending upon the size of the hospital and resources available separate areas of examination for the specialists should be provided.

This is the most important service provided by all the hospitals as it provides services to a large number of patients at a low cost. In ordinary hospitals, the same doctor examines all categories of patients while in secondary and tertiary hospitals, patients are examined by specialists. Successful management of out-patient departments can lighten the burden on the wards. Besides, poor people have to rush to private clinics and nursing homes because of the poor services provided in out-patient departments (OPDs). Based upon our discussion with the doctors, hospital administrators, nurses and patients, we mention the major problems being faced in the OPD.

I. Delays and Wastage of Time: Need of streamlining the procedures

Most of the patients complained that they have to waste a lot of time in waiting for their turn. They mentioned that sometimes it takes 2-3 hours for them to see the doctor concerned. The doctors, on the other hand, complain that patients visit most of the hospitals again and again without making use of the earlier records. Many of the patients were sore because

CHART 2.2

Procedure for an OPD

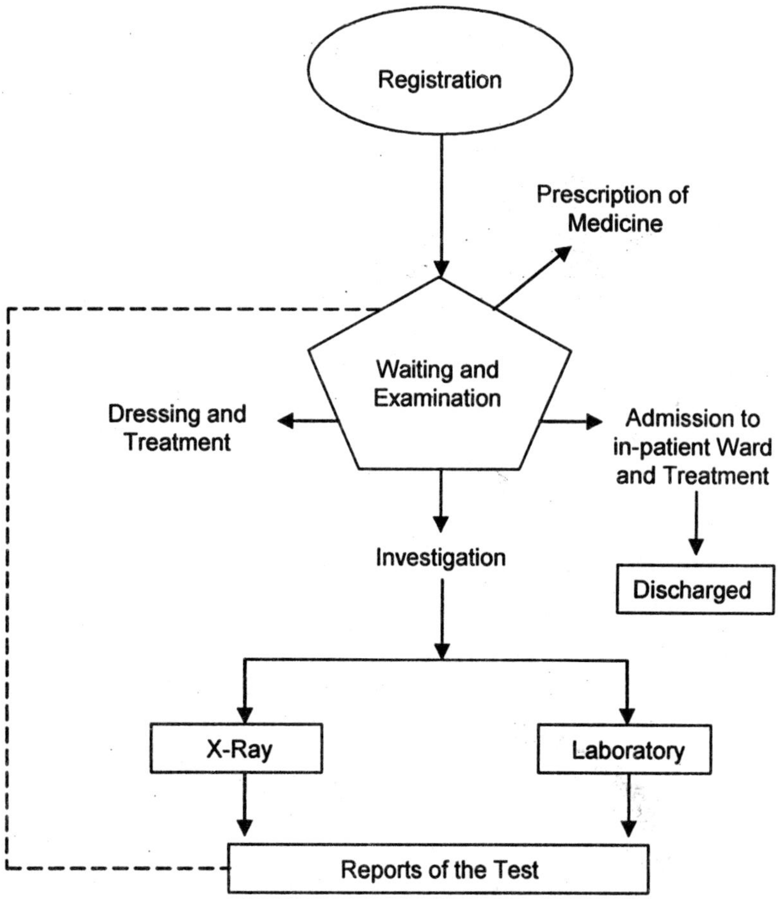

they felt that the doctors examine the VIP patients in preference to other patients. The delay can be avoided if the patients at the time of registration may be advised about the probable time of his turn. This can help the patient in chalking out his schedule. Besides, the patients from the village may be given preference so that they can go back to their village after examination and consultation and thus may not unnecessarily crowd the hospital premises.

2. *Laboratory Facilities Inadequate Resulting into Unnecessary Harassment: Need of rejuvenating laboratory services*

Most of the patients after examination by doctors in OPD are advised various test concerning urine, blood, stool, etc. Patients have to stand in long queues for every test and they find that it consumes a lot of time.

Because of the non-functional nature of equipment in many hospitals, patients have to get these tests done outside the hospitals at a very high cost. Some patients even mentioned that doctors in the hospitals are in collusion with the clinics outside and thus intentionally refer the patients to these clinics. Moreover, the results of these tests generally do not move automatically to the file of the patient, rather the patient or his relatives have to collect the results of these tests. These results are to be examined by the doctors after 3-4 days when his turn comes next time. There is also a lot of problem pertaining to the quality of these tests. Since most of the prescriptions by the doctors are based on these reports, it is necessary to manage the laboratory services efficiently. In this context, it is suggested that the tests of the results should be made available by evening the same day (as far as possible) so that most of the patients coming from out-stations can leave to their villages and avoid the exhorbitant cost of the city life.

3. *Lack of Co-ordination among Different Specialities: Need of integrating the efforts of the specialists*

It has been generally observed that patients visiting one speciality are referred to other facilities as well for checking and consultation. This is a time-consuming process and demoralises the patients as well. It is suggested that such patients may be examined by a board of specialists once a week so that they are examined from all the angles before the administration of treatment. It was observed that most of the hospitals are without medicines because of low budget and pilferage. The hospital authorities must keep a constant vigil on the pharmaceutical section so that the patients get the medicine of right quality. A list of medicines and their manufactures must be displayed outside the dispensary so that patients can check and be satisfied, otherwise they will spread the poor image of the working of the hospitals.

4. *Lack of Faith among the Doctors: Need of creating a good public opinion*

Most of the people in the catchment area of the hospital complain that the doctors in government/semi-government hospitals do not bother much about the patients and that is why there is mushroom growth of private practitioners or the coming up of a large number of nursing homes. This phenomenon is in contravention to the Directive Principles of the State Policy enshrined in the Constitution of India that the Government would ensure the provisions of decent health care for all at a cost that the people can afford. The behaviour of the doctors is rude and thus act as repellant to the patients. Thus. there is a need of educating the people about their rights *vis-a-vis* the hospitals so that the services available in the hospitals are utilised efficiently.

5. *Restricted Role of the Doctors: Need of broadening their vision and functions*

Most of the doctors think that their job is simply to examine the visiting patients and prescribe treatment. This is a negative approach. The doctors in OPD must utilise this opportunity to act as health and medical leaders to bring about revolution in the health status of the people. As stated in the issue of *World Health* (April 1988. p. 15) his role is much wider.

6. *Absence of leadership Qualities among Hospital Managers: Need of awareness*

Chief Medical Officers, Medical and other managers do not make use of the talent to get more work out of them if they are properly motivated. We may quote here from the Lao Tzu that enlightened leadership is service, no selfishness. The leader grows more and lasts longer by placing the well-being of all above the well-being of self alone. Paradox by being selfless, the leader enhances self. Sumedha Khanna in her Article, "Learning to Need," in *World Health,* April 1988, has rightly mentioned the qualities in health leaders which must be imbibed by our doctors to make the OPD efficient. These are concern for social justice; compassion for the under-privileged, dedication to the growth of self-reliance; strong commitment, ability to communicate, courage to take risks and make bold decisions, and faith in the people's potentials.

Functions	*Activities*
as a Physician	treatment of patients promotion of health at community and individual levels prevention of diseases and accidents rehabilitation
as an Educator	oneself, health staff, patients, community as a Manager-relationship with referral services (district, regional) relationship with the communities and their representatives development of PHC activities (including research) leadership of staff/teams
as an Agent of socio-economic development	participate in community development, committee meetings and activities advocacy for HFA/PHC

7. *Dull and Awful Atmosphere Outside the OPDs: Need of decorating the lounge with meaningful literature*

Most of the patients and their relatives who wait outside the OPDs feel insecure and are afraid of the consequences of the diseases they are suffering from. Moreover, the congregation of different categories of patients make the situation still more serious. It is suggested that the hospital authorities must decorate the lounges outside the OPDs and use the opportunity for providing health-education. Changing behaviour is a complex process cultural traits are intertwined and change in one area of life is linked with changes in others. This is what makes behaviour change difficult, complex; but given the right conditions, behaviour change can be accelerated. People's pragmatic wisdom moves them into action.

8. *Great Rush of Patients: Need of appointment of Doctors according to Need*

It has been seen that the OPDs are overcrowded and it becomes very difficult for the doctors to examine them, seriously resulting into superficial check-ups done hurriedly. However, there are some OPDs where doctors do not get even the minimum number of patients. It is suggested that statistics may be collected for 2-3 years and personnel may be appointed accordingly so that the decent medical care may be made available. We must work out some norms for appointment of medical personnel to optimise the use of qualified personnel.

9. *Records Management in a Bad Shape: Need of Introducing Modern Management Methods*

Patients are treated as cases and for a particular disease. No records are maintained for the medical check-ups done from time to time. It is suggested that people in the area may be provided with permanent pass-books which can keep a chronological record of the health of the individuals. This can help the doctors in administering right medicine. We can safely conclude that there is a need of far-reaching improvements in the management of out-patient services to ensure optimisation of resources and satisfaction of patients. In short, we can say that we should not contend merely with the availability and accessibility of health services in OPDs but rather in their acceptability and acceptance.

(c) In-Patient Services (Wards)

After the patient has been examined in the OPD or the emergency area, he may be advised admission in the wards. Wards are of different types—open general wards (rows of beds in a big ward area), 4-5 bed units, and private wards for paying patients. Each ward has generally a doctor's duty room, dressing room, central Nursing Staff Station and other essential items needed for patient care. The departments to which direct patient access should be provided are operating theatre suite, X-ray and physical medicine departments. The pharmacy and pathology departments should also be readily accessible from the wards for the staff

(d) Intensive-Care Unit

Some of the patients admitted to hospitals require acute, multi-disciplinary and intensive observation and treatment, e.g., patients of shock, coma, heart attack, lung, kidney, brain diseases, etc. It is desirable to have an intensive-care unit for such patients. Like the emergency services, this requires much better staffing pattern—one nurse for 11/2 beds per shift. The staff needs to be specially trained to work in this area. This is very costly and should be set-up only at the apex-hospitals.

(e) Operation Theatres

Each operating room set should have a pre-anaesthesia room and sterilisation room and a scrub room for nurses and doctors. There is trend to provide simple laboratory facilities within the operating area to serve the purpose during emergency.

Supportive Services

(a) Central Sterile Supply Services Management

The Central Sterile Supply Department is supposed to store sterilise, maintain and issue those instruments, materials and garment which are required to be sterile. This requirement may steadily decrease as the use of disposable items becomes more economical. The Central Sterile Supply Department should have direct lines of communication with all wards, operations threaters, out-patient and casually departments, and to a lesser extent, with X-ray and pathology departments. Air control in this department is essential to check contamination through air. Proper control with indicators for sterilisation procedures is essential.

(b) Diet Management

The catering department, which comprises the kitchen, bulk-food stores and dining rooms, supplies all meals throughout the hospital. Direct and easy access is required from the main kitchen to the wards. The food should be transported in heated trolleys. This department is required to provide: (i) general diet, (b) special diet for patients suffering from certain diseases. Food served in an attractive manner provides an incentive for the patients to eat.

(c) Pharmaceutical Services Management

The pharmaceutical services in most of the hospitals in India today represent the functions of procurement and distribution of medcaments by medical store and compounding and dispensing of medicine on doctor's prescription by persons hitherto known as compounders, generally under the control of Medical Officers. In OPD, drugs are distributed on prescription while in wards the drugs are sent either on indents collecting for all patients; or indents for individual patient. Besides, every good hospital has a manufacturing section for various formulations and intravenous fluids.

(d) Laundry

There is a need for an efficient mechanical laundry to ensure the availability of bacteria-free washed linen. The small hospitals may get the cleaning done from washermen with due care and supervision. The aim is to make available to the patients clean and disinfected linen.

(e) Laboratory and X-Ray Facilities

For proper diagnosis of ailments of patients it is necessary to have diagnostic laboratory facility properly manned. The success of medical prescription depends upon proper laboratory diagnosis. Laboratories for routine blood, urine, microbiology, X-ray, etc. should provide round-the-clock service. It is desirable to locate the laboratory block and X-ray block in between the OPD and indoor area to be able to serve both the areas. We must ensure that the technicians are really doing the job because a minor mistake on their part may ruin the life of the patients. There is a need for constant supervision over the functioning of these laboratory services.

(f) Nursing Services

Nursing services should be managed by a matron who is assisted by a sister in-charge of the wards and staff nurses. Nursing sisters control the ward and arrange the leave day-off of nurses. The accepted norms by Indian Nursing Council for a general ward is one staff nurse per live beds. This norm is never achieved in practice resulting in poor service. Besides, nurses are engaged in non-nursing activities which results in poor service to the patients. The Public Accounts Committee was critical of Nursing Services in three hospitals of Delhi. The Committee remarked:

In view of the fact that the nurse-patient ratio excluding the specialised departments, is 1:33 in the Safdarjung Hospital and 1:19 in the Willingdon Hospital as against the ideal ratio of 1:5, the Committee feels that there is considerable shortage of nurses for manning the emergency and casualty services in the three hospitals.

The same situation prevails in most of the hospitals.

Auxiliary Services

(a) Registration and Indoor Case Records

Registration is a must for a hospital to enrol new patients with proper entry in OPD cards and keep track of the revisits of the patients. Medical records help in regulating admission of patients. It helps in codifying the record according to internal disease index. It also collects statistics of hospital stay of patients, i.e. admission, discharge, average stay, etc. for future planning and management. According to Calender:

The hospital's admission procedure should be such that the patient is made to feel welcome and secure. Every employee who comes in contact with the patient should make him feel that each one is genuinely interested in his welfare. This experience is the patient's first introduction to the hospital and should be a pleasant one.[4]

(b) Stores

The Central Store receives, stores and issues bulk items which can, with advantage, be stored centrally. Stores are of different types—Pharmacy Stores, Chemical Stores, Linen Stores, Surgical Stores, Glassware Stores.

CHART 2.3

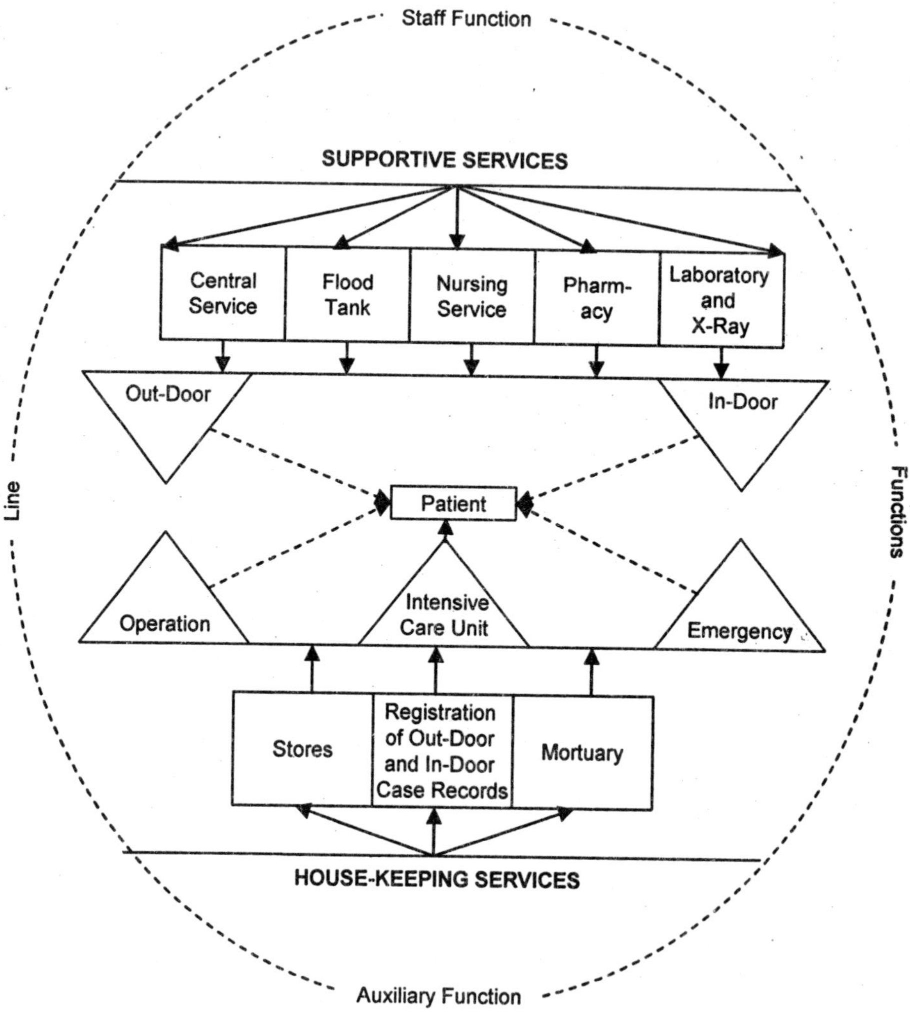

Stock policy should be devised in such a way that vital and essential items are always available. It should be managed by a competent stores officer.

(c) Transport

Transport requirements for the carriage of supplies and patients are:

(a) Trolleys;
(b) Stretchers; and
(c) Wheel chairs.

It is preferable to have a central transport gang to shift the patients. Supplies should also be distributed to all wards by the central areas.

(d) Mortuary

Each hospital should have a cold storage area or mortuary where dead bodies are kept before they are claimed by the relations. Sometimes post-mortems need to be done for medico-legal reasons. Unclaimed bodies should be disposed-off according to rules.

C. BRIEF DESCRIPTIONS OF SOME HOSPITALS OF DIFFERENT KINDS AND SYSTEMS

(i) Teaching-cum-Research Hospitals

Every teaching institution has an attached hospital which provides clinical material for teaching and training of the students. Such hospitals also provide facilities for research both for the teachers and the taught. The method of treating a patient in a teaching-*cum*-research hospital varies from that available in a general hospital. In the case of the former, apart from treatment, the patient is used for teaching and research. Here the patient is first handled by a trainee who examines him thoroughly, records his detailed history and suggests the diagnosis and treatment. The case is then presented by the trainee to the teacher (called consultant) who goes through the history recorded by the trainee and also examines the patient. The treatment is 'prescribed only by the consultant'. In this way the patient, beside receiving treatment also acts as 'material' for teaching. He is used for research by the teachers and the taught. It has to be accepted that the treatment in a teaching-*cum*-research institute takes more time than in a general hospital.

Let us describe briefly Post-Graduate Institute of Medical Education and Research, Chandigarh, to understand the organisation and working of such hospitals. The Post-Graduate Institute of Medical Education and Research, Chandigarh, was established by the Government of Punjab in 1962. It was declared an institution of national importance by an Act of Parliament with effect from April 1967.

The Nehru Hospital attached to the Postgraduate Institute of Medical Education and Research, Chandigarh provided tertiary care in all the medical and surgical specialists to the patients, who came not only from the neighbouring states but also from far off states like West Bengal and Bihar.

The total bed strength of the PGI has increased to 1412 beds. The number of patients who attended the outpatients departments and admitted during the last three years is as under:

A total number of 40,356 patients were attended in the emergency outpatients and 22,654 were admitted. In the emergency operation threatres, a total of 8280 operations were performed including 7284 major operations (which includes Labour Room Operations) and 996 minor operations. During the financial year 2005-06 Rs. 1,38,37041 was spent for subscription of 560 Journals and Rs. 4,69,569 has been spent for the purchase of books and including Book Bank Scheme meant for the SC/ST students.[5]

	2003-04	2004-05	2005-06
OPD Attendance	10,79,596	11,32,186	12,00,992
Admissions	54,430	46,723	50,216

Emergency and critical patients were attended to round the clock.

The administration of the institute including the Nehru Hospital is under the control of a Director, who is assisted by the Dean (for teaching purposes) and the Medical Superintendent (administrative purposes).

(ii) General Hospital

The main function of the general hospital is to provide treatment to the patient. No detailed history of the illness of the patient is recorded. Here the medical officer hears a verbal account of the illness of the patient, examines him and prescribes the treatment. The treatment is quick and less time-consuming. The only disadvantage of this system of treatment is that sometimes the serious illness may go undiagnosed properly.

Let us describe a Government General Hospital with reference to Civil Hospital, Ropar (Punjab). It is a 100-bed hospital (56 male and 44 female) with a provision for 10 extra beds. It provides the following special services:

Speciality	*Bed Strength*
Medical	30
Surgery	30
Eye	10
Paediatrics	10
Obstetrics and Gynaecology	20

It has been provided with all the facilities which can serve the patients. The affairs of the hospital are managed by the Chief Medical Officer (PCMS Class I); who has under him 12 Doctors, 5 Pharmacists, Radiographer X-ray Assistant, 4 Laboratory Technicians, 1 Matron, 2 Nursing sisters, 10 staff nurses. Besides, there are 10 members belonging to ministerial staff, 53 belonging to Class IV, one carpenter, one driver, one plumber and one electrician.

(iii) Working of the Special Hospitals

We shall explain this with the help of Chest Diseases Hospital, Patiala and the Punjab Mental Hospital, Amritsar. The Chest Disease hospital was started with the name, T.B. Clinic, in 1949, with ten beds only. It has been named as Chest Diseases Hospital. It has been serving as Training and Demonstration Centre as well since 1962. The hospital is under the control of Director of Research and Medical Education, Punjab. The day-to-day affairs of the hospital are looked after by the Deputy Medical Superintendent. The details can be seen from the Organisational Chart. (See Chart 2.4)

CHART 2.4

Structure of Civil Hospital, Ropar

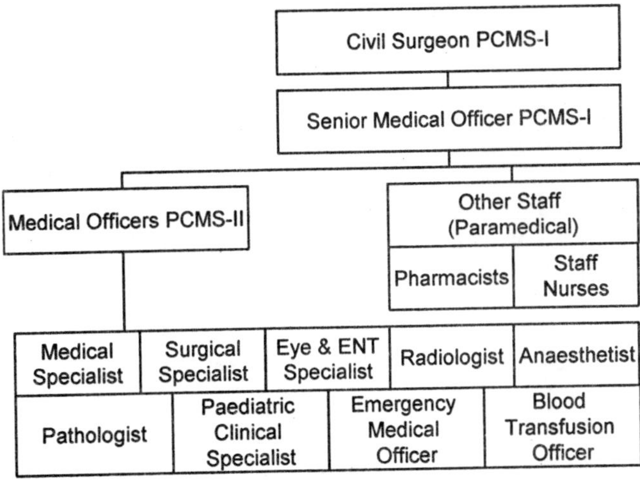

Services

The hospital provides patient care—out-door as well as in-door. It also provides community health services at all levels, i.e. (a) Primary prevention, (b) Secondary prevention, and (c) Tertiary prevention.

(a) BCG Vaccination is given to each child immediately after birth.
(b) The hospital has got mobile team, mobile X-ray plant and they move to places where they can detect cases. Such as at fairs where the public is gathered, at factories, industries, camps, schools, etc. through survey and screening of all the population.
(c) For this rehabilitation services are available. Rehabilitation includes everything that is done for the patient. It also serves as educational centre and provides:
  (i) Integration of tuberculosis course. In the general nursing 'A' Grade Diploma Programme.
  (ii) Tuberculosis course for the medical students.
  (iii) House job facilities for medical group.
  (iv) T.B. health visitors' training.
  (v) Multi-purpose worker's training.

Punjab Mental Hospital at Amritsar (See Chart 2.5)

The Punjab Mental Hospital, Amritsar, was set-up in 1949 with 50 beds. The present strength is 811 (512 male and 299 female). Treatment facilities are available at three levels in this hospital as given below:

(a) *The in-doors*: Certified patients are admitted at the in-doors of this hospital from the states of Punjab, Haryana, Himachal Pradesh and the Union Territory of Chandigarh.

CHART 2.5

Organisation of the Chest Disease Institute, Patiala

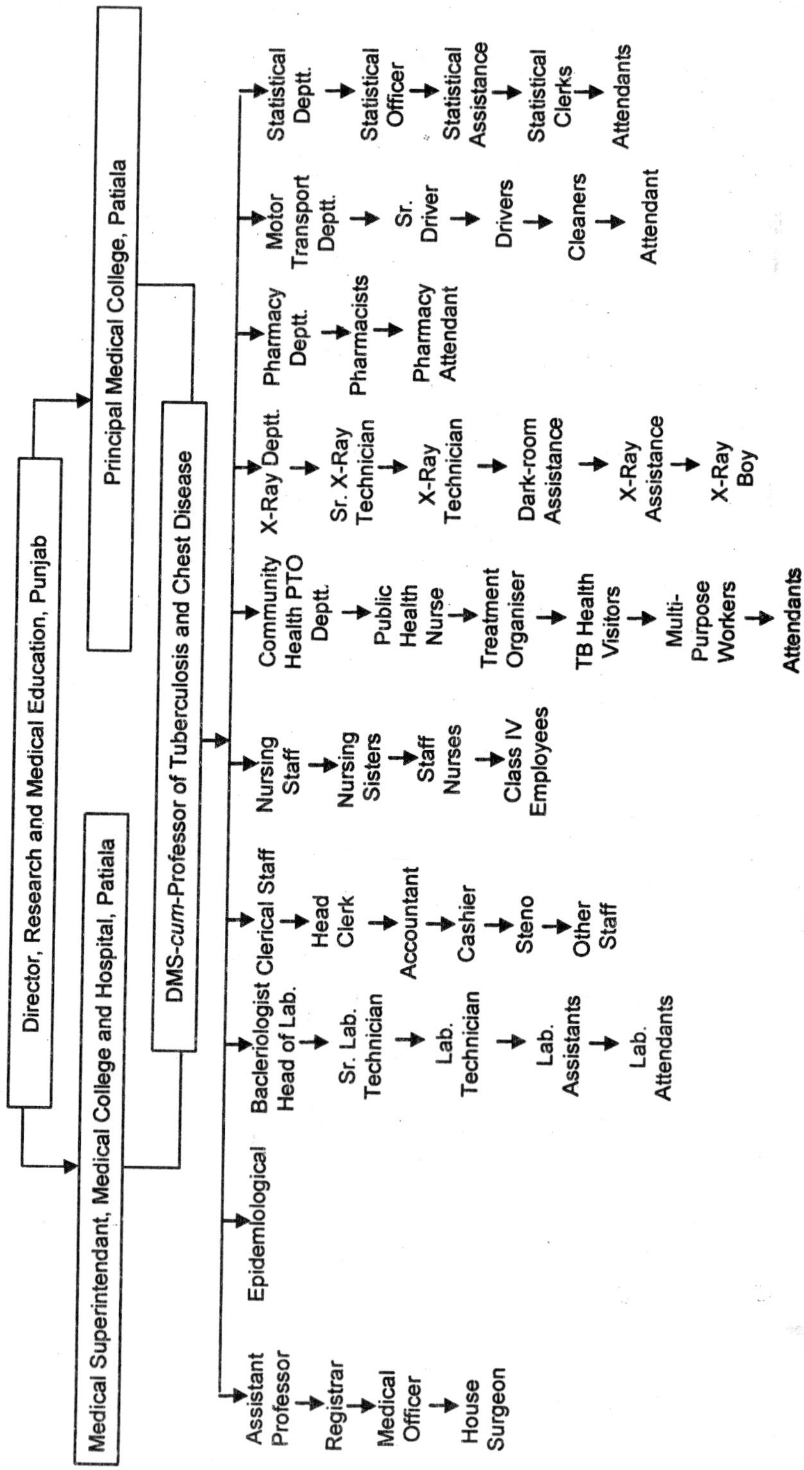

(b) The Out-Patient Department: Consultation facilities for the patients coming from Punjab, Haryana, Himachal Pradesh, Union Territory of Chandigarh and adjoining areas of Uttar Pradesh and Rajasthan are provided at the out-patient department.

(c) The Family Care Unit: This unit consisting of 70 ward-beds and 30 single-seat rooms provides intensive psychiatric treatment to the uncertified patients who need a short duration admission in the hospital. The unit is managed by a team consisting of 1 Medical Officer, 1 Clinical Psychologist and a Psychiatric Trained Nurse.

The hospital administration is looked after by the Medical Superintendent. The hospital staff consists of the following categories of employees:

Category of staff	*Sanctioned Posts*
Class I	6
Class II	8
Class III	83
Class IV	141
Wardens	332

The hospital besides providing patient care, also serves as a training centre for medical and para-medical personnel in psychiatry, clinical psychology, psychiatric nursing and mental health. Besides, the faculty carries out research on various aspects of mental health

(v) Working of a Hospital (Homoeopathic System of Medicine)

Hospitals in the traditional system of medicine are simple as they do not require costly equipments to diagnose the ailments. Let us now describe the working of a teaching-*cum*-patient care homoeopathic institution located at Chandigarh. It was set-up in 1974 under private management. It has a faculty consisting of 13 staff members-1 principal, 9 whole-time lecturers and 3 part-time lecturers belonging to the western system of medicine. The intake capacity of the college is 50 students and the course is of 4 years' duration.

The college serves as the hospital as well and provides both in-patient and out-patient services. The patient first of all is registered by the registration clerk who maintained the case history (backbone of the system) of the patients. After the registration, the patient is examined by the doctors/faculty members on duty. It takes about half an hour to record the case history of the patient. There is no referral system, since every doctor is competent to deal with all diseases as there is no classification of individual diseases, e.g., Cancer, Tuberculosis, etc. The chronic cases are admitted to provide in-door treatment. It has a simple laboratory structure and operation theatre. There is no para-medical staff. The hospital is visited by about 35 to 80 new patients and 100 to 150 old patients per day. It has 25 beds located in three rooms. The patients are administered medicine through a dispensary. Besides, there is a pharmacy section for the formulation of medicine.

The cost of such a hospital is negligible compared to that of hospitals based on the western system of medicine The setting up of such hospitals would lower the cost of medical care and would supplement the efforts of allopathic system of medicine.

Working of an Ayurvedic Hospital/Dispensary

The Ayurvedic system of medicine is also very simple. After the registration, the patients are examined by the doctor on duty. The patients are treated on the philosophy of vayu, pitta and kapha. We discuss now the working of an Ayurvedic dispensary located in Sector 37, Chandigarh, under the control of the government. It has 2 doctors—one male and one female. Both are qualified.

They have G.A.M.S./B.A.M.S. degrees. The patients are first of all registered by the Registration clerk and, thereafter, examined by one of the two doctors. It takes about 3-5 minutes to examine the patient. The doctors are taking the help of the stethoscope, manometer, etc. After the examination the medicines are prescribed. The patient gets free available medicines from the dispensary while he has to buy the rest from the market. There is no surgery and referral system. About 60 to 90 new patients and 150 to 200 old patients visit the hospital daily. The big Ayurvedic hospitals have in-door facilities as well, e.g., the hospital at Patiala has 100 beds.

These hospitals are very easy to operate and involve negligible expenditure. The government should encourage such hospitals to reduce the rising cost of medical care.

D. WORKING OF HOSPITALS

Hospitals are providing medical care only to those who approach them. Hospitals are not serving as the centres of total health care preventive, curative, promotive and rehabilitative Hospitals have poor linkages with the community and the family. They are providing expensive medical care and not comprehensive health care. The hospital has been described by Dorothea Sick as a "Self-chosen ghetto of the medical profession" and modern doctors as "Professional Cripples" useless without a hospital. Physicians in developing countries become estranged from their own people in the course of their training. The ablest men and women are not tackling the most acute and difficult problems. Besides, the faith of the people in the efficiency of hospital system is decreasing because of the negligence and indifference on the part of hospital authorities. Lawrence J. Sakarai is very critical of the role of most of the doctors in a hospital. He feels, barring some dedicated doctors, most of them are ruthless and says:

He (Doctor) exploits the gullible, conspires against the sick and cares little for medicine unless it makes him money. . . He could murder you through indifference, drugs or just sheer inefficiency all by masquerading under the garb of an ancient oath rendered superfluous in the business of our times.[6]

Dr. W.V. Rajan in his article, 'Men, Medicine and Misadventure' in *The Tribune* (Nov. 25, 1979) rightly mentioned that, "It is an unedifying fact, that we have no accurate recorded data on the occurrence and incidence of misadventures in drug administration, diagnostic procedures and surgical operation in hospitals. . . . In a complex hospital, negligence becomes error, scientific detachment and incompetence becomes a lack of specialised equipments. Medicine is still not an exact science in spite of the great advances in bio-chemical sciences. It is imperative for doctors, nurses and para-medical personnel to exhibit utmost precaution, care, judgement and skill in dealing with and treating patients, balancing the relative risk of the disease with the risk involved in the use of drugs, surgery or diagnostic procedures, apart from the cost-benefit consideration."

What can be done to prevent the erosion of the values among the medical professions? What can we do to maintain the confidence of the people in the hospital services? How can we improve the functioning of the hospital system? How can we coordinate the functioning of hospitals? How can we check the rising costs of hospital services? These questions are being raised even in the context of the developed world. The 1968 report of the Secretary's Advisory Committee on hospital effectiveness, US Department of Health, Education and Welfare, Washington, D.C., emphasised the need to improve the internal efficiency of the hospital as a functioning mechanism to provide decent health care to all. We shall discuss in the following pages the answers to these questions. The analysis is based upon the already published documents especially the reports of the Parliamentary Committee and the personal discussion of the author with the health experts, general administrators and the beneficiaries of the hospital services.

Improving Patient-Satisfaction and Harmonious Relationship between the Patients/Relatives and Hospital Authorities

Hospitals should try to establish cordial, equitable and, therefore, mutually profitable relations between the hospitals and their beneficiaries. The patients mostly complain of discourteous behaviour of hospital staff especially at the lower level. . . . This irritates the patients and their relatives. The test of the efficiency of a hospital is the satisfaction of the beneficiaries. The sympathetic and courteous behaviour of hospital staff would have a soothing and lasting effect on the patients and their relatives. It is suggested that all hospital personnel must inspire confidence and put the nervous patients and their relatives at ease.

The hospital today is more than the combination of medical and therapeutic treatment by specialists, greater and refined medical and surgical knowledge and ever better and more effective facilities and equipment. It includes these factors as the core of its efficient operation but an additional

CHART 2.6

Structure of Punjab Mental Hospital, Amritsar

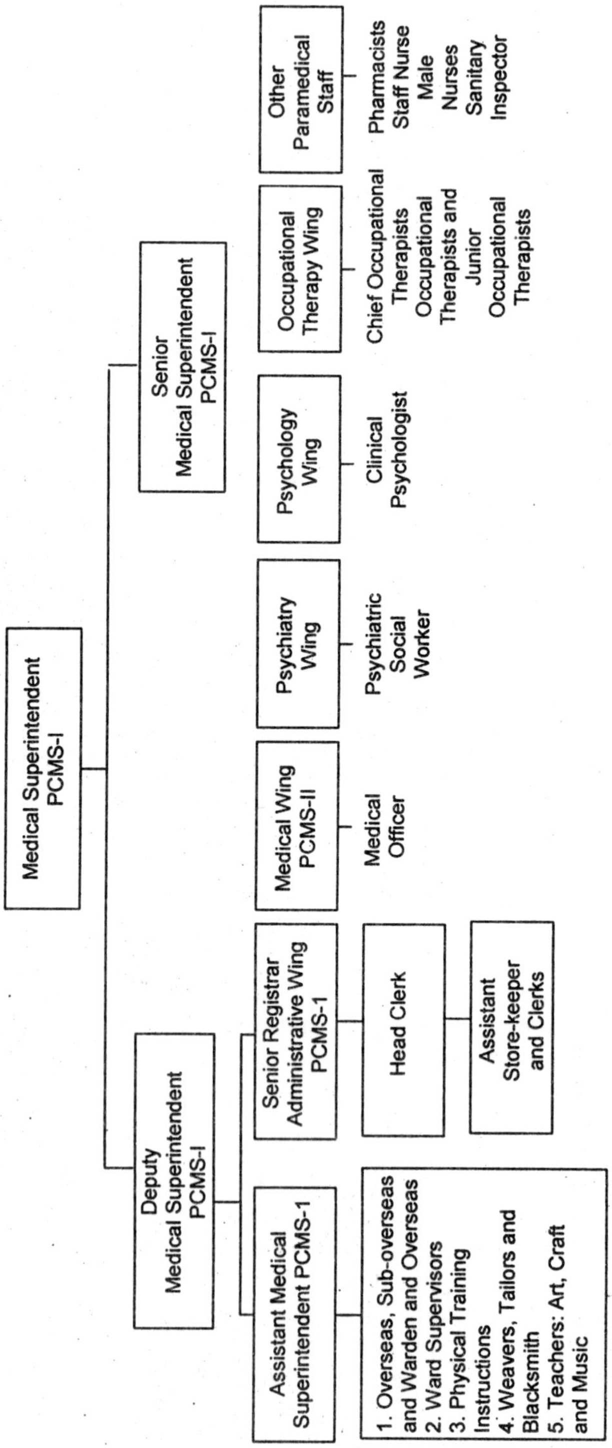

dimension—one which is too often ignored or at least minimized is the human and social element in the structure of the organisation.[7]

The ideal of service must be encouraged among the personnel responsible for health care. It is the responsibility of the hospital authorities to set the pattern for the philosophy of patient care. It was rightly mentioned by Gardner that, No society can reach heights of greatness unless in all fields critical to its growth and creativity there is an ample supply of dedicated men and women.[8]

Most of the patients complained of a great distance between the doctors and the patients. This gap between the doctors and the patients must be bridged through personal attention given by the doctors to the patients. According to K.G. Agarwal, "Hospital effectiveness which can be measured in terms of patient satisfaction does not depend on the improvement of hospital service aspect alone but on the medical care aspect. Hospital effectiveness has a positive association with the hospital social system. The hospital social system is almost the measure of its organisational health. . . . . some element of democracy must be introduced in the hospitals. This might take care of the alienation of hospital staff that we see all around these."[9] K.K. Kaul, Professor and Head, Smt. Patel Paediatric Centre, Government Medical College, Jabalpur (M.P.), has rightly said, to restore their reputation, hospitals need to develop a strong system of public relations and intimate involvement with the community they serve.[10]

Besides these, there are other areas which must be attended to by hospital authorities to build the image of the hospitals. The most irritating factor for the dissatisfaction of the patients is that they have to wait for a long time in the out-patient departments because of the poor planning and management of hospitals. Most of the studies conducted in this regard found the time to be excessive and intolerable, i.e. varying between 2 to 3 hours per patient. The Public Accounts Committee remarked that,

Although certain delays are inherent in the situation and thus are inevitable, yet to a certain extent these can be overcome by rationalising the existing procedures and strengthening the organisations where necessary.

The patients also complain of the preferential treatment being given to VIPs and influential people. Some of the patients were of the view that these big hospitals are meant only to serve the VIPs. B.L. Agnihotri, in a letter to *The Tribune,* mentioned about the unsatisfactory conditions in hospitals in Himachal Pradesh. He mentioned that,

After waiting for two hours we were told by some interns that senior doctors were not concerned about the general public and only attended to VIPs and persons with recommendations from the secretariat. The majority of the doctors agree that conditions in these hospitals are bad but they feel helpless in the matter.[11]

The patients also complained of the lack of coordination between supportive services and the medical services. Most of the patients complained of the non-availability either of their X-ray report or other laboratory reports. They go on wasting their time in tracing their reports. Besides, many patients complained that preferential treatment is given to friends and relatives of the hospital. Many patients complained of the non-availability of medicines. Besides, patients are referred to other departments which results in great delays for the treatment to be given to them because of unsatisfactory coordination among the various departments of the hospital. In order to improve this relationship, the Public Accounts Committee suggested the following:

(1) To encourage polite and courteous behaviour of the staff towards the patients, orientation and in-serve training opportunities should be provided to the staff.
(2) Out-patients should be properly guided by the doctors issuing prescriptions regarding the procedure to be followed to get their blood, urine, stool, etc. samples tested.
(3) Laboratories may be modernized and out-dated equipment replaced as early as possible to improve the accuracy of the test results because these tests form the basis of the medical treatment which the patients are to be imparted.

Further, it is suggested on the basis of the observations by the author that the patients may be issued the slips on arrival on which may be indicated the probable time of his examination by the doctor. The following steps could also be taken to improve matters:

(a) Effective coordination should be established between the medical services and the supportive services to ensure promptness and clarity.
(b) Effective coordination and cooperation must be ensured among the various departments of the hospital to help the patients in diagnosing their ailments. It is suggested that a medical board may meet once a week where all the specialities may be represented and the patients needing the attention of more than one speciality may be asked to attend the board.
(c) A receptionist well versed with the functioning of hospital system may be appointed to guide the patients to approach the hospital properly.
(d) There is a need of playcards and signboards to guide the patients and their relatives.
(e) Provision of cheap and quality goods to be used by the patients or their relatives.
(f) Arrangement of stay of the relatives in Dharamsalas specially constructed for the purpose.
(g) Hospital beds may be given to patients according to the severity of the disease rather than other trifle considerations like obliging the VIPs.

In brief, the functioning of the hospital should be organised and re-organised to serve the patients most efficiently. All the personnel engaged in patient care must keep the following definitions of the "patient" in their minds.[12]

- The patient is the most important in the Hospital.
- The patient is not dependent upon us—we are dependent on him.
- The patient is not an interruption of our work—he is the purpose of it.
- The patient is not an outsider to our business—he is our business.
- The patient is a person and not a statistic. He has feelings, emotions, biases and wants.

It is our business to satisfy him. The participation of people in the formulation and administration of local and national plans and programmes that affect their well-being is particularly important at a time when developing countries like India are rapidly widening the scope of public services and adopting technological advances for improving their administration. Both developments could make public administration increasingly complex and more difficult for the mass of citizens to understand. Imaginative measures are needed to promote and sustain the interest of citizens in the hospital administration to give them a sense of participation in the decisions of hospitals that immediately affect them and to enable them contribute to better administration. Citizen participation in hospital administration is also an important safeguard against the abuse of administrative authority. It is a method for tapping human and material resources for development that might otherwise remain inert. It is a means for communicating to people the results of hospital action in fields that are of interest to them. To quote Pt. Jawaharlal Nehru, "Administration not only has to be good but also to be felt to be good by the people."

Administration is manned by and meant for human beings. Administration does not exist for itself but for the citizens. Jawaharlal Nehru while delivering the inaugural address at the Indian Institute of Public Administration said, "Administration like most things is, in the final analysis, a human problem to deal with human beings, not with some statistical data. . . . there is the danger that pure administrators at the top (not so much at the bottom, because they come into contact with human beings) may come to regard human beings as mere abstractions . . ..the administrator may think in abstract of the people he deals with, come to conclusions which are justifiable apparently, but which miss the human element. After all, whatever department of Government you deal with, it is ultimately a problem of human beings and the moment we forget them, we are driven away from reality."

Thus, Hospital Administration is not to exist in some kind of ivory tower. The true test of Hospital Administration is the welfare of the people visiting the hospitals. The Administrative Reforms Commission has also observed in this very connect that, "If, in the prosperity of the people, . . . the strength of a Government, it is in their contentment that lie the security and stability of democracy." In the words of Sir Harold Scot: "If a wide general knowledge is useful, even more valuable is a knowledge of people. It is very important that the young administrator should not retire into his cell when he leaves his office, but should mix with all kinds and conditions of people. From them, he will learn things that are not in his files.

It, therefore, follows that all the citizens have a right to participate in administration at all levels and they should in the interest of efficient functioning of administration in a democracy exercise this right.

It would be improper to describe this participation as hindrance, nuisance, interference or obstacle to efficient administration. Citizen participation, on the other hand, is an important part of the unfolding democratic process and not only should it be understood and welcomed but the sooner we all learn to use it, the better it would be for us all. In the past, the beneficiaries of hospital services were passively receiving hospital services. In modern times, there is a trend wherein the beneficiaries and the community at large wish to participate in the programmes of delivery of hospital and related community services. The hospital authorities must be alive to this emerging change and develop their hospital service plan accordingly.

We must set-up the patients Complaint Enquiry Committee for all hospitals on the pattern of Patient Complaint Enquiry Committee set-up in the Directorate-General of Health Services to look into the public complaints regarding the services in government and other hospitals in the Union Territory of Delhi.

Lack of Managerial Training on the Part of the Hospital Administration

Hospital Administration is a science as well as an art. The hospital administration has become complex and requires administrative capability to solve its managerial problems to provide the optimum care to the patients. It is, therefore, necessary that the persons charged with the efficient running of the hospitals are trained in the managerial techniques and tools which may be applied by them for getting the best out of the resources available. A Diploma in Health and Hospital Administration was started by the PGI in collaboration with the Punjab University (Department of Public Administration). It continued for two years 1975-76 and 1976-77, and was discontinued later on. Similarly, refresher courses are arranged twice a year by the NIHFW. What has been the impact of this training? Such a training could not make much impact as the trainers were acquainting them with the problems of management without their applicability in the Indian context. It is suggested that,

(a) All the Governments, Union and the States, must ensure that the top officers are appointed in the hospitals after giving them managerial training. What happens is that the persons on promotion become hospital administrators, without any management background.
(b) The trainers in the art of hospital administration must be given intensive training before they start imparting instruction. They should not bewilder the participants, with glamorous managerial techniques applicable in advanced countries but should provide them with simple tools, useful and applicable in the Indian context.
(c) A model hospital run on the modern lines may be set-up. The participants may be taken to this hospital to let them observe the application of techniques being taught to them.
(d) Training may be restricted only to those who are to shoulder this responsibility at present or in the immediate future.
(e) A regular follow-up of the training programme must be taken upto ensure the utility of training.

The hospital administrators should not be taught merely as the art and science of managing formal organisation which would add to the efficiency of hospitals. Rensis Likert, in his article, "Motivational Approach to Management Development in *Harvard Business Review* (pp. 37-77, July-August 1959) has mentioned a number of such principles which when taught intensively to the administrators would add to the performance of an organisation. These factors are as follows:

(i) Extent of loyalty to the institution and identification with it and its objectives.
(ii) Extent to which the goals of units and individuals facilitate the achievement of the organisation's objectives.
(iii) Level of motivation among members of the organisation with regard to such variables as:
  (a) Performance including both quality and quantity of work done.
  (b) Concern for elimination of waste and reduction of costs.
  (c) Concern for improving the product.
  (d) Concern for improving processes.
(iv) Degree of confidence and trust among members of the organisation in each other and in the different hierarchical levels.
(v) Amount and quality of the teamwork in units and between units of the organisation.
(vi) Extent to which people feel that delegation is effective.
(vii) Extent to which the members feel that their ideas, information, knowledge of processes, and experiences are being used in the decision-making processes of the organisation.

(viii) Upward, downward, and sideward efficiency and adequacy of the communication process.

(ix) Leadership skills and abilities of supervisors and managers, including their basic philosophies of management and orientation towards leadership processes.

(x) Hospital Services Consultancy Corporation: We may mention here the recent development in India to improve hospital efficiency. The government have set-up a company in the public sector under the Ministry of Health and Family Welfare, called "Hospital Services Consultancy Corporation (India) Limited" with an equity investment of Rs. 50 lakhs to provide comprehensive consultancy services both within the country and in developing countries on all aspects of establishment and management of hospital facilities. It is to provide the following services:

  (i) carry out analysis of the requests for hospital services, conduct feasibility studies and prepare initial project reports,

  (ii) undertake preparation of architectural designs for hospitals,

  (iii) undertake hospital construction on turn-key basis,

  (iv) undertake supply of equipments needed for running the hospital services,

  (v) prepare and supply medical as well as para-medical manpower needed for the management of such hospitals,

  (vi) undertake administration of the hospital for a period of time on contractual basis, and

  (vii) provide consultancy services in building up low cost primary health services, family planning services, etc. in developing countries.

Hospitals should make use of this Corporation to improve efficiency.

Medical Audit not a Regular Feature in most of the Hospitals

The purpose of Medical Audit is to evaluate factor impinging on patient care. All the deaths in a hospital where cause of death are not certain are investigated by the Mortality Review Committee. This improves the knowledge of the medical personnel and enhances their capability of handling such cases in future. The Health Survey and Planning Committee (1959-61) recommended the use of medical audit in all hospitals. The Delhi Hospital Review headed by Dr. K.N. Rao (1968) also recommended the appointment of a Medical Audit Committee in each hospital. Such committee will ensure specific checks on the quality of work performed in the hospitals. We have found the following drawbacks in some of the hospitals where such committees are functioning:

(1) Poor recording of a case history.

(2) Sketchy documentation.
(3) Operation notes not properly recorded.
(4) Lack of inter-departmental coordination.
(5) Incomplete case-notes.
(6) Not proper follow-up by the senior faculty members.

Either mortality committees have not been set-up in hospitals or function irregularly. The Public Accounts Committee also mentioned that, "Although the recommendation of the review committee to carry out hospital mortality review periodically was accepted by the Government in February 1970, it was only after a lapse of six years (May 1976) that the mortality review committee started functioning in Willington Hospital (Rammanohar Lohia Hospital)."

The conditions are worse in hospitals under the control of State Governments in this regard. Thus, there is a need to set-up such committees to ensure efficient and effective medical audit.

Unsatisfactory System of Drugs and Medical Supplies

The efficiency of hospital services depends not only on the competence of medical personnel but also on the availability of drugs in right quantity and quality. We are witnessing a number of problems in regard to the drugs management in hospitals. Some of the important problems are:[13]

(a) Pilferage of drugs.
(b) Purchase of drugs at higher prices from the open market because of lack of advance planning.
(c) Use of adulterated drugs.
(d) Shortage of essential drugs.
(e) Corruption among the authorities in a hospital.
(f) Qualified persons not responsible for drug management.
(g) Absence of regular inspections to check the drug stores.
(h) Use of expired drugs.

The Committee on pilferage of drugs observed,

"Some government hospital authorities were in league with drug suppliers. By manipulating records and accounts, hospital stores returned part of their stocks to suppliers for a financial consideration, or sold them to chemists at rock bottom prices. Often drugs obtained under the Central Government Health Scheme or the Employees' States Insurance Scheme were found to be falsely indented and sold to chemists."[14]

The Public Accounts Committee in its (1977-78) report was very critical of the drug management in the Central Government in Delhi. The

Committee remarked:

> "Certain medicines consumed by patients in the hospitals were substandard. There have been periodical reports of shortage of certain medicines and it appears that no effective machinery exists to take notice of such shortage in time for remedial action in a coordinated manner."[15]

We give here some suggestions to remove these defects:

(a) Different colours and designs of medicines may be specially manufacture for the distribution through hospitals like the service stamps used in the Government offices.
(b) The machinery to ensure quality drugs in the States needs to be strengthened.
(c) Advance planning of the requirements of the drugs should be done to ensure regular supply.
(d) Cheap drugs may be manufactured by the Government and all multi-national drug companies may be either wound up or asked to manufacture cheap drugs.
(e) The working of medical depots under the Ministry of Health and Family Welfare needs to be streamlined so that the hospitals may not get the opportunity to purchase drugs from the open market.
(f) *Ad hoc* purchases may not be encouraged except under serious circumstances.
(g) The hospital authorities should ensure that only genuine and fully tested medicines are provided to the patients. Time-barred medicines may not be used. Timely action may be taken to ensure that medicines may not become time-barred through the exchange of such medicines from the firms.
(h) Drug stores should be under the control of qualified pharmacists and not semi-skilled compounders

Less Emphasis on Human Side of Medicine

Many people visiting the hospitals constantly turn to doctors without showing any sign of physical disorder. Most of the doctors do not bother to diagnose their problems and administer them sleep inducing drugs which are ultimately harmful. Tranquillizers and barbiturates are being dispensed on a large scale. "It is because medicine has become so accustomed to searching for technical answers to its dilemmas that quests for answers on the behavioural side continue to be deferred."

What can be done to make the doctors understand all this? The situation can be improved by providing courses in anthropology, sociology, and psychology to the doctors. According to Maureen A. Bailey, "In the face of a virtual epidemic of behavioural disorders, modern health care must place a new emphasis on solving the human side of medicine."[16]

Absence of Cost Consciousness among Hospital Authorities and Staff

The budgets of hospitals are increasing beyond proportions over the years which is beyond the capacity of poor countries like India. The whole of the health budget is spent in maintaining few hospitals neglecting the vast population needing health and medical care.

According to H.A. Goddard, "In the management or administration of any enterprise, the quality, quantity, timing, and cost of the work necessary to reach the objectives of the enterprise are inter-related factors which must be given constant attention. If the resources for health work, in trained persons and in finances, were unlimited the need for constant attention to these factors would not be so great. But the limitation in the number of trained personnel and the lack of adequate financial resources are major obstacles to greatly improved health in the world today. We must, therefore, husband our resources carefully to accomplish as much as possible with what we have available."[17]

A serious problem in health care administration is the absence of cost-consciousness among the staff of public health administrations. All over the world, health service staff-even of the highest professional cadre-are taught little about the economics of health services and know little about the costs of the equipment and supplies they use. Doctors tend to employ what is new without regard to cost. It is a fashion to prescribe costly drugs. They are also subjected to considerable sales pressure from manufacturing firms. A cheaper drug or cheaper equipment may give just as good a result for the vast majority of patients. Cost-consciousness is not just a matter for central administrators or planners but should be inculcated in all those working in health care.

More people can be provided with services if no service cost more than what is a must to provide the necessary level of care. The price paid for high-cost technology for a few is no technology at all for the many. Another aspect of this problem is the use of hospital non-judiciously. In the more developed countries, the majority of secondary care is generally given in hospitals, and increasingly the hospitals in which it is provided tend to be large, i.e. 500 beds or more. The larger hospital offers the opportunity for a high degree or specialisation and for achieving the fullest use of expensive specialised equipment. The larger the hospital and the more specialised its work, the larger catchment area it needs to serve. The higher average transport costs for staff and patients may be justified by the quality of service that a large hospital should be able to provide.

In the developing countries like India where the bulk of the population live in rural areas with limited public or private facilities for long distance travel, such transport is costly, except for the few patients who can be transported to hospital in vehicles travelling for other purposes. Moreover, in-patient care must be provided much more selectively if it is not to absorb an excessive share of the health budget. It must be confined to those with a high probability of deriving clear and lasting benefit from it. The emphasis should be on ambulatory services.

For these reasons, hospitals should on average be smaller in developing countries than in more developed countries and they should not be used to provide the most sophisticated technology. Costs can be saved if limited number of relatives accompany the patient and take responsibility for preparing food and providing basic patient care. But many developing countries have followed the example of more developed countries and concentrated on a high proportion of their health service expenditure on large urban hospitals, many of them teaching hospitals, equipped to provide tertiary care with high technology. These hospitals have been set-up before smaller district hospitals have been developed and as transport is not normally developed they tend to be used to provide secondary care to the urban population. Moreover, they are mainly used for patients who do not need their special facilities, e.g., the chronically disabled children suffering from malnutrition, and patients with minor illness who could be treated in a much simpler hospital or at home. In some countries, the out-patient department of a regional hospital is even used to provide primary care as there is no referral system and time of super-specialists is wasted on minor problems which could be dealt elsewhere. It is suggested that the referral system must be made statutory to screen the patients.

Absence of Proper Space Planning

A large number of hospitals in the country have come to be established and housed in buildings which were not originally designed for the present needs and technology. The new hospitals have also to undergo changes as new facilities are provided to the community. The planning of hospital facilities in such a changing situation within the constraints of the existing space availability is one of the biggest problems that any hospital faces.

> "Moreover, hospital development is often designed in an *ad hoc* way or based on 'type plans', with the result defects are repeated in new hospital construction and remains unremedied in the existing ones."[18]

There is also lack of coordination between the hospital authorities and transport authorities resulting in the poor transport facilities available to the patients. The buildings and equipment are not maintained properly. It is suggested that:

(a) Hospital Engineering section must be set-up in all big hospitals to take care of the building and equipment.
(b) Hospitals may be located at places wherefrom transport facilities are easily available so that the patients can reach back home the same day.
(c) Proper maintenance of hospital equipment should be ensured otherwise these would tell upon the efficiency of hospitals.
(d) Hospital planning and administration should receive greater attention.

(e) Operational studies on such aspects as the utilisation of hospitals, over-crowding and referral system would help to define requirements realistically and bring improvements and economy in hospital design.

Poor Management of Dietary Services

The dietary unit stands as the second major department of a hospital from the point of view of expenditure. It needs careful analysis and control. Most of the patients always complain of poor and costly diets served in the hospitals. There is a problem of excess diets issued as compared to the number of patients resulting in huge expenditure. Besides, many of the patients do not consume all that is served to them. Patients generally prefer food from their houses as they do not like hospital food. The Public Accounts Committee (1977-78) has mentioned in this connection:

"The Committee are constrained to note that whereas economy on expenditure on diet is being thought of by reducing quantum of diet, other measures to effect economy without diminishing the quality and quantity of diet such as plugging leakages of diet, have not been given the attention they deserve. In the opinion of the committee the leakage of diets may be possibly one of the reasons for issue of excess diets over the census figure. Therefore, it is necessary that institutional arrangements are made to watch that leakages of diet and dietary materials do not take place."

It is suggested that the efficient management of dietary services may be done to achieve economy and quality. The hospital authorities must compare the cost of dietary services with other hospital dietary services and thus try to locate the defects and remedy them.

Non-Availability and Non-Judicious Utilisation of Blood

There is a lot of resentment among the patients and their relatives regarding the availability of blood required for certain ailments. Most of the patients complain about the prevalence of corruption in the supply of blood to patients. Besides, it is mentioned that only high ups in the Government can get the required supply of blood while the poor people are denied this right. It is suggested that the supply of blood must be made according to the needs of the patients rather than on the basis of their status. This would motivate the general public to donate blood for saving the lives of the people—a noble cause. The present author was entrusted with the task of arranging a camp to donate blood. The people when approached were very critical about the use of blood taken from voluntary workers. This feeling prevents most of the potential donors of blood to contribute to this noble cause. It is necessary to manage the blood banks in the hospitals judiciously to inspire confidence among the people in general-donors as well as consumers of the service.

Absence of Effective Personnel and Materials Planning

In most of the hospitals, there is no personnel planning, resulting in the under-utilisation of resources. Expenditure on personnel is mounting high and care must be taken to ensure optimum utilisation of resources. After the personnel, materials constitute about 50 per cent of the total expenditure of an organisation. Optimum utilisation of these resources must be ensured to achieve high productivity. There have been many cases where articles lying in bulk quantities in one department were purchased by the other and sometimes in emergency at exorbitant price. The situation can be improved by designing a proper system of purchase, storage and utilisation. The hospital authorities must ensure whether the existing staff in the various departments has been deployed consistent with the work-load and are accordingly to prescribed norms.

Besides, they are to ensure economy by avoiding wastage, duplication through inventory control. A study may be carried out in every hospital after three years in the following areas to ensure optimum utilisation:

1. Corporate Planning.
2. Manpower Utilisation.
3. Materials Management Drugs Control.
4. Management Information System.
5. Organisational Planning and Development.

Thus, periodic studies of the functioning of hospitals are needed to enable the administrators to manage them efficiently.

Absence of Planned Regionalisation to Ensure Graded Patient Care

At present, all hospitals whether at the state, district or local levels are working in isolation and their services are not provided in a coordinated manner. Most of the patients visit all these hospitals and are examined afresh by all of them resulting in wastage of efforts and resources. The medical staff prescribe medicines to patients without having a proper awareness of his previous treatment.

Mrs Indira Gandhi, former Prime Minister of India, while presiding over a function at Lady Hardinge Medical College at Delhi, rightly mentioned (quoted by Late Dr. P.N. Chhuttani, Ex-Director, PGI, in his article "Decentralisation Needed" published in Medical View Point column of *The Tribune,* dated 4-5-1980) that "The referral system has entirely failed in almost all our larger towns and cities. Consequently, there is growing overcrowding at our major hospitals whose services stand diluted. In the larger cities there is the multiplicity of the controlling authorities—The Government, the Municipal Corporation, the Municipal Committee, Voluntary Organisations, Private Hospitals, etc."

She further stated that "there is no common meeting ground and hospital services have become almost totally unregulated. Consequently, the conditions in our capital city are chaotic. The poor and the needy flock towards the larger, better known hospitals in the hope of better treatment and care only to find that they have to wait for days to be examined, much less to find a place to stay. Patients wander from hospital to hospital. Besides, facing considerable inconvenience, their efforts to seek relief cause duplication of work and expenditure. It is thus necessary that every big city must have an apex body, perhaps called the hospital board, to establish referral hospitals for every zone."

Referral System

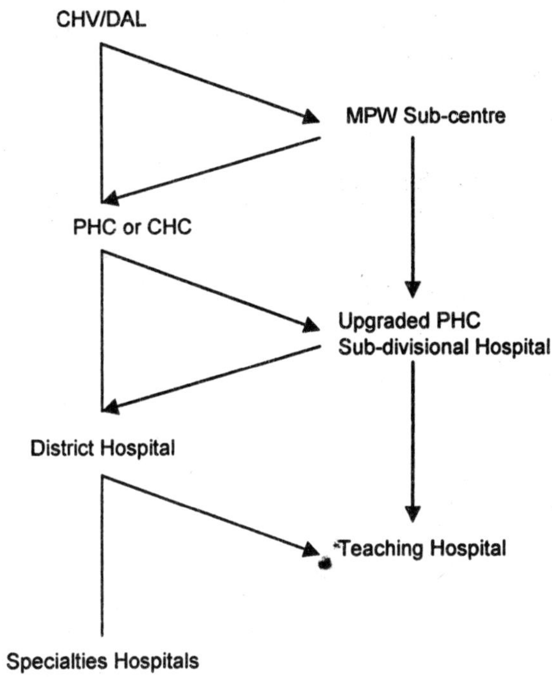

How can we get out of this chaos to design a system of patient care? The answer is-introduction of Regionalisation. Regionalisation connotes the development of graded patient care within a defined geographical or functional area from lower to higher levels adapting the health services to the characteristics and needs of the area and, thus, ensure the optimum utilisation of resources. The essential characteristics of regionalisation are:

(a) Two-way flow of patients,
(b) Two-way flow of records,
(c) Two-way flow of services,
(d) Two-way flow of personnel,
(e) Mobile units,
(f) Centralised administration and decentralised execution,
(g) Coordinating education programme for the region,
(h) Communication and transport between components, and
(i) Coordination with other community health services.

Thus, regionalisation would ensure the best utilisation of time of the specialists and provision of comprehensive health care to the patients nearer their homes with all the benefits of specialities. The regional area should neither be too large nor too small but should be such as to ensure adequate span of attention. It would also automatically develop referral system scientifically. The referral system presents the following five aspects:[20]

(a) It has to be built into the organisational structure of the medical services of a country. The file should be that only when one unit cannot provide what a patient needs should the patient be referred to the next higher unit in the chain.
(b) The referral system has to be organised both internally and externally. 'Internally' means that patients in the hospital have to be referred from the in-patients to the out-patients department just as soon as their health situation permits. The 'externally' referred system exists among the several institutions on different levels of the hierarchy.
(c) The referral system must be established for the purpose of diagnosis and treatment and used for both in-patients and out-patients.
(d) It is a two-way system. Patients should be referred to higher level institutions for diagnosis and treatment when necessary, but they should also be referred back to the referring institution as soon as possible.
(e) The referral system concerns not only patients and diagnostic facilities but also the personnel of the medical services.

This is also a two-way system, so that human knowledge and skills are utilised fully and are continually developed through consultations and the interchange of ideas and experience. The specialists from the regional hospital must come to the District hospital and the specialist from the District hospital to the health centre on a regular basis as consultants, to hold specialist clinics and give guidance; the medical and para-medical personnel should go to the higher level institution regularly for in-service training.

Absence of any Legislation for the Organisation and Functioning of Hospitals

At present there is no comprehensive legislation to guide the organisation and management of hospitals. There is need of a hospital legislation to ensure maintenance of standards, to define rights and duties of the hospital staff and to ensure the efficient function in of hospitals. It is suggested that the Government of India may set-up a body that is Development Council for Hospitals with its branches in the States like the Medical Council of India, to lay down policies to ensure that the hospitals have requisite facilities and provide efficient services to the patients. It has become a common practice to set-up nursing homes in the private sector. These so-called 'nursing homes' are often huge money-making projects devised by the specialists in league with one another. All these nursing homes must be under the control of the proposed council.

It should be the duty of the council to see that the specialities like the private industry do not fleece the people and provide medical care of right quality and at a reasonable price. Besides, the proposed council may attend to the complaints of the patients to ensure smooth relations between the hospital authorities and the beneficiaries and thus help in the building of a 'Welfare State, a cherished ideal in the constitutions of most of the states in the world.

We must attend to all these problems to ensure efficiency of the hospitals. These problems also emanate from a number of constraints on hospital authorities, e.g., shortage of staff at all levels, absence of proper accommodation to provide space to the ever increasing number of patients. shortage of equipment political and administrative inference, etc. which need to be attended to by the governments at the Union and State level to provide satisfactory hospital services. Besides, the patients and their relatives must cooperate with the hospital authorities to make the best use of the available resources. Thus, we shall have to have a three-pronged attack—increasing internal efficiency, mobilising government support and enlisting people's cooperation to ensure the reputation, prestige, credibility and viability of the hospital services.

Notes and References

1. WHO, Technical Report Series, 1968, 395, p. 6.
2. WHO, Technical Report Series, 1957, 122, p. 4. .
3. Punjab Government Memo. No. 118754-81-66/30459, dated 25.10.1977 (from the Secretary to Government of Punjab, Medical and Health Deptt. to the Director, Health Services, Punjab).
4. Tiny M. Calender, Unit Administration, W.B. Saunders Co., London, 1962, p. 66.
5. V. Ramalingaswami, "Medicine, Health and Human Development" in Health and Basic Services: Key to Development by UNICU, New Delhi, p. 10.
6. Lawrence J. Sakarai, 'The Hippocratic Oath: License to Kill" in *Sunday Standard*, Chandigarh, 12 August, 1979 (Sunday Magazine, p. 1).
7. Mary D. Shanks and Dorothy A. Kennedy, The Theory and Practice of Nursing Service Administration, McGraw-Hill, London, 1965, p. 95.
8. John W. Gardner, Excellence, New York, 1961, Harper and Brothers, p. 154.
9. K.G. Agarwal, "Managing Patient Satisfaction in Hospitals" in the *Indian Journal of Public Administration*, Vol. XXII, No. 2, April-June 1976, p. 277.
10. K.K. Kaul, "Hospitalisation of Children", Health and Population—Perspective and Issues, 2(1): 49-53, 1979.
11. *The Tribune*, Chandigarh, November I, 1979.
12. Edythe Alexander *et al.*, Nursing Service Administration (ed.), New York, C.V. Mosby Co, 1962, p. 63.

13. Based upon personal discussion with hospital staff at Chandigarh.
14. *Indian Journal of Hospital Pharmacy,* Vol. VII, No. 3-4/70.
15. Lok Sabha Secretariat, Public Accounts Committee, Forty-ninth Report, Sixth Lok Sabha, December 1977, p. 142.
16. Maureen A. Bailey, "The Human Side" in *World Health,* December 1975, p. 4.
17. H.A. Goddard, Principles of Administration applied to Nursing Service, *World Health* Organisation, Geneva, 1958, p. 84.
18. WHO, SEA/RC/21/2, p. VIII.
19. Timmappaya Regionalisation of Health Care (Mimeographed).
20. WHO, SEARO; SEA/RC 23/1, pp. 39-40.

3

CHAPTER

Organisation and Working of AIIMS

A Regional Tertiary Health Care Hospital

INTRODUCTION

The All India Institute of Medical Sciences (AIIMS) was established by an Act of Parliament in 1956 as an institution of national importance. Its main objectives are to develop patterns of teaching in undergraduate and postgraduate medical education in all its branches, so as to demonstrate a high standard of medical education to all medical colleges and other allied institutions in India; to bring together in one place educational facilities of the highest order for the training of personnel in all important branches of health activity; and to attain self-sufficiency in postgraduate medical education.

For pursuing academic programmes, the AIIMS has been kept outside the purview of the Medical Council of India. The Institute awards its own degrees. The AIIMS continues to be a leader in the field of medical education, research and patient care in keeping with the mandate of the Parliament. The Institute is fully funded by the Government of India. However, for research activities, grants are also received from various sources including national and international agencies. While the major part of the hospital services are highly subsidized for the patients coming to the AIIMS hospital, certain categories of patients are charged for treatment/ services rendered to them.

ORGANISATION

Institute Body

It consists of 20 members with Health Minister as Chairman, two Members from Lok Sabha, one member from Rajya Sabha, Secretary Health and Family Welfare (Ex-officio), Director-General of Health Service (Ex-

AIIMS
Organisation Structure

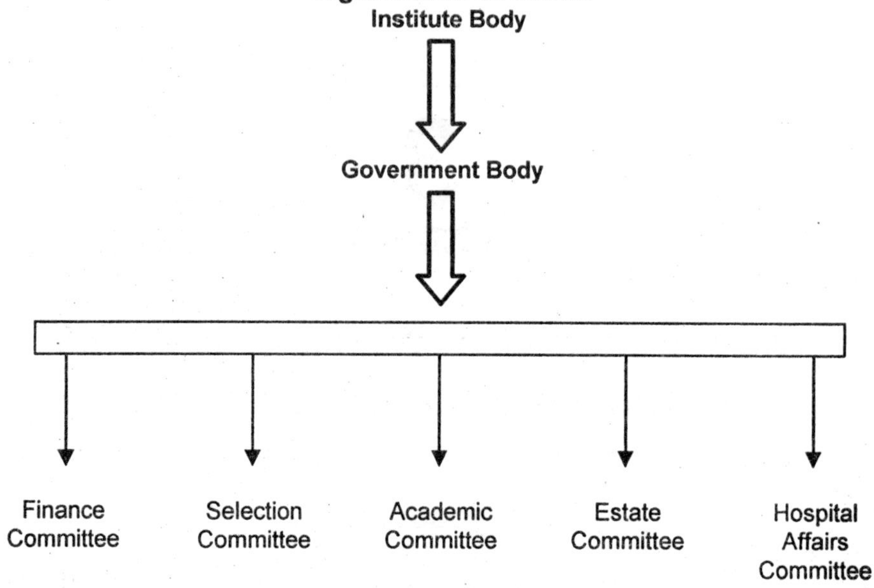

Office), Additional Secretary and Financial Adviser (Ex-officio) Ministry of Health and Family, one Joint Secretary, Ministry of health and Family Welfare, Sectary of Department of Biotechnology, Secretary Secondary and Higher Education and other Experts from AIIMS and other places. From the composition of AIIMS Institute body it appears that the body is dominated by Ministry and other Government functionary. Its composition should reflect top persons of health who can contribute to the development of the Institute. Minster of Health and Family Welfare, GOI, should not be put as Chairman as in his presence, other members' freedom is limited. Since this is top body of the Institute, it should be occupied by eminent persons in different areas of medicine. Same should apply to Governing Body and its Committees.

Governing Body has 10 members with Health Minister as the Chairperson with 9 other members including Director as Member Secretary. All the committees have nine members.

The Organisational structure of AIIMS appears to be under strict control of the Ministry of Health and Family Welfare. The development of such an apex institution of national importance need be granted autonomy otherwise there can very less innovation and creativity without which AIIMS cannot grow to International standard. The Ministry of Health and Family Welfare should exercise policy control and not interference in day-to-day affairs.

FUNCTIONS

1. Undergraduate Education

Academic section handles post-admission formalities for new students, develops and revises curricula, and administers teaching programmes including internal assessment of undergraduate students. the courses include MB, BS, B.Sc. (Hons.) in paramedical courses such as Medical Technology in Radiography and Ophthalmic Techniques, and B.Sc. Nursing (Post-certificate) and B.Sc. (Hons.) Nursing courses.

Every year 50 students are admitted to the MB, BS course. Out of 50 seats, 5 seats are reserved for foreign nationals and the screening and admission for these 5 seats is done on the recommendation of the Ministry of External Affairs, Government of India. For the remaining 45 seats (7 for Scheduled Caste, 4 for Scheduled Tribe and 34 general category candidates), students are selected on the basis of their performance in an All-India entrance examination. Further, 3% seats are reserved for orthopedic physically handicapped candidates on horizontal basis. During 2006 there were 52,798 applicants and 38,516 candidates appeared in the entrance examination for these 45 seats. The total number of undergraduate students as on 31 March 2005 was 260 including 54 interns.

In addition, 17 Students of B.Sc. Nursing (post-certificate) course including one foreign national, 51 students to B.Sc. (Hons.) in Nursing course including four nationals, foreign 12 students to B.Sc. (Hons.) in Opthalmic Techniques including one foreign national and 7 Students to B.Sc. (Hons.) in Medical technology in Radiography including one foreign national student.

The MBBS course is spread over five-and-a-half (5½) years, dividing the period to one year for pre-clinical, one-and-a-half (1½) year for para-clinical and two years for clinical subjects followed by one-year rotating internship. Para-medical courses like B.Sc. (Hons) in Nursing, Ophthalmic Techniques and Medical Technology in Radiography continued to be popular and attracted students from other countries also. The curricula of these courses are under constant scrutiny by the faculty of the Institute for purposes of improvement.

2. Post-Graduate Education

The Academic Section looks after all activities pertaining to admission, selection and training of postgraduate students including junior and senior residents. It also deals with all service matters relating to senior residents. It handles all activities of the Ph.D., DM, M.Ch., MD, MS, MDS, MHA, M.Sc. and M.Biotech courses in different disciplines.

The admission to all postgraduate courses is done by an All India entrance examination that is held twice a year. Foreign nationals are also admitted through an entrance examination. Postgraduate students from Nepal are admitted under a bilateral agreement between the Governments of India and Nepal.

During 2006-07 session (i.e. for the courses commencing in January 2006 and July 2006), 333 students were admitted to various postgraduate, post-doctoral and superspeciality courses, i.e. MD, MS, MDS, MDA, Ph.D., M.Ch. DM and M.Sc. in various specialities. 24 candidates belonging to Scheduled Caste, and 9 candidates belonging to the Scheduled Tribes got admission to the postgraduate courses. The Institute provides full time postgraduate and post-doctoral courses in 57 disciplines. In the year 2004, 193 postgraduate students including DM/M.Ch. for various degrees in December 2006 and May 2006 and 29 students qualified for Ph.D. degrees from October 2005 to September 30, 2006. The guiding principle in postgraduate training is to train them as teachers, researchers and above all as competent doctors to manage and treat the patients independently. 290 candidates from various organisations and State Government received short term training at various departments of the Institute during the year.

Following are the important departments of Excellence:

1. Dr. R.P. Centre for Ophthalmic Sciences
2. Department of Neuro-Radiology
3. Dr. B.R.A. Institute Rotary Cancer Hospital
4. Department of Psychiartry
5. Department of Radio-Diagnosis
6. Department of Forensic Medicine and Taxicology
7. Department of ENT
8. Department of Obstetrics and Gynaecology
9. Department of Urology
10. Department of Pediatric Survery
11. Department of Pediatrics
12. Department of Orthopaetics.

3. Continuing Medical Education

The Institute organized a number of workshops, symposia, conferences and training programme in collaboration with various national and international agencies during the year. Professionals from various institutions all over the country participated in these seminars and workshops and benefited with updated knowledge. Guest and Public Lectures were organized by visiting experts and faculty of AIMS.

4. Short and Long-term Training Programmes

The Academic Section handles activities regarding training programmes of short- and long-term duration for both medical and paramedical personnel. During the year, the Institute had 464 short- and 10 long-term trainees. In addition, 14 short-term trainees under the WHO fellowship programme and 18 foreign trainees and 53 (out of 72 candidates) fellows under the WHO In-Country Fellowship (2004-05) were imparted training in various departments. The elective posting of foreign undergraduate medical students is also handled by the section. During the year, 56 foreign undergraduate medical students underwent elective training.

5. Training for Scheduled Castes (SC) and the Scheduled Tribes (ST)

The SC and ST candidates are given due consideration and weightage in accordance with the Government of India guidelines in all selections. During the current year 32 SC/ST candidates were selected for various undergraduate courses, i.e. MBBS, B.Sc. Nursing (Hons), B.Sc. (Hons) Radiography. 33 SC/ST candidates selected for various postgraduate courses, i.e. MD, MS, MHA, M.Sc. (Nursing) and M.Sc. in various other disciplines during the year 2006.

6. Research

The All India Institute of Medical Sciences is a leader in the field of teaching and research which are conducted in 50 disciplines, having more than 1300 research publications by its faculty and researcher in a year 2005-06, besides publishing books. Over 385 research projects are continuing during this period. Research grants totaling to Rs. 8.20 crores (Approx.) has been received from various international and national funding agencies during the year 2006-07 (w.e.f. 01.04.2006 to 30.09.06).

7. Patient Care Services

AIIMS being a premier tertiary care hospital caters not only to the patients from India but also from neighbouring countries like Nepal, Bangladesh, Sri Lanka, Bhutan and other Asian Countries. At present it has an OPD attendance of over 16,30,479 in-patients admission of over 83,559 and conducts more than 86,081 surgical procedures in a year (2005-06).

8. Budget

During the year 2006-07 the Institute has been provided Rs. 205.86 crores under Plan and Rs. 283.00 crores under Non-Plan. Hospital is administered by Medical Suptd., Professor, Additional Professor and Associate Professor.

The AIIMS has been highly appreciated for contributing to the advancement of medical sciences. Dr. Uton Muchtar Rafei, Former Regional Director for WHO SEARO remarked that WHO in General and the South-East Asia in particular has had a long, productive and cherished relationship of close collaboration with AIIMS. Certainly the fact that we are located in the same great city helps. But the reason of our partnership goes for beyond this. We recognize AIIMS as one of the prestigious and eminent institution on medical education, health care and in health research. Several departments with AIIMS have been designated as WHO collaborative centres where research on "cutting edge" issues is called out in active collaboration with WHO" . . . We are also working on a number of projects in Nutrition. All of these will have significant effect not only for AIIMS and India, but for the entire region and in most instances, for the people of the whole world.

Inspite of some cases of negligence as the operation of a worng eye, leaving a place of cloth in stomach after operation in a woman's stomach, and others, there have been appreciation from all sections of society. Recently the AIIMS was in limelight because of the controversy between the Director and the Minister of Health, Government of India. However, AIIMS can still reach the heights of academic excellence and maintain international standards, we suggest the facts and suggestions.

Outpatient Department and Specialty Clinics

A total of 16,30,479 patients attended the general outpatient departments and specialty clinics of the main hospital. The details of the outpatient load profile is given in Appendix III.

Inpatient Services

The hospital had maintained its tradition of services and quality of patient care in spite of the ever-increasing number of patients that come to this hospital from all over the country as well as abroad. A total of 83559 patients were admitted during the year in the various clinical units of the hospital. 86,081 surgical operations are performed. Due to non-functioning of computers, some parameters such as unit-wise average length of stay, etc. could not be compiled. The state-wise and department-wise admissions are given in Appendices IV and V. The number of surgical procedures performed during the year in different surgical disciplines is given in Appendix VI.

General Information

Total number of beds	986
General ward beds	861
Private ward beds	125

Hospital Performance Indices

	Current year	*Past year*	*Comments*
Average length of stay (days)	5.2	5.4	Indicates effective utilization of beds.
Average bed occupancy rate (%)	83.2	80.5	Indicates fair occupancy
Net death rate(%)	2.7	2.8	Indicates a low mortality rate despite the fact that a large number of critically ill patients are admitted to the hospital
Combined crude infection rate (%)	8.92	9.5	

Please see Appendices I and II for details.

AIIMS is known all over the world for education, research, training, consultancy and tertiary health care. International specialized agencies like *World health* Organisation, World Bank and other bilateral agencies have rated AIIMS very high and that is why these agencies have made AIIMS their regional centres in many areas of medical sciences.

A landmark in Delhi, the Institute attracts 9,000 patients a day in OPDs and specialty clinics. It has 50 OPDs and 152 specialty clinics (Monday to Saturday) open 300 days a year. The emergency is open 24 hours round the year and caters, on an average, to 500 to 600 patients a day. A study done by AIIMS in 2003 inferred that 26,500 vehicles are parked in the Institute everyday.

Expansion Plans

As part of its redevelopment plan, the administration wants to go in for a multi-storey parking lot. The bed capacity of 2200 will be increased to 4500 when additional specialty centres come up. In the pipeline are centres for geriatric care, renal diseases, liver diseases, genetic and molecular biology, besides a surgical block and the school of public health.

AIIMS also runs a comprehensive rural health project in Ballabgarh to train MBBS students and resident doctors in community health. It also runs the National Drug Dependence Treatment Centre in Ghaziabad.

Rated as the best teaching institute among the medical colleges by two magazine surveys, AIIMS enrolls 50 MBBS students every year from the total of more than 75,000 who appear for the MBBS entrance examination. Of these, five seats are reserved for foreign nationals and 13 are reserved. In the postgraduate entrance examination, about 30,000 doctors appear for 270 seats.

CRITICAL APPRAISAL

I. Eminent Faculty Members feel frustrated and disenchanted and Leaving the Prestigious Institute: Need of Retention

AIIMS claims to publish 1300 to 1400 papers in national and international journals and 25 to 30 books every year. In its glorious days, till mid-1970s, AIIMS was compared to Mayo and Cleveland Clinic. Professor S.N. Mehta, former Head of the Department of Surgery at AIIMS says, "The Parliament and the government should take some concrete measures to preserve AIIMS. Such institutes are made once in the life of a nation."

A large number of poor and semi-literate patients, in the words of a former faculty member, "are kicked around", the hospital administration insists that the hospital is pro-poor. They cite *Newsweek's* report of October 2006 describing AIIMS as "an oasis for India's poorest," which says that 3.5 million patients were treated in AIIMS in 2005.

A former faculty member whose association with AIIMS is as old as the institute says, "AIIMS is still the best. There is overcrowding because we are paying the price for our popularity, credibility and professionalism. The image has suffered because of the number of patients. It has reached a saturation point in terms of the number of patients attending the OPD, emergency and the hospital for surgeries."

On the burden on AIIMS, Anoop Saraya, Convener of the AIIMS Front of Social Consciousness, says, "It is up to the government to create proper infrastructure at the periphery so that people don't come to the Institute for minor ailments, otherwise this tertiary care centre will crumble under the workload. Around 8,000 to 10,000 patients come to the Institute every day. At times, I examine 100 patients a day stretching the OPD till 3 p.m. So do other doctors."

In the last three years, more than half a dozen senior faculty members have left AIIMS. Last summer, three senior, high-profile doctors associated with AIIMS for nearly three decades, left. They left because they were disillusioned with the system.

Professor V.S. Mehta, Chief of Neurosciences Centre, and Dr Anoop Misra from the Department of Medicine, bid adieu to the institute in April last year. Four months later, Professor S.N. Mehta, Head of the Department of Surgery and Chief of Kidney transplant services quit and joined Indraprastha Apollo Hospital as a senior consultant. He said, "I had ceased to enjoy my work for almost two years and decided to consider the offers that were coming my way. In my 27 years of association with AIIMS, I had never seen an administration that was so indifferent to the needs of the department and the institute." In May 2005, Dr Sabyasachi Bal, lung surgeon quit his job as he felt he had not got a fair deal from AIIMS. Professor V.S. Mehta, Director of Neurosciences at Paras Hospital, Guragon left AIIMS on April 1 last year as he was "disgusted with the work environment." Dr Sandeep Vaishya, Additional Professor, Department of Neurosurgery, left AIIMS in March last year after 14 years of service to join Max Super-Specialty Hospital in Saket as Senior Consultant, Neurosurgery and Spine Surgery. "I wanted a fresh challenge. The gradual change in the work environment at AIIMS was disheartening." Dr Anoop Misra, Director, Diabetes and Metabolic Diseases Department, Fortis Hospital, Saket, quit the Department of Medicine. "When I joined AIIMS as an undergraduate in 1978, it offered a very good learning platform. The students were very bright. The caliber of students is now second rate. The best students are no longer opting for medicine."[1] We suggests here the following:

1. Faculty is the life of the Institute. AIIMS is known by its eminent faculty. The Ministry of Health and Family Welfare should provide incentives to faculty to retain their services.
2. Faculty should engage itself in its work and not engage in politics and try to be favorate to politicians and their relatives.
3. Faculty must attend to their teaching assignment whole-heartedly so that excellent doctors can be prepared.
4. Faculty should inculcate ethical values in students as medical

profession is coming under great criticism because of its material approach.

5. Faculty should keep themselves up-to-date and take the patient care seriously.
6. Faculty should not try to be popular with MD, MS students but should make them work serious as they would imbibe the approach taught to them.

2. No Political Interference

The medical experts working in AIIMS do not belong to any party except their discipline and specialisation. The faculty of AIIMS must be allowed to carry out their work without any political interference. Since AIIMS is located in the capital city of Delhi where VVIPS are in large number. There is no harm in giving best treatments to them but they should not ignore the poor patients who have come from long distances with some hope which should be fee filled otherwise AIIMS would become only a tertiary hospital of VVIPS. It is suggested that the personnel working in AIIMS must keep themselves away from politics and concentrate on their specialisation in theory and practice.

Politicians in India interfere in the day-to-day work of such an institution of national importance. Political interference demoralizes the Director and employs and ultimately ruin the institution and act as road blocks in the progress of the institution. During the last two years, AIIMS has been in the news and there has been bad news daily about the institute. Even courts have to interfere the protect the institute from deteriorating. However, political interference went on increasing causing a great damage to this institute.

A Case Study of the Director of AIIMS

For a long time, Health and Family Planning Minister, Government of India was determined to remove Director AIIMS on whimsical grounds. However, he failed to do so because intervention of the Court.

The bill was moved following a Delhi High Court ruling of March 29, 2007, which held that the appointment to the director's post was a tenure appointment and could not be curtailed except for justifiable reason and with prior notice to the director.

The court had also directed the centre and the AIIMS's governing body to formulate a policy covering the various facets and conditions of service of its employees, including the director, in accordance with law and to uniformly apply such policy in the future.

The Congress-led UPA government today forced its way and got the AIIMS Bill, which indirectly seeks to remove AIIMS Director Dr P. Venugopal, passed in the Rajya Sabha amid pandemonium and strong protest from the opposition.

Rajya Sabha Deputy Chairperson K. Rahman Khan had to adjourn the House twice as vociferous opposition members trooped into the well of the House to prevent the bill from being passed.

The opposition members belonging to the BJP, AIADMK, TDP and the Trinamool Congress shouted that the government was trying to destroy the premier medical institution by pushing through such a bill.

However, when the House reassembled, Khan allowed union health minister Ambumani Ramadoss to seek the passage of the bill through voice vote amid pandemonium and slogan shouting by opposition members.

The AIIMS and the Post-Graduate Institute of Medical Education and Research (Amendment) Bill, 2007 has now got the Parliamnet's nod as the Lok Sabha has already passed it.

The bill, seeking to amend the AIIMS Act 1956 and the Post-Graduate Institute of Medical Education and Research, Chandigarh Act, 1966, was introduced in Parliamnet on August 17.

Justifying the bill, Ramadoss who made his statement amid persistent slogan shouting from the opposition members said the bill would streamline the functioning of AIIMS, New Delhi, and the PGI, Chandigarh.

Earlier as soon as the House reassembled at 3.10 p.m. after two adjournments, opposition members rose on their feet, raising slogans: "Loktantra ki hatya band karo" (stop the killing of democracy), "sansad mein manmani nahi chalegi" (whims and fancies of government will not be allowed in parliament).

Amiddin, Samajwadi Party leader Amar Singh, who heads the Parliamentary Standing Committee on Health, regretted that the bill was introduced without consulting the committee.

"I am not opposed to the bill. I am only opposed to the manner, in which the bill has been introduced in the House," he said, and sought the projection of the Chair to ensure that it did not turn into a precedent.

Even as Ramadoss continued his reply on the bill, BJP member from Orissa Rudranarayan Pani moved menacingly towards the health minister, forcing members of treasury benches to stop him. Tore the copy of the bill of treasury benches to stop him. Some AIADMK members even tore off the copy of the bill.

The bill seeks to fix the term of the director for five years or till he/ she attains the age of 65, whichever is earlier.

Dr. Venugopal turned 65 in July this year, and with the director and the health minister not having a cordial relationship amongst each other, the bill has become an utmost priority for Ramadoss.

Once this bill becomes law, it will also empower the central government to terminate the services of the director even before his term expires for the sake of public interest.[2]

AIIMS does to resume strike, OPD shout today

Hindustan Times, Thursday, November 29, 2007, Jaya Shroff, November 28, New Delhi, said in his article:

"If the bill is signed, entire AIIMS will be paralyzed," said Dr. Harsh

> Kumar, president, RDA. "The situation is worse than Pakistan. There was a lot of resistance in Lok Sabha at the time of passage of the bill. Only selected information was made available to the public. Who says we are a democratic nation?"

Over 10,000 patients may have to return without treatment from the All India Institute of Medical Sciences (AIIMS) on 29th November 2007, as the Out Patient Department (OPD) will be shut.

The emergency ward too will close down when the AIIMS bill, seeking to limit superannuation age of directors of the institute, is passed in the Doctors Association (RDA).

> "it is an unfortunate situation as the battle between two individuals is going to affect thousands of helpless patients. But strike is absolutely inevitable." said a senior doctor of the institute.

Hindustan Times, Live Corresponding Chandigarh, November 28, 2007 "AIIMS, PGIMER Bill: Things Calm at PGI observed:

> "Everybody knows that the Bill is extension of an individual's whims and fancies and we extend support to our counter-parts at AIIMS.

On a clause of removal of Directory by the government if he is not acting in public interest, Dr. Banerjee, said this would end autonomy of two premier institutes of the country. "Director would not be able to function properly since he would always feel a sword hanging over his head."

In an Editorial of *The Tribune*: Targeting a doctor when ministerial pique becomes a policy.

The ostensible purpose of the All-India Institute of Medical Sciences (AIIMS) and Post-Graduate Institute of Medical Education and Research (PGIMER) Bill, 2007 passed by the Rajya Sabha on Wednesday and the Lok Sabha earlier may be to fix the age and tenure of the directors of these two premier medical institutions situated in Delhi and Chandigarh, respectively. But the real purpose is only to fix the head of AIIMS P. Venugopal by law or otherwise at the instance of the recalcitrant Health Minister A. Ramdoss who has been engaged in a running feud with the eminent surgeon. When nothing else worked, the minister has managed to bring in a Bill which will ensure that the heart surgeon will have to bow out. What is worse is that the minister, who is unable to swallow his pride bordering arrogance, and is hell-bent on throwing out Dr. Venugopal. That should be the first time that a Bill has been brought in to show the door to an eminent doctor who has given new life to thousands of people. That is a dangerous precedent unfit for a democracy. Dr. Venugopal has challenged the decision, saying that it smacked of mala fide and arbitrariness.

Politician's depredations have played havoc with the nation's leading institute. The only way to bring it back on the rails is by giving it autonomy, freeing it from ministerial whims. It should be run by professionals and the government should have nothing to do with its day-to-day affairs.

But the new Bill is a step in exactly the opposite direction. It will push AIIMS even further under the thumb of the minister who is not going to be in the saddle all the time. That is an unacceptable situation, particularly when the minister happens to be as erratic as Dr. Ramadoss. The PMK representative is not likely to understand on his own that AIIMS is not his personal fiefdom. The Prime Minister may have to intervene to ensure that an institute like AIIMS does not suffer. The doctors of the institute are agitated. But they too should not do anything, which inconveniences the public.[3]

S.S. Negi, Legal Correspondent, *The Tribune*, Chandigarh on Friday, November 30th 2007, "Venugopal Moves SC against new law."

NDA boycotts proceedings in RS observed:

> The BJP-led opposition NDA today boycotted proceedings in the Rajya Sabha for the entire day in protest against the manner in which the Bill fixing the age of retirement of the director of the All India Institute of Medical Sciences (AIIMS) was introduced and then passed yesterday.

Immediately after the House met for the question hour, deputy leader of the opposition in the Rajya Sabha Sushma Swaraj said her party was boycotting the day's proceedings in the House in protest against the Bill passed yesterday, fixing the age of retirement of AIIMS director at 65.

The NDA decision came despite chairman Hamid Ansari's assurance that the members could raise the matter after the question hour.

The passage of the Bill has paved the way for the removal of present AIIMS director P. Venugopal, who has been at loggerheads with health minister Ambumani Ramadoss over various issues.

There seems to be no end to the face off between AIIMS director P. Venugopal and health minister Ambumani Ramadoss as the noted surgeon today in a swift action moved the Supreme Court to challenge the new law curtailing the fixed five-year tenure of the directors of AIIMS and Chandigarh's PGIMER.

The powerful doctors body, Faculty Association of AIIMS, also in a separate petition challenged the AIIMS and PGIMER Amendment Act, 2007 passed by the Rajya Sabha yesterday after the Lok Sabha had passed it last week.

Both the petitions were filed in the Supreme Court Registry amid hectic activities by the lawyers of Venugopal and the faculty association of AIIMS governing body, which virtually went on tracking their move.

In a bid to strengthen his case, the noted doctor cited two rulings of the apex court pertaining to the AIIMS director's tenure in 1992 and 1996 holding it was a fixed tenure of five years.

Similarly, he also cited the two orders of the Delhi High Court of July 7, 2006 and October 18, 2006 while staying Ramadoss-sponsored AIIMS governing body's order sacking him.

Physicians, heal thyselves

In what appears to be a personal vendetta against All India Institute of Medical Sciences (AIIMS) Director Dr P. Venugopal, Union Health Miniser Dr. Anbumani Ramadoss has once again thrown the health facility into turmoil. The bone of contention this time is the AIIMS Amendment Bill 2007, which the minister has pushed through in both Houses of Parliament. The Bill sets the age limit for the director at 65 or limits him to five years in office. When the President clears the Bill, the eminent cardio thoracic surgeon, who will be 66, will lose his post, something the minister has been agitating for. The Bill also provides for the removal of future directors of AIIMS with three months notice. Dr. Venugopal has already moved the Supreme Court challenging the Bill. The result of this standoff would have been the closure of OPD facilities at the institute and enormous hardship to thousands of patients had Dr. Venugopal not appealed to the doctors to refrain from disrupting work.

The Delhi High Court has taken a very serious view of the situation and warned doctors that it will not stand by if patients are harassed. The Health Minister, who should be occupied with far more pressing issues relating to the health system, has been obsessed with wresting control of AIIMS. No one can have a grouse with a government facility dictating the retirement age of its director. But after the unseemly wrangle between the director and minister, it is difficult to believe that the amendment was motivated by professional considerations. The fact that there has been little political opposition to the minister's efforts could lie in the politics behind all this. The minister is the son of S. Ramadoss, the head of the politically powerful Patali Makkal Katchi party in Tamil Nadu, which is wooed by both the major parties in the state, the DMK and the AIADMK. In the era of coalitions, no one, not even at the Centre, can alienate regional satraps like Ramadoss senior.

The minister must realize that after these shenanigans, there will be less incentive for doctors to work in the public health system, even in urban areas. All talk of attracting doctors to work in the rural health system becomes meaningless. We are rightly proud of foreigners flocking to take advantage of Indian health facilities. But when it comes to the health of our own citizens, it would seem that the government's medicine is just not working. A bitter pill that we are forced to swallow.[4]

The Case of Dr. Venugopal: It's nothing but vendetta gone wild

Ordinarily, poets, writers, doctors and intellectuals should be treated with respect in every democratic country. The sacking of Dr P. Venugopal from the post of Director of All India Institute of Medical Sciences within minutes of President Pratibha Patil giving her assent to the AIIMS

(Amendment) Bill, however, cannot do the nation proud. Union Health Minister Anbumani Ramadoss can have the satisfaction that he could push his Bill through both Houses of Parliament to see the back of Dr P. Venugopal. In the process, he has caused harm to the medical profession and thrown to the wind all niceties in minister-AIIMS relations. It is, perhaps, the first time that an individual-specific law has been enacted by Parliament. Even if there was a case for fixing the retirement age of the Director, the government could have implemented it with prospective effect and not focused it on Dr P. Venugopal for satisfying the ministerial arrogance.

The heavens would not have fallen if Dr P. Venugopal, one of India's topmost cardiac surgeons, was allowed to complete his full term of five years for which he was appointed. But to expect such etiquette from Mr Ramadoss was not to understand the minister, who has been at the Director's neck for no other reason than that Dr P. Venugopal did not allow ministerial interventions to scuttle the autonomy enjoyed by the premier medical institute of the country. On the other hand, the minister expected the Director to dance to his whims. The standoff between the two has been adversely affecting the functioning of the AIIMS. Yet, the Prime Minister could not take any step to rein in the minister because of the compulsions of coalition politics, much to the annoyance of the staff, students and patients of the AIIMS.

Had the MPs, who gave their nod for the controversial Bill, cared to find out the minister's motive in introducing it in such a hurry when many other issues concerning the Health Ministry do not engage his attention, they would not have fallen for it. The lack of medicines and staff in government hospitals, the pathetic health delivery system in the countryside and the death of a large number of children even before they complete five years and the prevalence of HIV/AIDS are some of the issues the minister should have ideally been tacking. Alas, he was obsessed with getting rid of Dr P. Venugopal so that he could sleep well. That the Supreme Court will go into the question is one silver lining in the otherwise sad saga. But Parliament suddenly changing the law might cramp its inclination for justice.[5]

SC sore with Centre over Dr P. Venugopal's hasty removal

Describing the removal of AIIMS director Dr P. Venugopal as "very unfortunate", the Supreme Court on Monday shot searching questions at the Centre, asking what prompted it to rush through the controversial law fixing 65 years as the age of superannuation.

"Why such a reputed person is humiliated in this way", a Bench comprising Justices Tarun Chatterjee and Dalveer Bhandari asked while questioning the motive behind bringing out an amendment to the AIIMS Act when Dr P. Venugopal's tenure as director was coming to an end after six months in June next.

The Bench, which was inclined towards the arguments of Dr P.

Venugopal, however, said there was "difficulty" in staying the operation of the law passed by Parliament. "Was there any necessity of bringing the amendment at this stage?" the court asked when the Centre justified its act by saying Dr P. Venugopal was on contractual appointment and it was addressing the concern of Delhi High Court which wanted that the ambiguity in the appointment be removed by way of regulation or a stature. The Bench's annoyance over the turn of the events was further evident at the fag end of an hour-long hearing when it said, "on the facts of the case we are with Dr P. Venugopal."

The case came up before the apex court after a bitter turf war between Dr P. Venugopal and health minister Ambumani Ramadoss over the control of the prestigious institution. The Bench found strength in many of the arguments put forward by senior advocate Fali Nariman and Arun Jaitley, who appeared for Dr P. Venugopal and Faculty Association of AIIMS. The advocates alleged that the amended law as "hostile" and "discriminatory" against the distinguished cardiologist.[6]

3. Need of selection of the Director purely on merit to provide the leadership to the Institute

The Director of Institute should be selected on merit which is in the interest of the institute and no other extraneous considerations. It has been rightly said about the Chief Executive "Put a good man in a bad set-up, he will make the things go through, Put a bad man in good set-up he will make the mesh of the situation." The Director must be a person who can exhibit quality of leadership to lead the institution to academic excellence.

Swami Chinmayananda feels that it is scarce to find real leaders in today's world. To quote him: But the rare few that develop a universal love and constantly engage themselves in activity under the guidance of their superior intellect, are called "man-men" and they alone can claim the prestige, dignity and glory of man. The core of the human personality is the consciousness, which is the life centre around which all the activities of the body, mind and the intellect revolve. It remains ever changeless and immovable like an axle in the wheel, but causes all changes and movements to occur. When men succeeds in identifying with this changeless, immovable conscious principle within him, he is no longer victimized by the changing phenomena of perceptions, emotions and thoughts, but becomes the Supreme Lord of them all. The intellectual pursuits, emotional attachments and physical cravings of such a man naturally wither and fall away like petals of a flower when the fruit emerges.

According to A.H. Maslow: Self-actualizing people are without one single exception involved in a cause outside their own skin in something outside of themselves. They are devoted working at something, which is very precious to them—some calling it vocation in the old sense, the priestly sense. They are working at something which fate has called them to somehow, which they work at and love, so that the work-joy dichotomy in them disappears.

Swami Chinmayananda says that a life organized for the discovery of the potentialities already exists within ourselves, and the ordering of our behaviour so as to nurture and nourish them, is a life well spent. Herein our success depends upon the amount of transformation we can successfully bring about in our personality and character. The vital question is not how many talents each one of us has, but how much of our existing talents are we capable of exploring, developing and exploiting. An individual may have many talents, and yet, he can be a miserable failure in life. That person is successful who makes a practical use of at least one great talent that he possesses. Our present and future welfare thus mainly depends upon ourselves. Let us never look outside ourselves for help. Let us not fall into the delusion that the influence of others would enable us to do better or accomplish more. All our success entirely depends upon ourselves. Let us realize these fundamentals. We must.

Eminent Industrialist, Mr. Rahul Bajaj, observes, "To realize our goals and aspirations, we need outstanding leadership in every field and at every level. Leadership means that there is no substitute for excellence, no tolerance of mediocrity and no compromise with integrity. Leadership is not just charisma, not public relations, not showmanship. Leadership is performance, consistent behaviour and trust worthiness.[7]

We must remember that it is the top men in each department who set the tone of the administration. It is they who set the example for those under them to emulate. When the acts of those at the top become tainted, when their reputation becomes shady, they will not be able to enforce high standards of integrity in those below them. It is, therefore, imperative that men at the top should exhibit the highest standards of personal integrity, probity and rectitude. As Sir Ivor Jinninegs observed, the most elementary qualification demanded of a minister's honesty and incorruptability. It is, in addition, necessary not only that he should possess this qualification but also that he should appear to possess it.

4. Need of Personnel Motivation of Personnel

The most important task of an organisation must be to give abundant and constant evidence of its belief that personnel in an organisation are the key to development. This requires proper motivation of the employees which provides a base for the management functions of planning and organizing. It has been noticed that the performance of the personnel either as individuals or members of a group is less as compared to their capabilities in terms of skills, abilities and capacities. Finer, for example, states that demonstrated performance generally never exceeds more than fifty per cent of the individual's ability to perform. Most individuals tend to balance their efforts around an assessment of relative costs (time and energy) and benefits. A climate of creativity must be developed and maintained by management so that the performance levels know no bounds and growth becomes a way of life.

B. Rattan Reddy opines that there is no doubt that Indian

Administration needs a strong core of dynamic values to transform its ethos at all levels. Laws can be enacted and rules framed to this end. Enforcement agencies can prosecute and the system can punish. This will have an impact. Nonetheless, enforcement of morality through law will largely remain an external process that can at best delineate a framework for public behaviour that should not be transgressed. But beyond that, laws or rules have inherent limitations in addressing the question of societal and individual change. As such, lasting public morality and ethics can not be forced from outside. These must take roots and grow within the system itself. People have to understand and accept it so that change becomes organic.

Motivation is a tendency which keeps a person attentively and purposefully engaged to achieve his formulated goals. This, a sense of commitment occurs only when the enterprise becomes a perpetual vehicle for the satisfaction of the dominant needs of the employees, so long as the employees strives fully to achieve the goals of the enterprise. From the above discussion, it is clear that motivation as such cannot be observed, rather it is a concept derived to cover a number of relationships having their immediate point of origin within the organism

5. Not Effective Administration: Need of Good Governance

Though the progress in harnessing scientific and technological potentiality is good but not sufficient. There is a need of Good Governance to optimize the use of scientific and technological potentialities. Good governance can make India a knowledge super power. A brief description of scientific and technology development reveals that India is rich in her resources but these are not reaching the people and are not making much difference in enriching the life of the poor. Why? India lacks good governance and good government which cause poor delivery. The need is to promote good governance which can improve the growth of scientific and technological progress as well as can accelerate their reach to people to improve their standard of living.

A senior parliamentarian (Prof. Hiren Mukherjee) speaking of politics generally, bemoans. It will not be far wrong to say, sorrowfully, that there never was a time in living memory when politics and politicians were, almost rightfully, as denigrated, even degraded and sometimes detested, in the eyes of our people as they are at the moment.

The work and conduct of the legislature both at the Union and State level is increasingly becoming a matter of great shame for the legislators as well as the citizens who elected them. It has taken a more serious turn as citizens are viewing their performance on T.V. The legislature passes the law relating to good governance like Right to Information Act, 2005, Consumers' Protection Act, 1986 and other Important bills which are supposed to smoothen the life of the people. What can be the impact of the legislature when the members composing it are highly indisciplined, and possess no moral conduct and values? This is not specific to any party and individuals. The same behaviour is observed from the opposition to whatever party it may be.

6. **AIIMS was supposed to set the standards of undergraduate and post-graduate medical education but have not been able to achieve the same so far. Need of designing the curriculum as per the need of the country.**

The objective of a good medical education should be to produce general practitioners, specialists, teachers and research workers. The factors governing this are the curriculum, medium of instruction, duration of course, admission qualifications, the examination system, teachers-students relationship, prospects of teachers and, students, etc. Besides, it may be mentioned that the medical education should fit in with the needs of the country and the conditions prevailing there. For instance, 70 per cent of the population of India live in rural areas. The training given to the doctor should enable and motivate him to carry on his work among the vast masses in the villages. We have been designing our undergraduate and postgraduate medical education which can fulfil this basic aim. There, has been a big gap between aims and fulfilment, J. Gallagher, Regional Officer for education and training, WHO Regional Office for Europe has expressed concern about inadequate communication between educational systems for health personnel and the health administrations that use the products of these systems. There is very little understanding of how the manpower training and development needs of health administrations can be met in a systematic way."[8]

The Government of India launched the Re-orientation of Medical Education Scheme in 1977 with the objective of involving the various medical colleges in the country in the direct delivery of health care services to the rural and semi-rural population. Under the scheme, each of the 106 medical colleges in the country is to accept in the first instance, the total responsibility for promotive, preventive, curative health services in three Community Development Blocks in the districts in which the institution is situated. 318 mobile clinics at the rate of 3 per college have been provided to the medical colleges to render quality services nearest to the rural population. The objectives of the scheme are:

(i) To expose the Medical faculty, residents in terms and the students to the Rural Community;
(ii) To train the students, interns and Residents in Community Organisation and Community Participation; and
(iii) To render comprehensive health care services to the villages in collaboration with the local Primary Health Centres.

It has been expressed in the Fifth Plan document that teaching in medical colleges still requires a radical change for its orientation towards the need for community care. Medical education over the years, has been urban biased. It is hoped that in the Sixth Draft Plan (1978-83), it would be possible "to produce medical graduates who are aware of the health problems of the community, who have a sense of compassion and motivation to serve the public and who have ability to effectively meet the urgent needs of the health care problems of the rural masses and the urban-poor."

According to the Estimates Committee: "The National Policy should indicate in unmistakable terms the goals to be achieved and the method of accomplishment . . . . . . Such a policy especially in the context of health being a State subject will help in maintenance of the requisite standards of medical education throughout the country in keeping with the needs of the people."[9]

The Government of India has announced the National Medical Education Policy. There is a need to set-up a Health Care Medical Service Commission responsible for planning of medical manpower, medical education, research, training of all para-medical personnel would be a step in the right direction. This commission when appointed should use Health and Medical Educational Planning as a means of rationalizing the education of health manpower. Besides, the Commission may encourage the health administrations to provide the policy and planning backgrounds required for this purpose.

Medical Education must have Public Health Orientation—The pattern of medical education guided by market economy has concentrated on biological causes of the diseases and curative actions based on hospital care, drugs, surgery, etc. without any recognition of the socio-economic and environmental status of the population. Health problems in a country like ours cannot be solved only through marketing medical therapy and interventions with a curative bias by neglecting the preventive, promotive, environmental health and the community need orientation. The lack of a holistic and community-based approach to disease control over the years has further led to over emphasis on quantity rather than quality of health care resulting in erosion of trust on the quality of health care services provided by the public sector and increasing dependence of the population on the private sector. Thus, during the past five decades, despite the quantitative growth in terms of hospitals, health centres, health manpower, infrastructural support services and number of health and family welfare programmes, the public health situation has remained a cause of great concern as reflected in the mortality, morbidity, health status, urban-rural differentials and health-seeking behaviour patterns of the population. This calls for re-orientation and health-seeking behaviour patterns of the population. This calls for re-orientation and reorganisation of our medical and health education system with emphasis on holistic and community-based health care as well as effective and efficient administration and management of health care delivery services. Keeping in view the national needs priorities and goods for health for all, it is essential to upgrade the managerial, technological and professional skill of health manpower through appropriate changes in the course curriculums of medical and health education institutions at different levels with greater emphasis on epidemiology, computer and management disciplines.[10]

Even Health Policy 2002 also Siderites

In any developing country with inadequate availability of health services, the requirement of expertise in the areas of 'public health' and 'family medicine' is markedly more than the expertise required for other. clinical specialities. In India, the situation is that public health expertise is non-existent in the private health sector, and far short of requirement in the public health sector. Also, the current curriculum in the graduate/post-graduate courses is outdated and unrelated to contemporary community needs. In respect of 'family medicine', it needs to be noted that the more talented medical graduates generally seek specialization in clinical disciplines, while the remaining go into general practice. While the availability of post-graduate educational facilities is 50 percent of the total number of qualifying graduates each year, and can be considered adequate, the distribution of the disciplines in the post-graduate training facilities is overwhelmingly in favour of clinical specializations. NHP-2002 examines the possible means for ensuring adequate availability of personnel with specialization in the 'public health' and 'family medicine' disciplines, to discharge the public health responsibilities in the country.

Health policy 1983 also stressed:

It is also necessary to appreciate that the effective delivery of health care services would depend very largely on the nature of education, training and appropriate orientation towards community health of all categories of medical and health personnel and their capacity to function as an integrated team, each of its members performing given tasks within a coordinated action programme. It is, therefore, of crucial importance that the entire basis and approach towards medical and health education, at all levels, is reviewed in terms of national needs and priorities and the curricular programmes restructured to produce personnel of various grades of skill and competence, who are professionally equipped and socially motivated to effectively deal with day-to-day problems, within the existing constraints. Towards this end, it is necessary to formulate, separately, a National Medical and Health Education Policy which (i) sets out the changes required to be brought about in the curricular contents and training programme of medical and health personnel, at various levels of functioning; (ii) takes into account the need for establishing the extremely essential inter-relations between functionaries of various grades; (iii) provides guidelines for the production of health personnel on the basis of realistically assessed manpower requirements; (iv) seeks to resolve the existing sharp regional imbalances in their availability; and (v) ensures that personnel at all levels are socially motivated towards the rendering of community health services.

A. Rajasekaran, President National Board of Examination, New Delhi, in his convocation address in *University News*, June 5-11, 2006 observed that our present system of medical education was inherited as legacy of the British. Even though beneficial to our progress it has not fulfiled the aspirations and expectations of our people particularly rural poor. Starting from BHORE Committee (1946) there were several attempt at reorientation of medical curriculum to produce a basic doctor or community physicians. Reoreintation of Medical Education (ROME Programme) of WHO for Asian countries was aimed at developing Medical Education system responsive and relevant to the needs of our country by making necessary curriculum changes.

The medical students entering the medical college is not adequately briefed on compassion and care, and learns the communiation skills and moral values. Instead his first exposure is to a cadaver in the anatomy dissection hall. Here comes the need for a preparatory course. In the present under graduate medical education the preclinical years, which was two years earlier, has been reduced to one year to learn anatomy, physiology, Biochemistry with too much of information squeezed into the curriculum.

AIIMS can do a lot in this education but failed to do till its golden jubilee. It is high time for AIIMS to demonstrate its leadership in giving right direction to medical and health education.

7. Researches bear no Relevance to Practical Problems: Need Action Research

There has been a lack of co-operation and co-ordination among the institutions engaged in teaching and research. This resulted in disjointed, isolated and rank duplication of scientific research in several national laboratories resulting in waste of scarce resources. The Public Accounts Committee in its 40th Report of the 5th Lok Sabha emphasised the importance of collaboration and co-ordination among various agencies engaged in medical research with ICMR taking the lead and suggested that energetic steps may be taken to enlarge the scope of collaboration to avoid repetitive research.

Besides, over the years, for a variety of reasons the medical research programmes in the country could not follow the path of problem-oriented medical research in priority areas such as nutritional disorders, control of communicable diseases, operational research for providing health care to all, research in medical education, health manpower planning, utilisation of health personnel, research in indigenous system of medicine, etc. The Sixth Draft Plan (1978-83) was also critical of the research policy pursued so far. It was stated that:

> "Medical research in the past had, by and large, failed to lay emphasis on problems of immediate practical importance. Efforts were mostly towards collection of disjointed and isolated research work by individuals/agencies in the country."

The Estimate Committee in its 102 Report pointed out that "the purpose of medical research is to bring about results of practical utility in the fight against disease with the maximum expedition possible and that little purpose will be served unless the results of research can find immediate application in the field. . . It is unfortunate that resources and time and talent of the medical community of the country have not been meaningfully utilised over the years according to well thought out priorities."[11] Thus, there is a need of costing of research projects in terms of time and money likely to be required for their completion. The aim of the research should be to solve health problems of the social significance to the country.

The foreign sponsorship of research projects has not been examined properly before accepting the proposals. The Public Accounts Committee in their 167th and 200th Reports have been very critical of the research projects conducted in collaboration with foreign organisations, e.g. Genetic Control of Mosquitoes Unit Projects, the Bird Migration and Arbovirus studies, the ultra low volume spray experiments, the Pantnagar Microbial Pesticides project and some of the research projects undertaken in West Bengal and Narangwal in collaboration with the John Hopkins University. The Committees are not unwilling to concede the importance of research efforts, the projects examined revealed a rather casual attitude and indifference on the part of the authorities concerned towards foreign supported research in India. The Committee reiterated the imperative need for the utmost care, caution and critical scrutiny before approving foreign sponsorship of research projects undertaken in India, particularly when such projects have military or quasi-military implications of an almost incalculable character. Such researches must be got conducted by the Indian scientists. If the foreign collaboration is indispensable, research ventures should ensure the following:

(a) that such ventures are not only of potential value for the country but are of immediate productive utility;
(b) that the objectives of the projects are clearly spelt out and the research plans are notified in advance so as to avoid any ambiguity:
(c) that the collaborating Indian agency or institution has personnel with the requisite qualification and equipment to concurrently evaluate and monitor the progress of the research;
(d) that the technical and administrative control of the projects and determination of policies vest only with the Indian agencies and personnel concerned;
(e) that all data and materials collected are shared with the Indian collaborators;
(f) that any kind of secrecy in the conduct of research is eschewed and that the results of the research are made public; and
(g) that all research is conducted in accordance not only with the

> country's own environmental standards but the international environmental standards as well. In the new millennium, research must also be encouraged in the areas.[12]

AIIMS can take up such research which can solve the heath problems of the country.

8. **Good Relationship between Minister and Experts: AIIMS is a complex organisation which requires good governance to operate. There is shortage of staff, lack of facilities for patients, overcrowded. There is a need of good governance which can manage the problems of a complex organisation like AIIMS**

Since the minister occupies the top position in politico-administrative hierarchy. It is essential that he should have full legal and constitutional authority to administer with good governance the affairs of his department. Theoretically, it is feasible but in practice, he cannot achieve much whether it is policy-making or implementation or evaluation unless he gets due co-operation, help, participation, involvement of the personnel of his department. The volume of work with the Council of Ministers at the Union and the state levels is so large and the problems so complicated that it is impossible for any number of ministers to deal with all the matters themselves. The civil servants provide all the information and analysis for the guidance of the ministers and the cabinet. The channel through which a minister must operate is the secretariat. The secretariat acts as an institutionalized memory to enable the government to examine the feasibility of the proposed policy.

Sir Warren Fisher, in a memorandum to the Tomlin Commission (U.K.) defined the duties of the civil servant *vis-a-vis* the minister as follows:

> Determination of policy is the function of a minister and once a policy is determined it is the unquestioned and unquestionable business of the civil servant to strive to carry out that policy with precisely the same energy and precisely the same goodwill whether he agreed with it or not. This is axiomatic and will never be in dispute. At the same time it is the traditional duty of civil servants while decisions are being formulated, to make available to their political chief all the information and experience at their disposal, and to do this without fear or favour, irrespective of whether, the advice thus tendered by accord or not with the minister's initial view. The presentation to the minister of relevant fact, the ascertainment and marshalling of which may often call into play the whole organisation of a department, demands of the civil servant the greatest care. The presentation of inferences from the facts equally demand from him all the wisdom and all the detachment he can command.

The preservation of integrity, fearlessness, and independence of thought and utterance in their private communion with ministers of the experienced officials selected to fill the top posts in the service is an essential principle in enlightened government, as whether or not ministers accept the advice frankly placed at their disposal, and acceptance or rejection of such advice is exclusively a matter for their judgement, It enables them to be assured that their decisions are reached only after the relevant facts and the various considerations have, so far as the machinery of government can secure been definitely brought before their minds.

In the last three years, more than half a dozen senior faculty members have left AIIMS. Last summer, three senior, high-profile doctors associated with AIIMS for nearly three decades, left. They left because they were disillusioned with the system.

Professor V.S. Mehta, Chief of Neurosciences Centre, and Dr Anoop Misra from the Department of Medicine, bid adieu to the institute in April last year. Four months later, Professor S.N. Mehta, Head of the Department of Surgery and Chief of Kidney transplant services quit and joined Indraprastha Apollo hospital as a senior consultant. He said, "I had ceased to enjoy my work for almost two years and decided to consider the offers that were coming my way. In my 27 years of association with AIIMS, I had never seen an administration that was so indifferent to the needs of the department and the institute." In May 2005, Dr Sabyasachi Bal, lung surgeon quit his job as he felt he had not got a fair deal from AIIMS. Professor V.S. Mehta, Director of Neurosciences at Paras Hospital, Guragon left AIIMS on April 1 last year as he was "disgusted with the work environment." Dr Sandeep Vaishya, Additional Professor, Department of Neurosurgery, left AIIMS in March last year after 14 years of service to join Max Super-Specialty hospital in Saket as Senior Consultant, Neurosurgery and Spine Surgery. "I wanted a fresh challenge. The gradual change in the work environment at AIIMS was disheartening." Dr Anoop Misra, Director, Diabetes and Metabolic Diseases Department, Fortis Hospital, Saket, quit the Department of Medicine. "When I joined AIIMS as an undergraduate in 1978, it offered a very good learning platform. The students were very bright. The caliber of students is now second rate. The best students are no longer opting for medicine."

9. Faculty in AIIMS may follow code of ethics to maintain the diginity and prestige of the institution

The document prepared by Deptt. of Administrative Reforms and public grievances has chalked out a Code of Ethics which need implementation. The objective of Code is to prescribe standards of integrity and conduct that are to apply in the public services. The principles stated below underlie and supplement the rules and laws to regulate the public and private conduct of various public services.

Selflessness: Holders of public office should take decisions solely in terms of the *Public interest.* They should not do so in order to gain financial or other material benefits for themselves, their family, or their friends.

Integrity: Holders of public office should not place themselves under any financial or other obligation to outside individuals or organisations that might influence them in the performance of their official duties.

Objective: In carrying out public business, including making public appointments, awarding contracts, or recommending individuals for rewards and benefits, holders of public office should make choice on merit.

Accountability: Holders of public office are accountable for their decisions and actions to the public and must submit themselves to whatever scrutiny is appropriate to their office.

Openness: Holders of public office should be as open as possible about all the decisions and actions that they take. They should give reasons for their decisions and restrict information only when the wider public interest clearly demands.

Honesty: Holders of public office have a duty to declare any private interest relating to their public duties and to take steps to resolve any conflicts arising in a way that protects is the public interest.

Leadership: Holders of public office should promote and support these principles by leadership and example.

These principles apply to all aspects of public life. The Committee has set them out here for the benefits of all who serve the public in any way.

10. Time Management

Tertiary hospital like AIIMS must concentrate their time on vital issues. Time is not thought of as a source. However, it is the most important and crucial factor as time is inelastic and non-renewable. An event cannot take place unless there is a time for it. Time and tide wait for none. We may keep in mind that time is neutral, i.e. it is neither good not bad by itself. Therefore, to blame the time for any inaptitude for failure will be quite unfair.

11. Lack of Effective Inter-personal Relations—Need of Harmonious Relationships

Manager of today need to be trained in understanding the inter-personal relationship and their management to insulate the organisation from internal behavioural disturbances. There are three inter-personal needs, (i) inclusion—need for interaction and association, (ii) control—the need for authority and power, and (iii) affection—the need for being loved and cared. Developing a successful inter-personal relation, conducive to achievement of organisational goals, is a challenging task and a slow process. It requires a deep psychological understanding of oneself as well as of others, with whom one comes in contact in various organisational capacities.

12. Researchers have no impact on hospitals

AIIMS must develop modules which can be used for practicing

doctors through video conferencing so that good medical education as well as continuous medical education can be spread among doctors so that people can be benefited of modern medicine at an affordable cost. There is not doubt about the excellence of AIIMS in academic achievement. However, AIIMS failed in its mandate of making medical education suitable for rural and poor people in the country. The leadership role of AIIMS was not put into practice.

13. Recruitment of Medical Personnel, not based on merit

The success of any institute depends on its highly talented medical personnel. To quote The Telegraph dated 22 Dec. 2007 (Report covered by Charu Sudan Kastrui) clearly observed that The All India Institute of Medical Sciences (AIIIMS) used unfair practices "designed to regularize" in-house teachers to fill posts for an entire decade, a health ministry inquiry has found.

The finding suggests several candidates from outside the campus were deprived of a chance to work in India's premier medical institute.

If the ministry decides to risk charges of witch-hunt and a possible backlash, upto 70 faculty members who were promoted between 1993 and 2003 could be demoted. The AIIMS authority, called the Institute Body, accepted the inquiry report yesterday.

Government rules and court orders were flouted in appointing teachers at the institute from 1993 to 2003 under two different directors, the committee has found.

Standard government rules require institutes to publicly advertise for vacant posts, and treat outside applications on a par with those from their own teachers seeking promotions.

From 1993 to 2002, AIIMS did not advertise outside the campus for posts, instead promoting *ad hoc* appointees to full-time jobs as teachers.

During this period, 152 out of 219 *ad hoc* posts were filled "in an arbitrary manner", the committee said in its report, a copy of which is with *The Telegraph*.

"It is sad to see the manner in which the rules were flouted by successive administrations to secure a coterie that would back them under all circumstances", a senior official on the five-member inquiry team said.

In 2003, advertisements were issued in newspapers for 170 associate professors at the institute. In all 762 people cleared the preliminary selection criteria and were called for interview. These included 151 assistant professors (a grade lower than associate professors) and 611 applicants from outside the AIIMS.

Among the 611 outside candidates were 209 reserved category candidates, the report says. But in the final selection, only 19 per cent of the seats went to applicants from outside the AIIMS, despite being "equally suitable candidates", the committee has said. "The committee concluded that the selection process lacked fairness and was designed primarily to regularize the existing *ad hoc* assistant professors in large numbers", the report said.

Seventy of those selected between 1993 and 2003 were found to have poorer credentials than many other applicants who were not picked, the committee has said. But the ministry is treading with caution on the 70 for fear that it may be accused of vindictiveness—a charge leveled by an associate professor who was promoted from an *ad hoc* post in 2003.

"This is vindictiveness at its peak. . . nothing else. The health ministry is not satisfied with removing (former director), P. Venugopal, they want to remove anyone else who can challenge them", the doctor from the pathology department said.

Several of the 70 faculty members are said to be close to Venugopal, who was expelled recently as director after a turf war with health minister Anbumani Ramadoss. Although the controversial selections were made in the period just before Venugopal was appointed director, cases against the appointments were filed soon after he took over. The panel was set-up in January.

This is highly serious as it encourages in house breading and merit becomes a secondary consideration. It becomes a closed door entry, suicidal to the growth and development of an institution of National Importance.

CONCLUSION

AIIMS is doing excellent work in medicine. Its students are spread throughout the world and occupying eminent positions. In India AIIMS has contributed in making available medical faculty, eminent doctors and other paramedical staff. Even taking the name of AIIMS brings before a person an idea of excellent institution. However, AIIMS must see that this institution must benefit the common man and not remain only in ivory towers. AIIMS must meet the needs of common man at a cost which he can afford.

Notes and References

1. Tripti Nath in *The Tribune,* Oct. 7, 2007, Spectrum "AIIMS: Ailing Institute."
2. *The Tribune,* Chandigarh, Thursday, 28th November 2007, p. 2.
3. *The Tribune,* Chandigarh, Friday, November 30th 2007, p. 10.
4. *Hindustan Times,* Chandigarh, Friday, November 30, 2007, p. 12.
5. *The Tribune,* Chandigarh, Monday, December 3, 2007, p. 10.
6. *The Economic Times,* Tuesday, 4 December 2007, p. 2.
7. AIU, *University News,* March 13, 2000.
8. Lok Sabha Secretariat: 102nd Report, Estimates Committee, (Fifty Lok Sabha), p. 4.
9. Lok Sabha Secretariat, 102nd Report, Estimates Committees, Fifth Lok Sabha, p. 4.
10. Madhu S. Mishra, Health Policy and Management of Health Care delivery services in India—Issues and Challenge in Public Health in India—Five Decades, 50th Anniversary of India's Independence, pp. 27-28.
11. Lok Sabha Secreariate: Estimates Committee, 102nd Report, (5th Lok Sabha), New Delhi, 1975, pp. 92-94.
12. Lok Sabha Secretariat, Public Accounts Committee: Fifth Lok Sabha, 200th Report, 1976, New Delhi.

APPENDIX I

Yearly Statistical Health Bulletin

1.	Total patients admitted	80,140
	a. Adults and children	77,803
	b. Newborn infants	2,337
2.	Total number of patient care days in hospital (as per daily census)	15,931
	a. Adults and children	409,462
	b. Newborn infants	6,469
3.	Daily average number of patients	1,140
	a. Adults and children	1,122
	b. Newborn infants	18
4.	Average bed occupancy ratio (BOR)	83.2
	a. Adults and children	83.4
	b. Newborn infants	72.0
5.	Average length of stay (ALS)	5.2
	a. Adults and children	5.3
	b. Newborn infants	8.8
6.	Births in hospital	2,337
	a. Male babies	1,261
	b. Female babies	1,073
	c. Intersex	3
7.	Total deaths (including newborns)	2,908
	a. Death under 48 hours	768
	b. Death over 48 hours	2,140
	c. Gross death rate (%)	3.6
	d. Net death rate (%)	2.7

Source: 49th Annual Report, 2004-05 of AIIMS, New Delhi, p. 36.

APPENDIX II

Inpatient Crude Mortality Statistics

S. No.	Department	Admissions	Deaths			Death rate (%)	
			Total	Under 48 hours	Over 48 hours	Gross	Net
1.	Anaesthesiology	785	-	-	-	-	-
2.	Cardiology	7790	235	72	163	3.0	2.1
3.	Cardiothoracic and Vascular Surgery	3269	233	19	214	7.1	6.6
4.	Dental Surgery	209	-	-	-	-	-
5.	Dermatology	3738	8	1	7	0.2	0.2
6.	Endocrinology	474	5	2	3	1.1	0.6
7.	Gastroenterology	1868	240	49	191	12.8	10.5
8.	Gastrointenstinal surgery	701	38	2	36	5.4	5.2
9.	General surgery	6325	180	46	134	2.8	2.1
10.	Haematology	5943	113	47	66	1.9	1.1
11.	IRCH (Private ward)	449	87	43	44	19.4	10.8
12.	Medicine	3519	575	180	395	16.3	11.8
13.	Nephrology	3394	147	46	101	4.3	3.0
14.	Neuro-anaesthesia	10	-	-	-	-	-
15.	Neurology	2514	211	30	181	8.4	7.3
16.	Neurosurgery	4322	405	103	302	9.4	7.2
17.	Newborn	2337	51	23	28	2.2	1.2
18.	Nuclear medicine	476	-	-	-	-	-
19.	Obstetrics and Gynaecology	9364	22	4	18	0.2	0.2
20.	Orthopaedics	4207	35	4	31	0.8	0.7
21.	Otorhinolaryngology	4546	17	7	10	0.4	0.2
22.	Paediatric surgery	2210	62	10	52	2.8	2.4
23.	Paediatrics	6187	189	63	126	3.1	2.1
24.	Physical Medicine and Rehabilitation	29	-	-	-	-	-
25.	Psychiatry	377	-	-	-	-	-
26.	Radiotherapy	188	36	15	21	19.1	12.1
27.	Urology	4909	19	2	17	0.4	0.3
	TOTAL	80140	2908	768	2140	3.6	2.7

Source: Ibid.

APPENDIX III

Attendance in OPDs and Specialty Clinics

Department	*New Cases*	*Old Cases*	*Total*
ANAESTHESIA			
Specialty Clinics			
Pain	1,795	5,208	7,003
Pre-anaesthesia	7,045	1,349	8,394
DENTAL SURGERY			
General OPD	29,714	27,234	56,948
Specialty Clinics			
Combined cleft palate	81	346	427
Oral prophylaxis	2,112	7,456	9,568
Orthodontics	1.094	7,215	8,309
Prosthodontics-*cum*-maxillofacial prosthesis	174	2,569	4,743
Restorative-*cum*-endodontic	7,648	4,810	12,458
Trigeminal Neuralgia	128	402	530
DERMATOLOGY			
General OPD	32,907	26,517	59,424
Specialty Clinics			
Allergy	445	870	1,315
Dermatological surgery	305	665	970
Leprosy	336	1,742	2,078
Pigmentation	550	1,619	2,169
Sexually transmitted disease	1,039	1,730	2,769
ENDOCRINOLOGY	9,537	16,215	25,752
GASTROENTEROLOGY	17,925	26,161	44,086
HAEMATOLOGY	4,206	14,121	18,327
MEDICINE			
General OPD	67,000	63,389	130,389
Specialty Clinics			
Chest	1,836	4,011	5,847
Geriatric	186	813	999
Rheumatology	233	5,957	6,190
NEPHROLOGY	5,628	14,357	19,985
Renal Transplant	79	4,536	4,615
NUCLEAR MEDICINE	1,644	2,007	3,651
OBSETETRICS AND GYNAECOLOGY			
General OPD	32,749	45,511	78,260
Specialty Clinics			
Antenal	1,059	5,955	7,014
Endocrine gynaecology	154	207	361
Family welfare	3,020	5,188	8,208
High-risk pregnancy	1,741	9,462	11,203
Postnatal	181	90	271
ORTHOPAEDICS			
General OPD	81,337	147,112	288,449
Specialty Clinics			
Club foot (CTEV)	248	1,164	1,412
Follow-up	-	6,703	6,703
Hand	801	1,080	1,881
Polio	73	31	104
Scoliosis	498	1,131	1,629
Tuberculosis	-	2	2
OTORHINOLARYNGOLOGY AND RUAS			
General OPD	5,305	32,227	77,532

Specialty Clinics			
Audiology	179	104	283
Hearing	675	871	1,546
Rhinology	118	58	176
Speech	1,340	851	2,191
Vertigo	109	107	216
Voice	461	573	1,034
PAEDIATRICS			
General OPD	33,493	32,208	65,701
Specialty Clinics			
Chest	478	3,256	3,734
Follow-up TB	235	1,235	1,470
Genetic and birth defects	1,287	936	2,223
High-risk neonatal	232	1,264	1,496
Neurology	1,760	4,418	6,178
Renal	492	3,265	3,757
Well baby	658	19	577
PAEDIATRIC SURGERY			
General OPD	7,486	10,624	18,110
Specialty Clinics			
Hydocephalus	31	334	365
Intersex	33	33	66
Urology	268	2476	2744
PHYSICAL MEDICINE AND REHABILITATION	12,698	9,570	22,268
PSYCHIATRY			
General OPD	1,227	-	1,227
Specialty Clinics			
Child guidance	428	205	633
Walk-in	12,783	22,999	35,782
RADIOTHERAPY			
General OPD	1,425	57,962	59,387
Specialty Clinics			
Radiotherapy in gynaecology	701	11,282	11,983
Radiotherapy in surgery	1,351	10,606	11,957
GENERAL SURGERY	34,408	24,042	58,450
UROLOGY	10,004	19,236	29,240
OTHERS			
Casualty	156,217	-	156,217
Employees Health Scheme	105,871	70,577	176,448
Marriage Counselling clinic	2,449	2,705	5,154
Nutrition	5,196	1,046	6,242
Total	756,806	790,024	1,546,830

Source: Ibid.

APPENDIX IV

Region-wise Distribution of Inpatients

Region	*Number of Patients*
Delhi	43,271
Uttar Pradesh	12,863
Haryana	9,058
Punjab	689
Rajasthan	1,548
Bihar	5,840
Other states	6,556
Other countries	315
Total	80,140

Source: Ibid.

APPENDIX V

Department-wise Distribution of Inpatients (2004-05)

S. No.	*Departments/Sections*	*Numbers*
1.	Anaesthesiology	785
2.	Dental Surgery	209
3.	Dermatology	3,738
4.	Dr. B.R. Ambedkar IRCH	449
5.	Endocrinology	474
6.	Gastroenterology	1,868
7.	Gastrointestinal surgery	701
8.	Haematology	5,943
9.	Medicine	3,519
10.	Neonatal	2,337
11.	Nephrology	3,394
12.	Nuclear Medicine	476
13.	Obstetrics and Gynaecology	9,364
14.	Orthopaedics	4,207
15.	Otorhinolaryngology	4,546
16.	Paediatric Surgery	2,210
17.	Paediatrics	6,187
18.	Physical Medicine and Rehabilitation	29
19.	Psychiatry	377
20.	Radiotherapy	188
21.	Surgery	6,325
22.	Urology	4,909
	Sub-total (MAIN)	62,235
23.	Cardiology	7,790
24.	Cardiotheracic and Vascular Surgery	3,269
25.	Neurology	2,514
26.	Neurosurgery	4,322
27.	Neuro-anaesthesia	10
	Sub-total (CNC)	17,905
	Grand Total	80,140

Source: *Ibid.*

APPENDIX VI

Surgical Procedures

S. No.	Department	Major	Minor	Total
1.	Casualty	5	8,106	8,111
2.	Dental Surgery	1,831	8,633	10,464
3.	Gastrointestinal Surgery	466	19	485
4.	Gynaecology	1,756	5,156	6,912
5.	Obstetrics	1,021	1,488	2,509
6.	Orthopaedics	2,439	1,559	3,998
7.	Otorhinolaryngology	1,603	21,770	23,373
8.	Paediatric Surgery	1,308	3,088	4,396
9.	Surgery	3,439	10,182	13,621
10.	Urology	1,636	8,269	9,905
	Sub-total (MAIN)	15,504	68,270	83,774
11.	Cardiothoracic and Vascular Surgery	3,641	5	3,646
12.	Neurosurgery	2,920	498	3,418
	Sub-total (CNC)	6,561	503	7,064
	Grand Total	22,065	68,773	90,838

Source: Ibid.

4

CHAPTER

Organisation and Working of Rajendra Hospital, Patiala

A State Level Tertiary Hospital

PROFILE OF PATIALA

One of the famous princely states of erstwhile Punjab, Patiala forms the south-eastern part of the state. It is surrounded by Fatehgarh Sahib, Roopnagar districts and its capital city of Union Territory of Chandigarh in the north, Fatehgarh Sahib and Sangrur districts in the west, Ambala and Kurukshetra districts of negihbouring state of Haryana in the east and Kaithal district of Haryana in the south. It was Maharaja Bhupinder Singh (1900-1930) who gave Patiala state a prominent place on the political map. The area of Patiala is 3,627 sq. km., with the density of 419 per sq. km., having nine towns, five tehsils, nine blocks, five sub-tehsils. The population in its rural area is 10,55,230 and urban area 4,66,100 with the sex ratio being 881 females per 1,000 males. Map of Patiala is shown in Chart 1.1.

As Rajindra Hospital is at a tertiary level therefore it has the Government Medical College attached to it. The hospital serves an approximate population of 15,21,330 people from Punjab, adjoining stations of Haryana, Himachal Pradesh, Rajasthan, Jammu and Kashmir, Uttar Pradesh. It is spread over a wide area of 70 acres and the foundation of its present premises was laid by Maharaja Yadavindra Singh of Patiala on April 15, 1950 and was inaugurated by Pt. Jawaharlal Nehru on February 12, 1954. This hospital was attached to the Government Medical College on December 21, 1953 and its opening ceremony was performed by Rajkumari Amrit Kaur, the then Health Minister of India on February 4, 1953. The hospital and the college face each other and are on either side of the road. The college building consists of an administrative block (Principal's Office) and an adjoining building for the departments of Anatomy, Physiology, Pathology and Pharmacology. It has a library for staff as well as students.

Map I

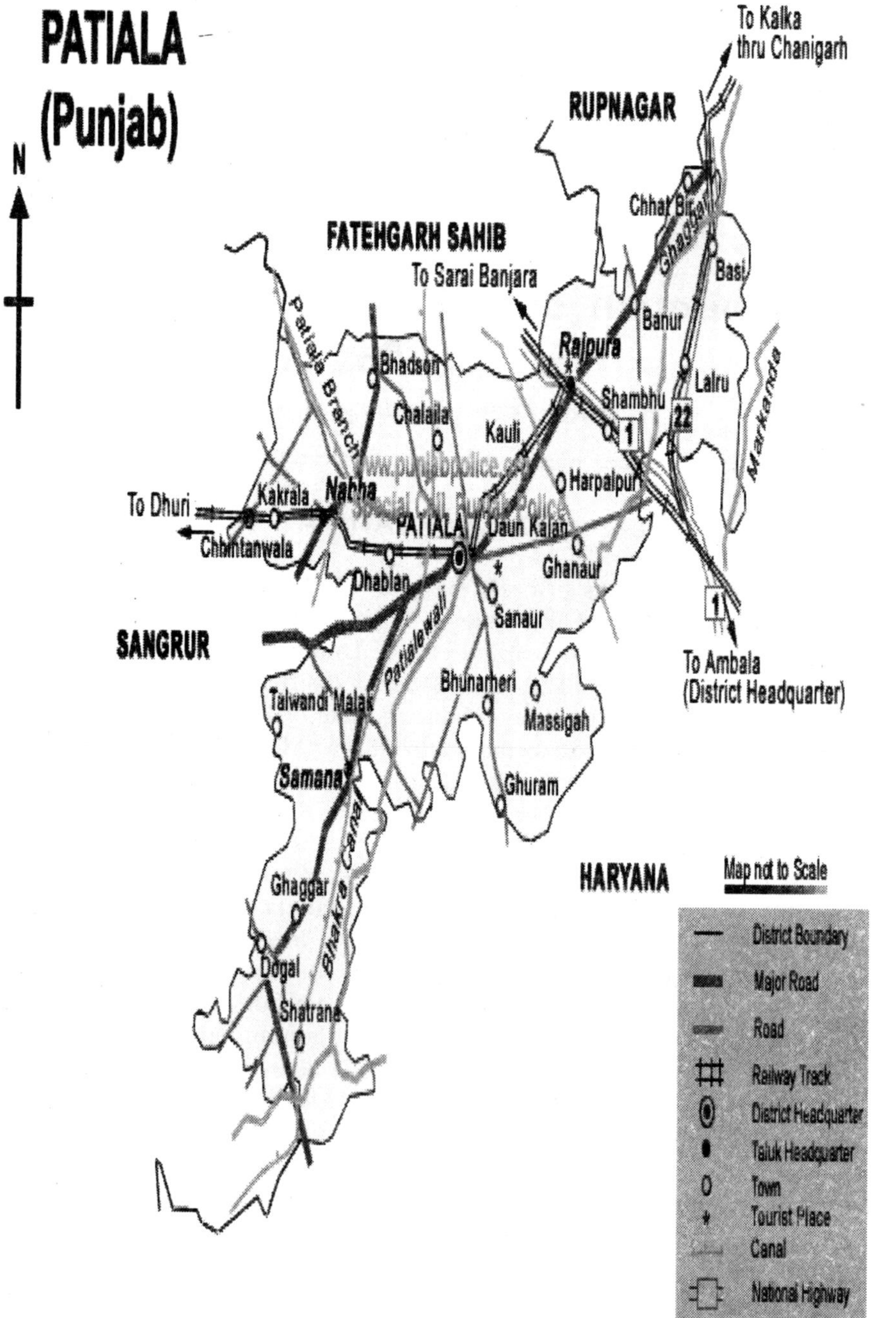
PATIALA
(Punjab)
N
To Kalka
thru Chanigarh
RUPNAGAR
FATEHGARH SAHIB
To Sarai Banjara
Chhat Bir
Ghaggar
Basi
Banur
Rajpura
Patiala Branch
Bhadson
Lalru
Shambhu
Chalaila
Kauli
1
22
Markanda
Harpalpur
To Dhuri
Kakrala
Nabha
PATIALA
Daun Kalan
Chhintanwala
Ghanaur
Dhablan
Sanaur
1
SANGRUR
Patialewali
To Ambala
(District Headquarter)
Bhunarheri
Talwandi Malak
Massigah
Samana
Ghuram
HARYANA
Map not to Scale
Ghaggar
Bhakra Canal
District Boundary
Major Road
Road
Railway Track
District Headquarter
Taluk Headquarter
Town
Tourist Place
Canal
National Highway
River
Dogal
Shatrana

The other side has an administrative block (M.S. Office) and the outdoor wing has various OPDs along with the laboratories for investigations. Besides the Superintendent's Office is the Emergency OPD.

To give impetus to the development of quality medical education institutes Baba Farid University of Health Sciences was established under B.F.U.H.S. Act, 1998. For the setting up of the University about 123 acres of land has been acquired at Faridkot. Then Rajindra Hospital was transferred to this University.

Function

(1) The institute imparts medical education to students for attaining the degree of MBBS and Postgraduate training leading to MD, MS and Super specialization. Teaching includes theory and practical training.
(2) Research in the medical field.
(3) Training in paramedical courses including Medical lab technology, Basic Nursing and Pharmacy.
(4) The institute imparts tertiary health care to people living in and around in this region.
(5) Emergency service including trauma and disaster management.

The power and duties of its officers

Principal

1. He is the overall In-charge of the administration of the Institute. He may delegate powers to heads of department and other members of institution as and when need arises.
2. He is responsible for proper management of the administrative machinery like various sections, units, etc.
3. He has to manage the budget of the Institute and to see that funds are properly utilized.
4. He is the controlling Officer for various sections like establishment, personnel, accounts, general stores, etc. and he has to see that these sections function properly.
5. He has the power of recruitment, transfer, dismissal or terminate of class IV employees.
6. Maintaining Annual Confidential Reports of Officers and Staff.
7. He has to complete the Annual Accounts of the Institute for submitting before the Audit.
8. He has to complete the Annual Reports of the Institute for approval.
9. He has to implement various policy decisions taken by Committees taken by Governing Body and Government orders.
10. He has to arrange for the Meetings of Governing Body and Standing Finance Committee.

11. Preparation of 5 years plans and Annual Plans.
12. He is the overall In-charge of the academic activities of the Institute like conduct of regular classes, teaching, training, practical classes and other education activities.
13. He has to see and arrange for the conduct of regular and timely annual examinations by the University.
14. He has to make coordination among the University and the institute with regarded to syllabus, curriculum, admission, examination, etc. for smooth conduct of various courses.

Deputy Medical Superintendent

1. He is responsible for the overall management of the Hospitals having OPD and IPD.
2. He has to supervise and control the Hospital Staff for the smooth functioning of patient care activities.
3. He has to allot duties and responsibilities to the Hospital Staff like Nurses, Pharmacists, and Group-D, etc. for the smooth functioning of the Hospitals.
4. He is responsible to see that the Hospital services are rendered to the patients satisfactory including availability of medicines, diet, linen, etc.
5. He has to arrange duties and responsibilities of the PG and Ph.D. scholars in the Hospital.
6. He has to see that the Hospital premises and facilities are properly maintained and the cleanliness is provided.

Accounts Officer

1. He is overall In-charge of the Accounts Section.
2. He has to supervise and control the budgetary allocations and to see that they are properly utilized for which it is provided.
3. Preparation of Annual Accounts and conduction of Audit on time.
4. Financial advice on purchase and budgetary utilizations.
5. Preparation of Annual Budget requirements.
6. Compliance of Reports of Audit.
7. Checking and passing of bills and co-signatory for fund operations with the Bank.
8. To supervise and checking of cash.

Punjab realized the need for a referral system and has been working on it since long but the present referral system of the state is inadequate. 'It is estimated that nearly one-third of all patients treated at tertiary level could be treated at the first referral facilities at lower cost if these referral facilities received adequate input. Patiala district was studied to see the efficacy of referral system. Table 4.1 shows the number of beds available at different levels in Patiala district.

TABLE 4.1

Beds at different levels of Health Care at Patiala District

Level	*Area*	*No. of Beds*
DH	Rajindra Hospital, Patiala	1300 (907)
SDH'	M.K. Hospital	200
SDH	Rajpura	50
SDH	Nabha	100
SDH	Samana	25
CHC	M. Town	30
CHC	Dudhan Sadhna	30
CHC	Kalomajra	30
CHC	Dera Bassi	30
CHC*	Ghanaur	30
CHC	Badhson	30
CHC	Bhadshahpur	30
CHC	Shutrana	30

Source: Reporting Performa for Referral Services, Punjab Health System Corporation, March 2002.

Number of patients referred to tertiary health care institutes in Patiala district in the month of March 2002 in following tables. Tables 4.2, 4.3, 4.4 and 4.5 show the patients who have been referred to high level of the health care services for emergency treatment, in various specialized OPDs and for investigations.

TABLE 4.2

Number of Patients Referred in Patiala District to higher levels of health care for emergency.

Medicine	35
Surgery	26
Gynae/Obst	36
Pediatric	07
Others	54

Source: Reporting Performa for Referral Services, Punjab Health System Corporation, March 2002.

The Reporting Performa's of Punjab Health Services was studied and patients referred in various medical specialties were calculated for the month of May in 2002, it was seen that 35 patients required emergency medical treatment, 26 patients required emergency surgeries, 36 were emergency gynecology patients, 7 children required emergency pediatric services, 54 patients from miscellaneous category required emergency services. They are shown in the following tables:

Table 4.3 indicates that 8 patients were sent for admission from lower levels of health care to higher level of health care for medical treatment 22 patients went for surgery, 11 were gynecology patients and 11 patients belonged to miscellaneous category that went for admission to the hospital.

TABLE 4.3

Number of Patients Referred in Patiala District to higher levels of Health Care for Admissions

Medicine	08
Surgery	22
Gynae/Obst	11
Pediatric	00
Others	06

Source: Reporting Performa for Referral Services, Punjab Health System Corporation, March 2002.

Table 4.4 indicates that 10 patients went for advance medical treatment in the medical OPD, 14 went to the surgical OPD, 8 children went for their further check up in pediatrics OPD and 10 from miscellaneous category went for their check up in various other OPD's to the higher level hospital.

TABLE 4.4

Number of Patients Referred in Patiala District to Higher levels of Health for OPD Services

Medicine	10
Surgery	14
Gynae/Obst	13
Pediatric	08
Others	10

Source: Reporting Performa for Referral Services, Punjab Health System Corporation, March 2002.

Table 4.5 indicates that 3 patients were referred for laboratory tests 8 went for X-rays and 1 went for E.C.G. to higher levels of health.

TABLE 4.5

Number of Patients Referred in Patiala District to Higher Level of Health for investigations

LAB	08
X-Ray	08
ECG	01

Source: Reporting Performa for Referral Services, Punjab Health Systems Corporation, March 2002.

FIGURE 4.1

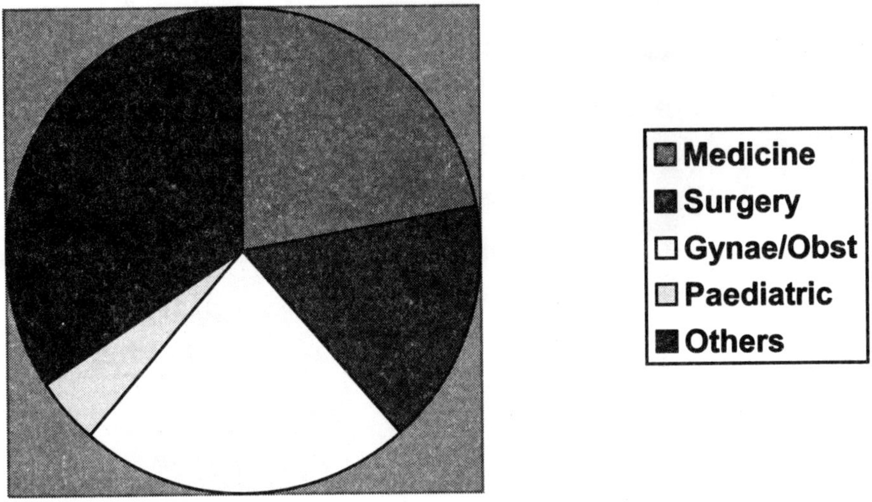

The report shows that 207 patients out of 256 referred patients were referred to Special Hospitals, 116 were referred for emergency services and 140 were referred for various OPD services and 12 for advanced investigations. Only one feedback was sent from Samana. Refer to Table 4.6.

During an interaction with the medical experts of Punjab Health Services, it was found that presently there is no well defined referral system in Punjab.

While discussing the referral procedures, the officer explained that the patients are being referred daily from one health institute to another.

FIGURE 4.2

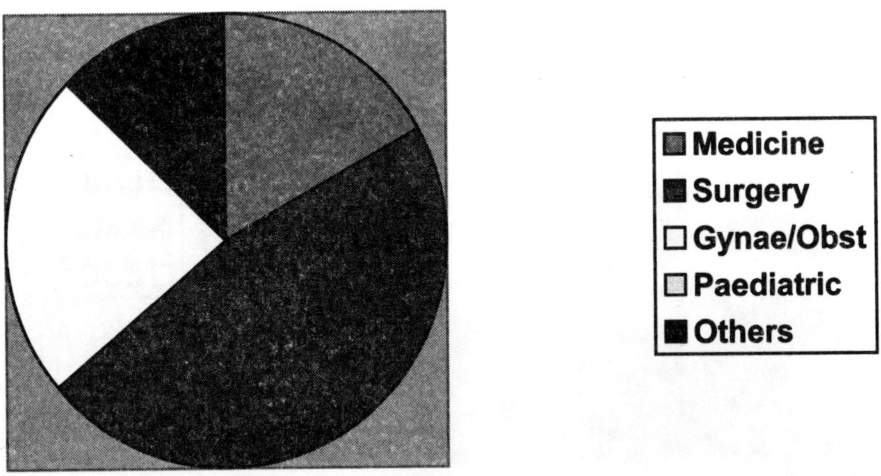

FIGURE 4.3

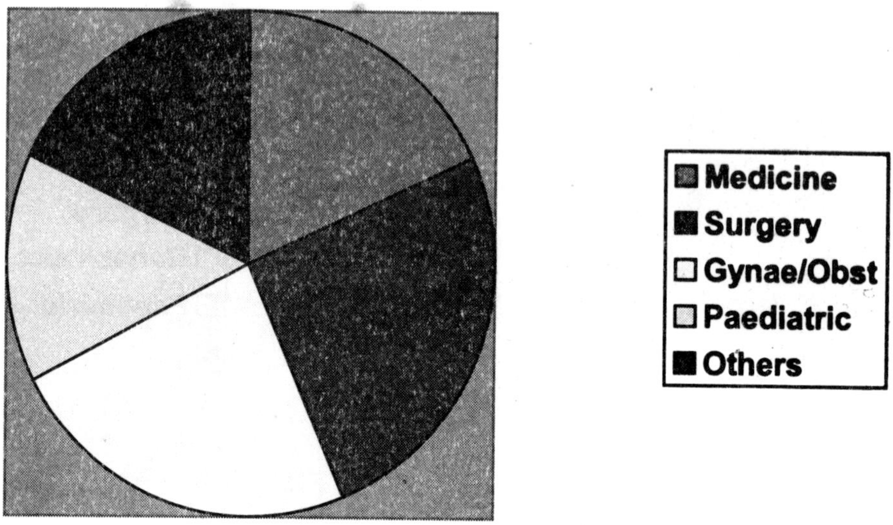

There is need for Referral system because most of the time, the patients from primary health centers are directly referred to tertiary hospitals. The patients report to tertiary hospitals on their own. Such a practice increases the workload on tertiary hospitals, thus bringing down the quality of services at lower level. Patients may not be aware of the type of services available at each level and may perceive lower level facilities providing lower quality of services. He further explained that the objective of the referral system is to see that the patient gets appropriate medical care as

FIGURE 4.4

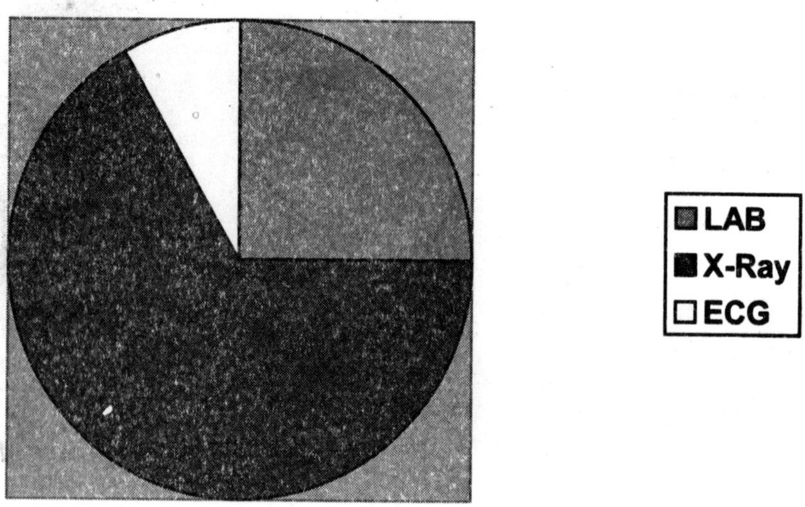

TABLE 4.6

Referred patients to and from in the Patiala district

	Emergency (referred)	*Others (referred)*	*Received*	*Referred Total No.*	*Feed Back Sent*	*Feed Back Received*	*Referred to Special Hospital*
M.K. Hospital	14	0	2	14	0	0	14
Rajpura	26	6	3	32	0	0	32
Nabha	9	9	3	18	0	0	18
Smana	12	4	1	16	1	0	16
M. Town	18	0	29	18	0	0	18
Dudhan Sudhna	0	3	0	3	0	0	3
Kalomajra	2	10	—	12	0	0	1
Dera Bassi	9	60	116	69	0	0	69
Ghanour	0	3	1	3	0	0	3
Badhson	10	11	6	21	0	0	11
Bhadshapur	—	20	11	20	0	0	10
Shutrana	—	—	13	—	0	0	—
Banur	16	14	1	30	0	0	30
Total	116	140	186	256	1	0	207

Source: Reporting Performa for Referral Services, Punjab Health Systems Corporation, March 2002.

early as possible and therefore, it is not a procedure to pass on or shirk the responsibility by shifting the patient from one hospital to the other. But, it is definitely not advisable to a doctor to continue treating a patient at his level when it is beyond his capability especially in view of the infrastructure available.

Whenever a patient is referred, his name has to be first entered in the referral register. The format for referral register is shown in Annexure 4.1.

Before referring the patient, counseling of the patient/relatives is a must, such as the patient should be informed as to why he is being referred to higher level of care. The patient needs to be assured that referral is for his benefit and that he will be taken care of at the referral units. The patient should be informed about the location of the referred hospitals, its timings and the likely cost of medical care. They should also be aware of the physical condition of the patient, in case of emergency. If the condition of the patient is unstable, first the patient must be stabilized and then transferred. Referral system should never be sued as means to shirk responsibility, but a tool to provide best possible medical care to a patient under any given circumstances.

In the referral procedure, there are two types of referrals—(i) Emergency, (ii) Routine referral. In the latter, the patient has to arrange for transportation but proper counseling needs to be done in both the cases. The patient is given a referral card and regular hospital hours, i.e. 8 am to 2 pm in summers and 9 am to 3 pm in winters are to be followed. For investigations, the best suitable timings are 9 am to 12 noon. However, emergency patients are attended to round-the-clock.

In Rajendra Hospital, the principal heads the college as well as the hospital and is assisted by a Medical Superintendent in the hospital. The college has a vice-principal, heads of the departments, professors, associate professors, assistant professors, senior lecturers, senior residents, junior residents. Principal is the overall in-charge of the Hospital and the college his functions are mentioned. The functions of the other person mentioned in the Hierarchy of Medical College are stated as below:

Professors and Heads of the Departments

1. In-charge of the respective teaching departments and its units.
2. Responsible for carrying\out teaching and training activities concerning the respective departments.
3. Responsible for Hospital treatment of both OPD and IPD concerning their discipline as well as beds allotted.
4. Supervising the teachers under them like Associate Professors, Assistant Professors and Lecturers for smooth and regular conduct of classes, teaching, training and patient care activities.
5. Supervising subordinate staff like technical staff, clerical staff and other Group-D employees.
6. Supervising and carrying out various research subjects allocated to PG and Fellowship scholars.
7. To arrange for practical classes in departments, laboratories, hospitals, etc. as required in the teaching and training programs of students and scholars.
8. Participating in seminars and conferences in the Institute as well as outside Institutions.
9. To conduct training and preparation of training modules for teachers and physicians training in the respective subjects.

Associate Professors, Assistant Professors and Lecturers

1. To carryout various duties and responsibilities of teaching, classes, practical, etc. allotted in the respective teaching departments and its units.
2. Responsible for carrying out teaching and training activities concerning the respective departments.
3. Responsible for Hospital treatment of both OPD and IPD concerning their subjects as well as beds allotted.
4. Managing for the smooth and regular conduct of classes, teaching training and patient care activities.
5. Managing the subordinate staff like technical staff, clerical staff and other Group-D employees.
6. Supervising and carrying out various research subjects allocated to PG and Fellowship scholars.
7. To arrange for practical classes in departments, laboratories,

hospitals, etc. as required in the teaching and training programs of students and scholars.

8. Participating in seminars and conference in the Institute as well as outside Institutions.
9. To conduct training and preparation of training modules for teachers and physicians trainings in the respective subjects.

FACULTY DEVELOPMENT THROUGH HUMAN RESOURCE DEVELOPMENT

A responsive administration to provide effective, efficient and good governance will remain a dream unless it has a motivated, trained and developed work force in the form of medical professional. An immediate need, therefore, is an appropriate HRD approach at the micro-level with an in-built system of training, career development, job enrichment and employee participation to improve the quality of work life and in the process attain quality governance. The government organisations and departments will have quality governance. The government organisations and departments will have to replace the traditional power and authority culture and adopt an effective HRD system and strategy. In the changed context, the present form and practice of recruitment and personnel polices for civil service personnel may not be workable and effective. Systematic career planning from the entry stage, coupled with planned training and

Hierarchy in Medical College

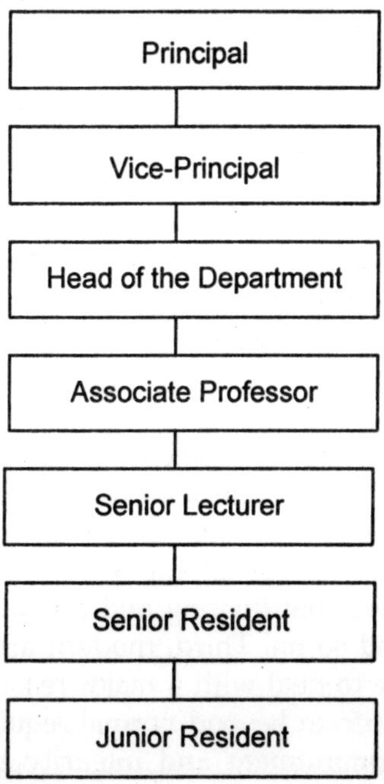

development programmes, will definitely ensure a satisfying growth for the employees in the government. In this context, human resource management in the government will assume an entirely different priority as it would emerge as the key factor for practice of good governance of the country.

HRD in brief is transformation of Potential Human Resources into Kinetic Human Resources for optimization of the potential capacity of employees. It has been rightly said in a study of the Capacity of United Nations Development System that "Human rather than capital is the key to development.[1]" Development is not a mechanical process. It is a human enterprise and its success will depend ultimately on the skill, quality and motivation of the persons associated with it. As professor Iris Claude has commended:

> "In a very significant sense, the identity of every organisation . . . is lodged in its professional staff. Members, stockholders, or citizens may control the organisation but they can not do it, the staff is the organisation.[2]"

It is therefore, by increasing the efficiency, integrity and the intelligence of its personnel that the organisation will give itself the real means for advancing towards growth and productivity. The constant improvement of the efficiency of an employee is as much the responsibility of the employee himself as of the organisation.

Critical Examination

Need for a full time Principal: Clear-cut policies regarding the functioning of every department should be framed, compiled in a Departmental Policy Book and circulated to every department with copies supplied to each staff. For effective functioning of the hospital, there is need for a full time Principal. It is essential to have proper flow of communication—be it vertical or lateral. For this, regular staff meetings may be arranged between the Principal and the available administrative staff. It is recommended, that the Principal should devote more time to manpower planning and development of staffing norms for various categories of technical and non-technical staff working in hospitals. Principal must possess leadership qualities.

EROPA has emphasized the following qualities

First, there are certain specialized fields of knowledge and skill which are programme-relevant, such as substantive knowledge of health administration. Second, managerial expertise and skills are paramount in effective implementation, coordinating and scheduling work, planning and allocating resources, and so on. Third, modern administrative leaders need human relations' ability to deal with a major resource in organisational life. Motivating people to perform beyond normal requirements to instill a strong sense of programme-commitment and integrity and to incite programme personnel to unfetter the suffocating bonds of anachronistic administrative values, traditions and practices are additional requisite skills. Finally, there are certain 'political' skills required to sustain, support and co-operation from the volatile public (legislation and ministers), mass media, clientele, local, political notables, etc[3].

Need for Hospital Administrator Competent is the Art and Science of Hospital Administrator

There should be Professionalization of Hospital Administration and compulsory training for the administrators of the hospital. Hospital administration needs to be developed, as it is a much bigger challenge and has to face two maladies: one of the patients other of the administration. Thus, there is a need of a technical hospital administrator and need to develop hospital administration by providing courses in administration to doctors and nurses who have to assume administrative responsibilities. They can be taught in the area of decision-making, leadership, motivation, supervision, planning, etc. The main functions of supervision say Roethlisberger and Dickson is to "maintain order and control." Hospital administration is a full-time job, which requires the services of a person who is free from clinical responsibilities.

Hospital Administration is a science as well as an art. The hospital administration has become complex and requires administrative capability to solve its managerial problems to provide the optimum care to the patients. It is, therefore, necessary that the persons charged with efficient running of the hospitals are trained in the managerial techniques and tools which may be applied by them for getting the best out of the resources available.

Hospital Administrator should Promote Medical Ethics

We suggest here some points to make ethical standards practicable and feasible:

(i) Top leadership should follow ethical standards to serve as bacon light for the health functionaries at the lower level.
(ii) We should encourage professional standards to inject in the medical team the spirit of service.
(iii) New entrants need be supervised properly so that wrong behaviours may be corrected in the initial stages.
(iv) There should be code of ethics which should be followed by all.
(v) Environment of the hospital should be such which can inspire confidence and loyalty.
(vi) Medical team should be respected and given due status.

Neglect of Hospital Maintenance: Need of Maintenance and Beautification

The first impression of the visitors to the hospital depends upon the proper upkeep of buildings, equipment, water-supply, electricity supply, etc.

A visit to a number of hospitals revealed the following which should be taken care of in the new millennium:

(i) The surroundings of the hospitals are covered with congress grass and is full of dirt. Even in many hospitals there are no boundary walls. It is suggested that green grass and plants should be grown to make the hospitals clean and greener.

(ii) Buildings of the hospitals are in bad shape. Because of the shortage of funds, these are not maintained properly. These become the breeding ground of insects and cause infection. In the hospitals, buildings must be maintained properly at regular intervals of time to avoid deterioration.

(iii) Sweepers and ward boys must be encouraged to keep the hospital clean. They must be told that cleanliness is very important for the recovery of patients.

(iv) Lavatories are in bad shape and even stinking. Hospital authorities must attend to it seriously otherwise the foul smell make the whole environment of the hospital unpleasant.

Delegation of Authority and Responsibility

Participative style of decision-making for issues concerning personnel should be practiced. Participative management encourages team spirit because it gives a feeling of belongingness among members, who otherwise may belong to different segments of the hospital. This would lead to a better decision-making process thereby ensuring proper and quick implementation of policies. For proper and effective management, the span of control should be reduced and more powers delegated to the lower level. This can be done by creating few administrative positions answerable to the Principal. This will leave the Principal with enough time to formulate policies and interact with the different agencies, who directly or indirectly are involved in managing the hospital.

Revision in Financial Powers—for the funds required for daily basis

Adequate funds and financial flexibility should be given to various departments so that emergency works should not suffer.

Delegation of More Financial Powers to Lower Levels

A necessary adjunct to performance budget is the delegation of adequate financial powers, commensurate with the functions and duties, entrusted to various levels of operating officials. This is necessary for the accomplishment of targets at various operational levels of performance. The delegation of powers to the operating officials should be the maximum possible and not the minimum necessary, in order to enable them to fulfil their assignment without frequent reference to the higher authorities.

Consistent Supervision

To ensure that hospital meets challenges in a befitting manner, there is need for effective supervision. Supervision does not mean control only, rather, "it is the extension of leadership functions applied to the direction of work at all levels." It is telling the staff what to do and helping them to do it, it is the principal means through which coordination is achieved. Nevertheless, supervision helps maintain control as well. "Through supervision a basis is laid for controlling results. So that Principal can understand the needs of the institute and can supervise effectively and rounds could be taken frequently with occasional surprise visits.

Medical audit at shorter interval: Medical audit be made a regular feature, the very aim of medical audit is to evaluate patient care. All the deaths in the hospital where causes are not certain be investigated by mortality review committee. This will add to the medical knowledge of the doctors and keep them abreast and accountable to general public for their action and deeds.

To sum up, we can say that Rajendra Hospital need more attention especially in matters of administration. It requires to motivate the staff to bridge gap between administration and work force through interaction with them at regular intervals. Hospitals involve high-costs and thus be administered sensibly enough to have fuller utilization of expenditure incurred on these, otherwise these will turn out to be den of corruption and junkyards of rotten material and equipment.

Recommendations regarding Teaching Services

1. The lecture theatres should be adequately lit and properly ventilated to induce an atmosphere of studying and the sitting should be comfortable.
2. It is important to have a hygienic canteen in the hospital to avoid wastage of time of students.
3. Hostels should have rooms with adequate lights and fans. They should have rooms white-washed on a regular basis. Almirahs should be provided for keeping the luggage and the toilets should have washbasins.
4. Proper teaching aids are a must. Methods of teaching, therefore, require introduction of innovations: integrated approach, multidisciplinary methods and laying stress on essentials, helping students to learn for themselves, modifying the curriculum to be in consonance with the aim of medical education, and appreciation that the aim of the curriculum is to help the learner to educate himself and develop the necessary skills, knowledge and critical faculties, computer, internet facilities, should be readily available.
5. Research facility should be good, as pursuit of research is an essential function of a teaching hospital. Any teaching hospital

that fails to encourage research fails in its duty towards humanity and will quickly cease to attract or retain professors and medical teachers of adequate caliber. Postgraduate students would cease to apply for admission. As a result, it would lack eminent supervisors for research projects. Moreover, the pursuit of research by all university teachers is necessary to undergraduate teaching, both because it ensures that teachers are actively pursuing their subjects in depth and because it is a further means to interest students in the scientific aspects of medicine.

6. Library should have the latest books and journals as medicine research has no end.

Recommendations Regarding Patient Care Services

Hospital services are for those who approach them. In modern times, we heavily depend on these hospitals but it needs to be seen how much health care the hospital and the hospital administration is providing to the Community. A hospital and its working is under great stress and often these institutions are accused of not providing for what they are created. There is the need to bridge the gap between the users and the servers.

Following are a few suggestions to improve the patient care services in Rajendra Hospital:

1. The waiting area should be neat and clean. There should be proper benches for the patients coming from the interiors of Punjab. Stray dogs should be kept away from the hospital; otherwise dog bite may cause an added problem. Spittoons should be kept at regular intervals, so that the patients do not spread infections. Dustbins should also be provided to help keep the area neat and clean.
2. Various departments/sections should be marked in Punjabi language at regular intervals, so that the patients coming from rural areas are also able to locate the concerned OPD. An enquiry booth/room should be made specially to help patient reach the right place without wasting any time.
3. proper lighting and examination tables should be provided in the OPD. The rooms should be adequately lit so that the doctor can examine the patient thoroughly and proper beds should be available so that an adult patient can also lie down comfortably.
4. Proper cards should be made for those visiting the OPD and record of the same should be kept in the hospital, as a single sheet slip is difficult to maintain for follow-ups.
5. Adequate rooms and proper facilities for the patients and their relatives should be provided in the hospital premises. There is an urgent need for sarai, as people reach this place from far-off areas for specialized care and investigations.

6. There is the need to have adequate and modern equipment with annual maintenance contracts with the selling company, as this will help reduce expenditure incurred on heavy repairs and save the patients from the inconvenience of going to private clinics for specialized tests.
7. To ensure delivery of efficient and proper health care services, adequate staff strength needs to be posted in hospitals as per the norms of National Health Department.
8. Availability of right quality and quantity of medicines is not the only thing to be ensured by hospitals. They have to ensure that they are not stocking irrelevant or outdated medicines. Buying a life-saving drug at heavy cost for select patients is necessary, but at the same time common drugs should also be available in the hospital.

To sum up, a lot of changes are required to improve the patient care services in Rajindra Hospital. It is important that being a tertiary hospital, Rajindra Hospital should lay a lot of stress on long-term treatment and should have a well-equipped rehabilitative department with well-qualified personnel to offer the best healthy care facilities which are not available in the interiors of Punjab.

Following improvements will make Nursing services efficient:

(a) to treat the nursing personnel as partners along with the other members of health and medical team;
(b) to help the nursing personnel reach self-actualization and thereby help release their creative energy for the promotion of health;
(c) to create facilities for continuous growth, development and training of nursing personnel to make them fit for higher jobs;
(d) to ensure adequate working arrangements and maximum participation in management and decision-making of the health system by nursing personnel;
(e) to provide institutional safeguards for redressal of grievance by nursing personnel;
(f) setting good professional standards by senior nursing personnel; and
(g) development of unity, energy, initiative and loyalty among nursing personnel.

If all these factors are improved, the nursing personnel will be satisfied Internally as well as externally at their jobs and will be proud of their choice of the profession. They will feel encouraged to come forward and to meet challenges in which high standards of performance will be maintained to yield best possible results in terms of achievement of goals.

Needs of Planning Hospital Services—Rajendra Hospital faces a number of problems which can be lessened through planning

Cyril, L. Hudson has given a comprehensive definition of planning in the following terms:

> "To plan is to produce a scheme for future action, to bring about specified results, at specified cost, in a specified period of time. It is a deliberate attempt to influence, exploit, bring about, and control the nature, direction, extent, speed and effects of change. It may even attempt deliberately to create change. It is a carefully controlled and co-ordinated activity.

Planning is the exercise of intelligence to deal with facts and solutions as they are and find a way to solve problems. Planning is in essence, an organized, conscious and continual attempt to select the best available alternatives to achieve specific goals. Planning is the phase of the total process, which leads from the policy statements to the concrete identification of the population whose needs and demands will be served; the indication of the types of activities that will be performed for these populations with their general attributes, and the specification of the type of instruments that will be required to carry out the activities.

John E. Laing has mentioned the following essentials of planning, which need to be kept in mind:

Rational

Much of what passes for planning in executing programmes is based on unconscious or at best, unexpected though process of the decision-maker. Such decisions, based on hunches, intuition or past experiences should play an important role in the planning process but only in conjunction with rational consideration of cost benefits and alternatives.

Deliberate

Planning should not involve hurried decisions except in special emergencies.

Specific

Whereas policy provides broad guidelines for action, planning should be more specific, breaking each task into its component parts, defining each individual's functions and responsibilities, specifying programme goals in measurable, quantitative terms.

Comprehensive

Planning should cover such diverse components of the programme as framing, resource allocation, research and evaluation, information and motivation, delivery of services and programme effects.

Systematic

Planning for each component should be both internally consistent and consistent with the plans for the other components.

Continuous

Plans should continuously undergo revision in response to changing conditions and to the findings from programme evaluation.

The success of socio-economic development in a developing country like ours depends upon the degree to which plan strategy has been carried out. The essence of development involves the setting up of planning machinery with a view to utilizing the resources in an economical and efficient manner, so as to promote the well being of the people and to increase the Gross National Product. The process of development planning can help us to get the benefits of modernization which depends upon "Systematic, sustained and purposeful application of human energies to the rational control of man's physical and social environment for various human purposes[4].

It is clear that poor Planning may upset the programme results. However, we may keep in mind that excessive Planning can divert valuable managerial resources from the present utilization. Rigid enforcement of the detailed plans can kill the programme by stifling initiative. Deviation from detailed task specifications should be allowed, if high-level targets are achieved. Therefore, there is a need that planning itself must be clearly anticipated in advance, so as to ensure that it will make a positive contribution to the programme.

Inadequate Facilities for Record Management

Since it is one of the oldest hospitals, it is very important that all the records should be maintained properly. Unfortunately, it was found that there was not proper system of record management. There are no adequate facilities for record management.

Need of Training to Medical Personnel in the Art and Science of Administration

Training is essential for building confidence, commitment and competence among medical personnel. Mahabir Singh Kasana, rightly observes, "Training is very important component of Human Resource Development. It is, perhaps the most cost effective method of improving competencies amongst the manpower of any organisations. Training has been defined as a planned process to impart knowledge, develop skills and modify attitude of the work force through learning processes to achieve the effective performance in any activity or range of activities. The right mix of knowledge, skills and attitudinal components in a training course or a training programme is essential for performance improvement. Performance calls for upgrading confidence, competence and commitment of the persons to enable them to handle the situation and show the results on the ground.

Whereas, increase in knowledge, arguability imparts confidence, the skills contribute to enhancement of competency of individuals. The attitude primarily leads to commitment to job. Possessing of the right attitude, combined with appropriate knowledge and skills is required to be assured through training efforts. It is, therefore, necessary that a systematic approach to training linking it with performance is necessary. Developing confidence, competence and commitments require enriching learning experience consisting of Tell, Show, Do, Check and Act through systematic approach to training.[5]

Inadequate Research

Research is one of the primary aims of the teaching and research institutes. It is the crux of development and without it everything comes to a standstill. The referral system are set, so that adequate time to carry out research at the tertiary health care level and minor ailments can be overcome at the primary and secondary levels. It is through research that we can overcome the challenges in the health sector. This hospital being a tertiary hospital has a primary role to carry out research. But it was found during the visit that neither the doctors nor the students were satisfied with the research work at the hospital. The lack of research work was owing to various factors as pointed out by the doctors working in the institutes. One of the major factors hindering research was lack of finances—the hospital doesn't have adequate diagnostic equipment to carry out the research work. Another factor that affected the research was lack of work culture in the hospital. People working in the hospital were busy in their private business rather than working sincerely in the hospital.

Regarding Medical Records not in good shape

Since, medical records are of great value and it is important that there should be a proper Central Registration Department to keep track of all case records of patients whether inpatient or outpatient filed together under one unit number. There should be more manpower to handle the records computer should be introduced for efficient record management.

CONCLUSION

We must attend to all these problems to ensure efficiency of the hospitals. These problems also emanate from a number of constraints on hospital authorities, e.g., shortage of staff at all levels, absence of proper accommodation to provide space to the ever increasing number of patients, shortages of funds, shortages of medicine, shortages of equipment, political and administrative inference, etc. which need to be attended to by the governments at the Union and State level to provide satisfactory hospital services. Besides, the patients and their relatives must co-operate with the hospital authorities to make the best use of the available resources. Thus, we shall have to have a three-pronged attack-increasing internal efficiency, mobilizing government support and enlisting people's cooperation to ensure the reputation, prestige, credibility and viability of the hospital services.

NOTES AND REFERENCES

1. UN: A Study of the Capacity of the UN Development System, Vol. I, Geneva, 1969.
2. Inis Claude, Swords into Plowshares, New York, Random House, 1964, p. 174.
3. ERORA: Summary Report of the Seventh General Assembly and Conference on 'Implementation: the Problem of achieving Results', Vol. II, pp. 1-8.
4. Quoted in Marrico B. Jansen, ed., Changing Japanese Attitude towards Modernization, Princeton, 1965, pp. 23.24.
5. Mahabir Singh Kasana, "Systematic Approach to Training for Rural Industrialization" in Management in Government, January-March, 2000, pp. 56-57.

5

CHAPTER

Secondary Health Care Administration

A Case Study of Jalandhar District in Punjab

PART I

SECONDARY HEALTH CARE ADMINISTRATION—A CASE STUDY OF JALANDHAR DISTRICT IN PUNJAB

Districts used to be very large but the recent trend is to make smaller district. Districts have multiplied three times. District is now not very far off from the people.

A district hospital is a hospital complex mainly engaged in curative services for the population of the district. The size of the hospital varies from 50 beds to 500 beds depending upon size and population of the district. Most of district hospitals are housed in old buildings while new buildings have been constructed in the new districts or upgraded the existing civil hospitals. However, old buildings have been renovated with extensions of OPD, wards and other facilities.

Nature

Since many health problems require a level of medical treatment and personal care that extends beyond the range of services normally available in the patients' home or in the office of the physician, modern society has developed formal institutions for patient care intended to help meet the more complex health needs of its members. The hospital, the major social institution for the delivery of health care in the modern world, offers considerable advantages to both patient and society. From the standpoint of individual, the sick or injured person has access to centralized medical knowledge and technology so as to render treatment much more thorough and efficient. From the standpoint of society, hospitalization both protects the family from many of the disruptive effects of caring for the ill in the home and operates as a means of guiding the sick and injured into medically supervised institutions where their problems are less disruptive for society as a whole.

Today, a hospital is a place for the definition and treatment of human ills and restoration of health and well-being of those temporarily deprived of these. A large number or professionally and technically skilled people apply their knowledge and skill with the help of complicated equipment and appliances to produce quality care for patient. The excellence of the product—the *raison d'etre* for a hospital, therefore depends on how well the human and material resources are applied to promote patient care.

The authority structure in a district hospital is based on hierarchical system, which leads to bureaucratization and rigidity. The Medical Superintendent/SMO heads the district hospital. Each unit is under the charge of a senior specialist who is assisted by junior specialists and general duty medical officers and almost works as independent units without even essential linkages.

Presently, the district hospital provides for both ambulatory (OPD) and in-patient care in most of the general specialties like medicine, surgery, orthopedics, ENT, ophthalmology, skin and STD, pediatrics, emergency and dental care, etc. The districts where there are no separate women's hospitals also have obstetrics and gynecology units as well. Most of the district hospitals have a post partum centre as well. The beds are allocated to each specialty but there is no rational system for its distribution.

These hospitals generally have very rudimentary, outdated, primitive and inadequate facilities for basic radiological and pathological laboratory services and blood bank facilities. Modern technology is to available and whatever is available is not of good quality. The typical district hospital totally lacks modern diagnostic and therapeutic equipments, adequate emergency care facilities, intensive care units, drugs and supplies, referral support and resources. The management and provision of even other supportive and ancillary services in these hospitals like medical rectors, dietary, contract laundry, housekeeping and nursing care services are totally inadequate and ineffective. The central sterile stores department does not exist. The units have their own autoclaves for the purpose. Many district hospitals do not even have qualified anesthetists on their rolls. All this does tell upon the quality of the care provided by the hospitals.

There is no trained staff for hospital management or for the management of other supportive or ancillary services as they have undergone only professional courses. They find difficulty in managing resources—men, money and material leading to a number of problems. High infection rates and death rates are common. The hospitals though treat patients from rural areas, but lack in organisation of an out reach mobile care on a regular basis of an effective referral service and thus its linkages with primary health care are weakened. These district hospitals further are divorced from the responsibility of coordinating the basic specialty care provided by the community health centres and utilizing them for follow up services of rural patients after being discharged from the hospital in-patient care. The linkage and supervision by district senior specialists of the CHCs, which are 30-bedded hospitals, is very essential to impart professional training.

The health system based on primary health care stipulates the strong back up support of a district hospital and an efficient system of patient referral for specialized care, which could not be made available at first point of contact of health care system. However, in the existing set-up of district medical care, the referral system is practically non-viable and lacks even basic elements of it. The question of having a good or efficient system does not arise at all.

Let us now mention the important functions of a district hospital.

Functions

(a) Patient Care

The first and foremost function of a hospital is to give care to the sick and injured and restore the health of diseased persons. Ethically, this care should be given to all without discrimination of social, economic or racial nature.

(b) Training

The education and training of doctors and nurses have traditionally been carried out in hospitals. It is a workshop wherein the students learn by seeing what his superiors and peers do. Radiology, laboratory, radiotherapy, highly advanced surgical techniques demand a variety of skills and knowledge, all of which cannot be mastered by the doctor specialist. These activities are today the vital support to the specialist whether he is the surgeon, physician, diagnostician or therapeutist. These people are indispensable for the all round excellence of all specialist work. To develop these technical skills, a programme should be organized by the hospital under the direction of people who have the required experience, knowledge and aptitude to teach others. The purpose of in-service education and training programme is to develop such knowledge and skills in all categories of paramedical personnel as are required to make them fit for the job they hold and keep them attuned to the growing needs of their jobs.

(c) Medical Research

The third important function of hospital is to give support to medical research, which is at present non-existent. A good hospital where the quality of professional work is excellent is an ideal ground for medial research. As a matter of fact, excellent professional care of patients largely results from the fruits of research into new problems. An attitude of enquiry and investigation should permeate through the day-to-day care of patients.

The hospital can develop facilities for research with comparative ease and speed if the staff and administration are properly motivated. True, elaborate research is expensive. There, nevertheless, remain clinical investigations of applied nature that call for little capital investment. Responsibility for creation of new knowledge is that of any enlightened profession. It is in a hospital that opportunities exist, for organized as well as individual initiative for research.

(d) Health Education

The fourth and final object is to support and assist all activities carried out by various public health and voluntary agencies to prevent disease and promote positive health attitudes in the community through health education. Social and economic rehabilitation are some of the many activities for which the hospital may provide assistance in terms of physical facilities and advisory services to staff. As a matter of fact, in the western countries, this aspect of the hospital as a community health centre is being emphasized more and more. Many ways are being devised to integrate the hospital with the activities of community health agencies.

The main function of a hospital is to promote the health of the community, which it serves. It has been stated in a WHO document that the hospital in an integral part of a social and medical organisations, the function of which is to provide for the population, complete health care, both curative and preventive, and whose outpatient services reach out to the family in its home environment, the hospital is also a centre for the training of health workers and for bio-social research[1] and an institution that provides in-patient accommodation for medical and nursing care. The hospital has a notable purpose expressed in the phrase "Promotion of health and welfare of the people." Hospitals have now become indispensable to the proper care of the broad spectrum of health problems. However in India, a district hospital provides a curative service within the hospital. It does not provide complete health care as defined by WHO.

Administration of such a complex organisation requires blending of technical and administrative competence in the right quantity, at the right time, at the right place, by the right man and in the right way or process. We should look at district hospital as a part of district health system to ensure success of integrated primary health care system. Viewed in this broader concept, the district hospital is supposed to ensure the following:

(a) provide curative services to any person approaching directly or through referral system;
(b) provide guidance, support, supervision to primary health centres and community health centres so that there may not be unnecessary rush at the district hospital because of the inadequate services in these centres;
(c) provide in-service training to personnel from CHC, PHC, sub-centre and its own staff since district hospital is equipped with modern gadgets;

(d) to act as a referral centre both to the patients and the personnel working in PHC and CHC;

(e) providing technological support to different levels of health care system in the district;

(f) extending specialists services to out reach areas in order to understand and prioritize community health problems;

(g) to act as a centre for immunization programme;

(h) District hospital should support promotive, preventive, rehabilitative services besides curative and strengthen the primary health care system; and

(i) District hospital should keep a continuous track on surveillance of diseases and keeping the CHC, PHC and sub-centre well informed in this aspect.

A case study of District Hospital in Punjab: Civil Hospital Jalandhar

In Punjab, District Hospitals are headed by Medical Superintendent (Senior rank officer) in case of big hospitals and an SMO in case of small hospitals. In some other states like Karnataka, these are headed by Civil Surgeon. Let us explain in brief the biggest district hospital in Punjab (400 bedded), that is Civil Hospital, Jalandhar. Other district hospitals are mostly 100 bedded. Personnel staff strength of this hospital is 418 comprising of specialists, supporting staff, administrative and other staff, and Class IV (Sweeper, etc.). These are shown in Table 5.1. It is good to note that all the posts were filled up. The building with the addition of five floors is sufficient to meet the present need.

TABLE 5.1

A. Specialists	*Sanctioned*
1. Medicine	3
2. Surgery	2
3. Ophthalmology	1
4. Gynae	2
5. Skin	1
6. Psychiatric	1
7. BTO and ENT	1
8. Radiologist	2
9. Child Specialist	1
10. Orthopedic Surgeon	1
11. Dental Surgeon	2
12. Anesthetist	2
13. GDMO	1
14. Pathologist	1
15. Microbiologist	1
16. EMO	4
17. EMO Revmp.	3

B. Supporting Staff Pharmacist	
Pharmacist	10
Matron	30
Sisters	23
Staff Nurses	76
Lab. Tech.	11
Total	150

C. Office Staff Helpers	
Office Superintendent	1
Senior Assistant	2
Clerk	6
Care Taker	2
Cashier	2
Storekeeper	6
Typist	1
Stenographer	1
Assistant Dietician	1
OTA Hawaldar	1
ECG Tech.	1
Ophthalmic Assistant	1
Radiographer	1
Dental Mechanic	2
Physiotherapist Barber	1
Plumber	1
Carpenter	4
Electrician	1
Total	**37**
D. Class IV	**200**
Grand Total	**418**

Finance

Besides the normal budget which is in the range of 3 crores per year, there are allocations from different schemes. The finances are hardly sufficient to meet the needs of such a big hospital. Salary itself takes away 60 per cent of the money. Let us explain with the help of expenditure incurred during the last five years (See Table 5.2)

MAP I

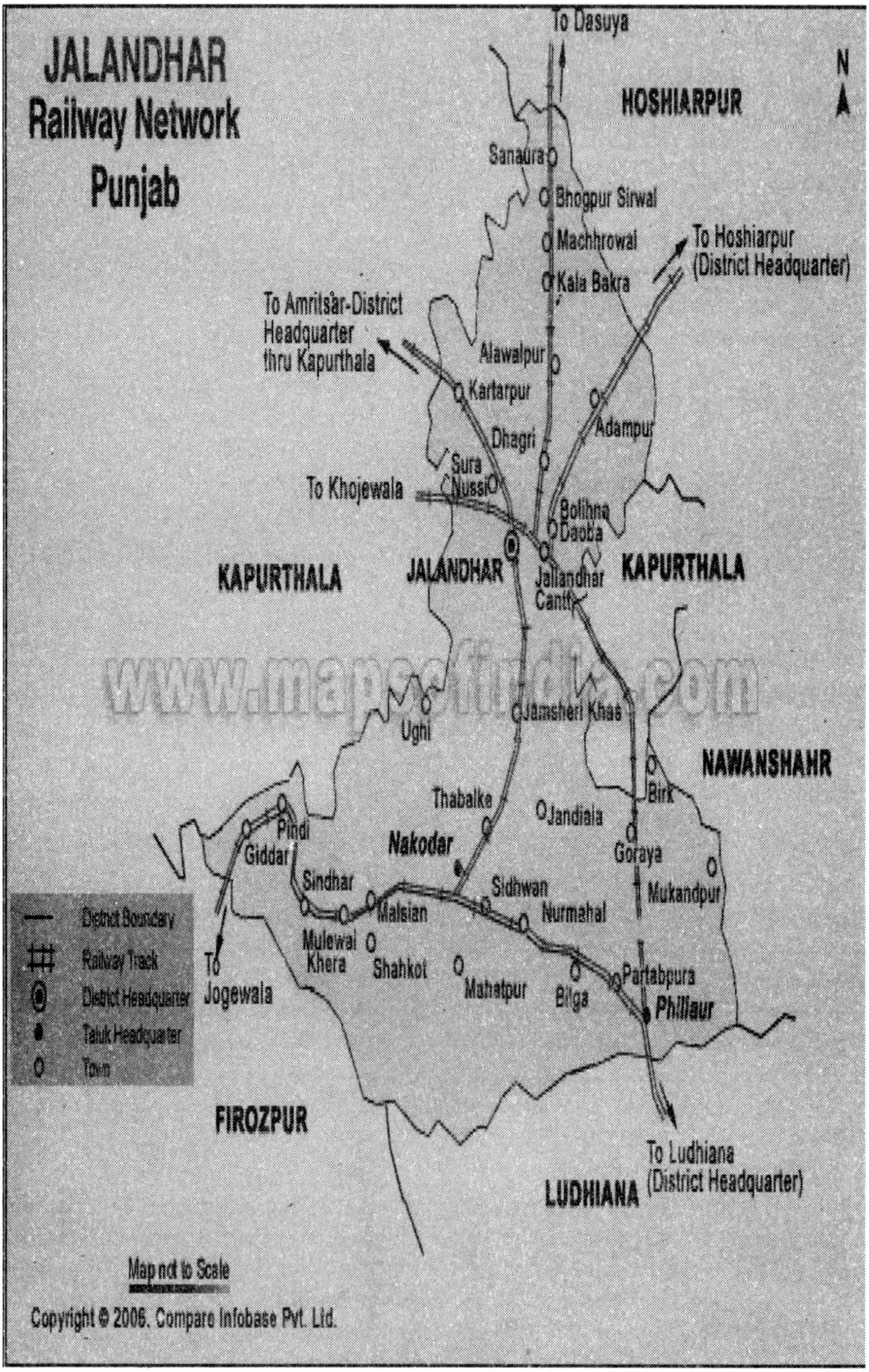
JALANDHAR
Railway Network
Punjab
N
To Dasuya
HOSHIARPUR
Sanaura
Bhogpur Sirwal
Machhrowal
Kala Bakra
To Hoshiarpur
(District Headquarter)
To Amritsar-District
Headquarter
thru Kapurthala
Alawalpur
Kartarpur
Adampur
Dhagri
Sura
Nussi
To Khojewala
Bolihna
Daoba
KAPURTHALA
JALANDHAR
Jallandhar
Cantt
KAPURTHALA
www.mapsofindia.com
Ughi
Jamsheri Khas
NAWANSHAHR
Birk
Thabalke
Jandiala
Pindi
Giddar
Nakodar
Goraya
Sindhar
Sidhwan
Mukandpur
Malsian
Nurmahal
District Boundary
Railway Track
District Headquarter
Taluk Headquarter
Town
Mulewal
Khera
Shahkot
To
Jogewala
Mahatpur
Bilga
Partabpura
Phillaur
FIROZPUR
To Ludhiana
(District Headquarter)
LUDHIANA
Map not to Scale
Copyright © 2006. Compare Infobase Pvt. Ltd.

TABLE 5.2

(Figures in Rupees)

Year	*Salaries*	*For other Purpose*	*Total*
1993-94	1,57,84,993	61,76,690	2,19,61,683
1994-95	1,74,98,871	55,18,142	2,28,17,013
1995-96	2,03,56,569	22,62,025	2,26,18,594
1996-97	2,62,22,741	20,93,973	2,83,16,684
1997-98	2,98,24,808	10,38,636	3,08,68,444
Nursing Facilities (Plan)			
1993-94	4,24,568	3100	427,668
1994-95	4,26,963	2,763	4,29,726
1995-96	5,36,179	4,485	5,40,664
1996-97	5,74,776	1,886	5,74,662
1997-98	6,31,593	3,029	6,34,612
T.O. Scheme (Plan)			
1993-94	4,20,973	28,624	4,40,597
1994-95	4,19,892	32,720	4,52,612
1995-96	5,74,005	18,782	5,92,787
1996-97	8,22,749	15,423	8,38,242
1997-98	9,83,481	41,975	10,25,456
Revamping Scheme (Non-Plan)			
1993-94	5,61,435	2,05,169	7,66,604
1994-95	6,46,374	31,784	6,78,160
1995-96	8,33,350	1,15,375	9,48,725
1996-97	9,42,315	958	9,43,273
1997-98	7,59,842	—	7,59,842
Dental Clinic (Non-Plan)			
1993-94	—	—	—
1994-95	5,187	2,798	7,985
1995-96	30,407	984	31,391
1996-97	58,654	4,453	63,107
1997-98	33,930	2,736	36,666

Equipment

The hospital has most of the essential equipment but some of the equipment was not functional. There was only one bus, which was functional. Ambulances were condemned. There is a need of new ambulance.

Activities

The hospital provides both curative and preventive services. In curative, it provides all types of services, OPD, ward, operations, laboratory examination, etc. Let us explain he services provided by the hospital during the last seven years (refer Table 5.3). An analysis of the table reveals that referral services are not a great success, which should be the main function of a district hospital.

TABLE 5.3

Hospital Performance Indicators

(Rs. in lacs)

	Year						
	1998	*1999*	*2000*	*2001*	*2002*	*2003*	*2004*
OPD	159836	136183	111679	124681	153961	178523	203970
IPD	7639	8235	8112	8551	11005	11374	13465
Delivery	426	421	377	413	382	592	631
X-ray	10962	11391	10695	13788	16445	19642	25436
Lab. Test	99667	53585	50972	63597	61161	83041	104570
User Charges	15.06	20.01	6.96	41.05	55.56	65.09	86.39

Before we discuss District Hospital Administration of Ropar, let us discuss the profile of the District Health System of Ropar.

Working of District Hospitals—We have covered a large number of issues in discussing hospital administration in General. Here, we shall concentrate on some other and important issues:

1. Lack of Proper Utilization of Resources

A major factor affecting the efficiency and quality of care provided by the secondary and tertiary care hospitals in the government sector is the mismatch between requirements and the provision of buildings, number of beds, equipments, laboratory and other facilities on the one hand and the actual human (medical, dental, nursing, allied health professionals and support services) and material resources.

The reasons for the mismatch are very many.

- The availability of staff was not as per the norms for the provision of buildings, inpatient beds and other facilities.
- Positions were created but not filled up.

- Equipment was purchased but trained and qualified technical personnel not available. It could be the reverse also: trained personnel available but there was no equipment or the equipment was not in working order for every long periods.
- Equipment is available but consumables like chemicals, reagents and X-ray films not available.

It is essential to ensure better match. Planned efforts are needed to address these issues effectively to improve the performance quantitatively and, more importantly, qualitatively.[1]

2. Gap between availability of resources and demands of the people

Financial and other resources are limited. But there are ever increasing demands. People are aware of the developments in diagnosis and therapy in the affluent parts of the world. Medical personnel trained in the use of sophisticated technology in those countries also demand the costly equipment, so that they could carry out such interventions here also. Ethical and other dilemmas occur in decision-makings. Even when the equipment is purchased at high cost, the equipment may remain non-functional, if it needs maintenance or repairs and there is no one to set it working[2]. Even patients in emergency do not get a bed and remain lying on floors. Staff strength is less while pressure on them is very high. In addition staff also do not devote the required time. The situation is compounded by many patients with vague symptoms and requiring primary health care come to secondary care hospitals. They are directed to one specialist unit or another by a non-medical person. The patients go from one queue to another, wasting considerable time of themselves and of the specialists before a diagnosis is made and treatment given. One way out is to have only patients referred from a primary health centre (or equivalent unit) to be seen at the secondary care hospital. But this can cause inconvenience to patients from the neighbourhood of the secondary care hospital, unless there is a general practice unit at the secondary hospital. The general practice unit can work in the outpatient department, manage a large proportion of the patient and refer others to the specialists, who can devote their greater attention to these patients.[2]

Administrative improvement means the act or the process of improving the administration. As stated in a United Nations Report: "Management improvement comprises of planning implementation and evaluation of various measures conducive to the increase of organisational effectiveness and efficiency.[3]

Simple commitment by management is not enough. The improvement process must become as basic and continuous as our concerns. There is no magic approach or solution to be gleaned from either a text-book or a consultant, although either of these can help management discover an effective programme for carrying out its required responsibility. But, the manager remains the key to tapping the most underutilized resource people.[4]

Administrative reform is still widely regarded as a special type of improvement activity, even when it is often closely connected with other activities. The concept of the 'administrative reform', as it is applied in practice, also has its weaknesses.

Efforts at administrative reform too often stop with the preparation of reports or promulgation of laws. Unless administrative reforms encourage macro-level improvement of performance and their micro-level self-evaluation with a view to providing a managerial feed-back loop for bringing about further improvement in performance, any elaborate machinery for external evaluation can only degenerate into evaluation for evaluation's sake. In fact, performance itself often becomes a casualty. It also helps to "pass the buck" upwards and reduce accountability from those who should perform to those who supervise.

Administrative reforms are not only to be planned but implemented as well, with sincerity at all levels, to achieve the desired results. There has to be a genuine desire to ensure just and impartial administration. Making improvements in procedures and practices, form and techniques of administration are only partial remedies. These along may not give the desired results unless the human elements incharge of running the administrative machinery show genuine commitment to bring about good governance. Unfortunately he deteriorating quality of leadership adversely affected the quality of administrative machinery as well. For, unless the top is clean and truly dedicated to the well-being of the people, other layers of administration are unlikely to behave any better. The lower ones generally follow the footsteps of the higher ones.[5]

In the case of teaching hospitals, there is an added advantage if there is a general practice unit. The patients with the vague symptoms and requiring primary health care can be very useful for teaching/learning about the common types of patients met in the community.[6]

3. *Emergency Services are not taken seriously*

The emergency department provides round the clock services but the rush of patients in very high while the availability of equipment and personnel are limited. It is a scene of Chaos. It appears as if crowd is lying without any proper arrangement. It is worse than the animals.

Emergency departments need be strengthened

These departments should be oriented to manage the persons requiring immediate treatments. They should not be 'traffic policemen', directing emergency patients to various inpatient departments. The staff of emergency departments must be capable of giving the treatment, calling the specialists as necessary. Once the patient is stabilized, the patient may be transferred to the respective departments for further definitive therapy.

Triage System

It is necessary to have sorting of patients, based on need for immediate attention, when there are more patients. We should have a practical triage system, with a rapid provisional assessment. This will lead to efficient and effective management.

We must minimize:

- patient waiting and process time;
- administrative activities of staff and patients; and
- movement of patients and relatives (attendants).

Communication

The role of communication systems (apart from the ambulance services) must be emphasized. Electronic data communication must be in place to facilitate transfer of information

- from place of accident or emergency illness to ambulance, and
- from the ambulances to the receiving hospitals.

This will ensure that the hospitals are alerted early of the arrival of the patient and delay can be avoided. Use of the police department communication system will be useful. It can also help in networking available agencies and personnel.

Quality Management

Hospitals must maintain performance standards. There can be many indices of performance:

1. *Operational Index*: Ability of the emergency department (hospital) to provide quality service. A part of it is patient turnaround rate—the average number of patients seen over an hour period.
2. *Service Index*: Personalized service to the patient. This can be assessed through patient satisfaction rating.
3. *Organisation Development*: This can be assessed by the degree of satisfaction of the staff.
4. *Clinical Quality*: This is based on outcome studies;
   - ability of the emergency department to manage patients well;
   - ability of the department to diagnose and admit accurately;
   - ability of the department to discharge the patient accurately; and
   - average length of stay of the patient.[7]
5. *Emergency Health Services*: Develop Emergency Medicine and Trauma Care Centres to provide comprehensive medical care, including medical, surgical, obstetric, paediatric and trauma care.[8]

We can thus say that there is a need to develop both human and modern technology to improve efficiency. We must, however, give priority to human development. As stated in a UN Report: "There were two aspects to development—technical and human. Organisations had usually been more sensitive to possibilities offered to them by the achievements of modern technology than to the refinements of human behaviour as revealed by the sciences of Sociology and Psychology. On the other hand, lessons drawn from experience showed that technical innovations driving from the engineering sciences encountered considerable resistance unless supported by corresponding changes in human attitudes and behaviour. In an era of rapid change, the improvement of management in its human aspect had become a critical issue. It was important to make full use of the findings of social sciences which endeavoured to be instrumental in giving guidance in behaviour of individuals and groups in varying circumstances. Organisations should, therefore, be conceived as complex, socio-technical systems whose management required both technical skills and insight into the motives of human behaviour.[9]

It is widely agreed that manipulation and lack of integrity produce strong negative side-effects and reduce organisational effectiveness. With this important value commitment the organisation may shift their styles and climate from one of direction, control and surveillance to one of providing help, support and instruction. Mutuality and collaboration between the leaders and the led, self-organisation . . . Left the newcomers strive to set-up organized society with social democracy and high human values settings up ideal societal or public management institutions and if such timely warnings are not accepted, social upsurges are bound to develop in a mild or a violent form[1.0]

Let us have a great ideal, an ideal that will startle us with its greatness. That is the only kind of an ideal to hold before our minds; eye and to work for. Little by little our imperfections and difficulties will vanish and instead of regarding life as a drudgery, instead of shrinking from it, we shall bless this life which offers so many opportunities. We shall find joy even in the little daily tasks and wherever we are placed we shall know happiness.[11]

4. Minimization of Hospital Infection

Because of great rush of patients and lack of cleanliness, there is a danger of hospital infection. Even relatives who go with the patients get hospital infection and come in the grips of one or more diseases.

Hospital acquired infection is a source of danger to the patients and to the staff working in the hospital. All personnel in the hospital must take adequate measures to prevent spread of infection.

All health care workers should be given systematic training programmes regarding the risks and precautionary measures to be taken to prevent infections, which may be transmitted through blood and body fluids.

Minimum standards of cleanliness and tidiness should be instituted.[12]

Hospital Waste needs to be disposed properly

Infectious waste from health care facilities poses a risk to the environment and to the people. Medical waste should be scientifically and hygienically managed from the point of generation to final disposal. Inappropriately managed medical waste can spread fatal disease like Hepatitis B and C and HIV/AIDS.

The Bio-medical waste (management and handling) rules of the government of India has been effected from July 1998 with a view to ensure safe and effective disposal of infectious and hazardous waste. These rules define the role of administrative medical officers of health facilities in waste management. Segregation, treatment and disposal options for different categories of waste have been specified based on location and size of hospitals. While hospitals located in towns and cities with population less than 5 lakhs may have simple disposal options like deep burial for infectious waste, hospitals located in towns with more than 5 lakh population will require to use other options.[13]

5. Corruption Prevalent at all Levels in Hospital: Need of Curbing Corruption

The prevalence of corruption in the health services is a serious issue. Corruption in any official agency is deplorable and must be eliminated. However, its presence in an essential social sector such as health is particularly obnoxious because it increases the costs of the services the public is entitled to and quite often determines both availability and quality of the services provided. It is pernicious and pervasive and operates at different levels in different manner. It could range from: (a) demanding payment for services which are free or even paid for and for carrying out the legitimate duties of the personnel involved; (b) direct diversion of supplies meant for patients or from hospital supplies; (c) carrying on private practice when this is prohibited; (d) deliberately treating patients outside stipulated hours and charging personal fees for such services; and (e) diverting patients to private clinics with which one is associated and charging fees or obtaining commissions. In particular, corruption in government hospitals has a serious effect on the availability of medical services to the poor.[14] It needs to be curbed to ensure efficient care.

Corruption has become constitutionalized and is ruining the very basis of the polity built with abounding faith and sincerity by Gandhi and Nehru. The average citizen finds himself helpless and is swept along with the tide. An atmosphere is which countless public servants even at senior levels, think that they must not miss any opportunity to make money because everyone else does, is a sorry reflection on those who rule the country. Corruption is now one of the major threats to Indian democracy and it in rapidly eroding the social structure. J. Dobel has rightly said in this connection that, "Once corruption becomes widespread, there is very little possibility of successful, significant reform of injustice in the State (and) even a successful violent revolution becomes almost an impossibility. Any significant legal, political or even economic change will be quite irrelevant since the citizens will either frustrate the goals or use the new arrangements for their own radically self-interests benefit. Without the consensual loyalty and trust of the citizenry, the new reforms will simply be shams to rationalize the continuation of corrupt practices."

Good Governance cannot function unless and until the Government itself is firmly committed to the task of the weeding out dishonest and corrupt officials, irrespective of rank and status. All government employees, irrespective of rank, whose integrity and honesty are even slightly in doubt, should be dealt with severely. Punishment for corruption should be exemplary, the least being dismissal from service. The Government should also ensure that anti-corruption agencies are manned by personnel whose integrity and spirit of dedication can never be questioned.[15]

The real remedy for the evil of corruption practices lies in creating a clean and healthy atmosphere in which every person holding a prominent position in the political, social, religious and even educational spheres shall follow a certain standard of conduct, a life of austerity and simplicity, and imbibe the good values of our country.[16]

A corruption-free environment is bound to improve the quality of governance. Checking or controlling corruption is an effective means of better governance. The rights, guaranteed under the Constitution, lose all their relevance especially, if a citizen cannot have good governance. Corruption gives a slant to the working and favours those, who become a party to talk of good governance and ensuring the enjoyment of fundamental human rights can be relevant if the citizens can be ensured corruption-free service.

Prime Minister Manmohan Singh on the concluding day of the 16th biennial conference on anti-corruption organized by the CBI called for a comprehensive strategy to reduce the scope for corruption and an integrated approach to deal with it. "The anti-corruption machinery in the country should create deterrence against by aggressively pursuing cases of high-level corruption to their logical end. Rapid, fair and accurate investigation of allegations of corruption against public servants at all levels should remain a priority." "We must recognize the need for an integrated approach to deal with corruption. Agencies like your's cannot operate in isolation. You must have the resources to take a broader view of individual cases and be able to make a distinction between a 'bonafide mistake'. Not only must the guilty be brought to book more speedily, but the innocent must be spared the trauma of delayed justice.

There are large number of cases against eminent doctors in the courts relating to corrupt practices.

6. Need of Homogenous Structure at State and District Levels

There should be integration of preventive and curative at district level as at state level.

7. Transfer Policy

Continuing the proposal for two main cadres namely Public Health and Medical at the District level, it is proposed to have a similar structure at the Directorate. Thus, the key preventive, promotive and curative functions of the Directorate of Health and divided among two directors, i.e. Director—Medical (for curative and clinical services) and Director—Public Health (Preventive and promotive services). This will ensure equal commitment from the Directorate to the District for both Public Health as well as Medical. Further, it will provide focused supervision in each of the areas. It will also address the promotional opportunity to each cadre to be their respective Directors.[17]

8. Good Governance Need be Assured through Hard Work rather than mere Paper Planning by the Health Executive

Words, written or spoken, are of no use unless put into action. The emphasis should be more on performance rather than paper planning. Khalil Girban has rightly said that "Believing is a fine thing, but placing those beliefs into execution is a test of strength. Many are those who talk like the roar of the sea, but their lives are shallow and stagnant, like the rotting marshes. Many are those who lift their heads above the mountain tops, but their spirit remain dormant to the obscurity of the caverns."[18]

Thus, the future of this budding developing democracy depends upon the attitudes of its political and administrative elite. There is no substitute for hard work, which would be reflected in better life of the people especially in the service sector like health. Nevertheless, without a concerted attempt to make the administration much more action-oriented than at present, these may not yield enough results. Kalibara Ekken, the Japanese sage has nicely put it as: If by study, enquiry or thought, we have learned the truth, we should then put it into practice in both our speech and action. Let what we say be true and what we do discreet. Regulate the emotions, and suppress anger and selfish desires. Shake off evil and cling to good. Discovering our faults, let us not hesitate to correct them. Towards others let us be considerate. All this is the way of true action. . . Without putting what we have learned into practice, it bears no fruit. Good Governance thus requires sincerity and faithful action from medical personnel.

9. Drugs Control

Patients are prescribed costly drugs, which are sold back by doctors to the chemists. There is a collision between doctors and chemists.

The main objectives of Drug control is to ensure that all the drugs that are made available to people who use them for prevention, mitigation, treatment and cure of diseases and disorders, are of standard quality, purity and strength.

The philosophy of drug control is that unless quality control discipline embracing ancillary requirements are imposed by law at all stages of import, manufacture, storage, sale or distribution, people cannot be assured of the quality and safety of medicines used by them. Besides, these medicines are required to be sold at reasonable prices fixed by the Government and also to ensure that unwary public are not mislead by objectionable advertisements in respect of drugs for certain ailments, diseases and disorders.[19]

Medical Profession must work with a sense of dedicated service to gain the confidence of people as well as improve their life.

In any developmental and welfare administration, that is the only right attitude. The administration takes money from the people as taxes; only to restore it back in hundred fold and in thousand fold measure to the people as welfare measures. How is the administration able to perform this miracle? Because the men who handle that money have that yoga-bala, energy of yoga, within them; they have imaginative sympathy; they have efficiency; they have dedication; they are always conscious that they are basically citizens of free India, who are called upon to perform a tremendous national function and mission. That attitude achieves a revolutionary miracle within them; they become dynamic persons instead of remaining static individuals. In such an environment, good governance can flourish.

10. Need of Protecting the Interest of the People

Good Governance in health administration can help in accelerating health promotion of the people provided it is run in the interest of the people. The contents of Good Health Administration for Good Governance are:

- (i) Openness in the sense of having wide contact with the people administered;
- (ii) A sense of justice, fair play and impartiality in dealing with men and matters;
- (iii) Sensitivity and responsiveness to the urges, feelings and aspirations of the common people;
- (iv) Securing the honour and dignity of the human being, however humble he or she might be;
- (v) Humility and simplicity in the persons manning the administrative machinery and their easy accessibility;
- (vi) Creating and sustaining an atmosphere conductive to development, growth and social change; and
- (vii) Honesty and integrity in thought and action.

11. Quality, Equity, Norms and Access to Medical Services

Quality, equity, norms and access can be improved by:

(i) Improving the referral system;
(ii) Improving the quality health and delivery system;
(iii) Upgrading and expanding physical capacity;
(iv) Service norms for health institutions.
(v) Staff norms for health institutions.
(vi) Upgrading clinical effectiveness and quality of services at Community; Block and District hospitals.
(vii) In respect of scheduled caste and scheduled tribes access can be improved through a system of annual health check-ups.
(viii) Granting autonomy to hospitals/health institutions.
(ix) Quality assurance and redressal mechanism such as Consumer Protection Act and citizens charter for hospitals are to be set-up.
(x) Patients below poverty line who cannot afford high cost treatment for serious ailments such as oncologic and cardiac disorders can be assisted through a specially constituted society for providing medical care.

12. Need of Promoting Value-based Governance in Health Organisations

The health organisations of tomorrow will crave for self-ordered self-controlled, self-disciplined and self-motivated employees to survive amidst a dynamic, competitive and changing global economic environment. Employees with commensurate human values to that of organisational values can meet such exacting demands. Such value system can create and sustain perennial satisfaction level and can develop human resources. We have to transform our personality and that of our health organisation by improving following value systems in our health organisations.

- Gaining knowledge
- Hard work
- Spirit of service
- High goals of integrity
- Sense of responsibility
- Positive attitude towards work.

A personal visit a number of times to District Hospitals in Punjab and discussions with experts reveals the following:

1. Patients and their relatives are not received properly staff at all levels is non-operative. A person who is not already well becomes worse seeing all this work procedures.
2. The patients have to wait long for their turn. They are not aware when their turn would come. It only takes 2-4 hours.
3. Doctors are not serous and their dealing with the patients is not sympathetic.
4. There is no proper arrangement of their sitting and lavatory facilities;

5. Most of the basic diagnostic Equipment is mostly out of order inspite of the fact that these hospitals were equipped with latest equipments with the help of Punjab at Health System Corporation.
6. There is lack of co-ordination among doctors' laboratory technicians and diagnostic personnel. Patients have to on the move to collect the reports.
7. Patients are advised to visit home and get better treatment as per payment. Dental department is notorious in this regard.
8. There is pilferage of drugs.
9. The knowledge of the doctors is out dated.

13. Use of Information Technology in Decision-making

In these high tech times, marked by a revolution in informatics and electronics, an effective administrator has to be a 'knowledge worker' in the service sector, which is 'knowledge' or 'information industry'. In such an industry, we receive information, process information and produce information as an output of decision-making. The time has come where there is hardly any scope of 'arbitrary' and 'ego-based' decision-making. The behaviour of subordinates will be controlled not perhaps through the code of conduct rules but through better knowledge and information on the part of the boss. Hence, the information skill of the decision-maker in getting information, in storing information and using information is going to be the crux and future decision scenario.[20]

T.K. Ramachandran in his Article, "Information and Systems Management in Government" in the *Administrator*, October-December 1997 rightly suggests the role of information system in decision-making. He says that millions of man-hours and rupees are lost because the right information is not available to the right person at the right time. Decisions are therefore, based on half-baked information and is perhaps out of date; inaccurate or misleading. . . During a drought a few hundred bore wells were to be dug and a proposal to purchase some drilling rigs was put up for urgent clearance. When he asked as to how many bore wells were in existence, nobody seemed to know. Then he wanted to know how many rigs were already available and their locations. Again nobody knew however the purchase had to be made and there was no alternative but to go ahead with the order. Here was a case of decisions having to be taken without necessary and sufficient information being available with all the concomitant implications in terms of higher cost and inefficiency of resources use that the nation can ill-afford.

CONCLUSION

"Any society should consider that a high quality life and happiness of the people which can only be obtained through a sufficient level of health is not a basic pre-requisite of development but should be the basic objective of any developmental effort." Development of health ultimately leads to National Development. Health, both as an input and output, is directly linked with development.

Inspite of the realization that all the people are not getting health care due to poor administration of health care delivery system, it has been the focus of the State Government and the people of Punjab.

Health is such a vast subject covering so many areas. Many new issues are emerging. Now we have telemedicine coming in, computerization which is changing the entire way of looking at things including medicine, we also have the other very critical issues on social side of delivery of health systems to poor, to the below poverty line (BPL) people. While there is some sensitivity in the system of delivery to below poverty line persons. We really have not been able to crystallize a mechanism for the same. Even the government delivery system really do not provide good services despite the fact that it is a system which is supposed to reach out for the poor.

Empowerment of patients will lead to medical uprising of the society by creating a class educated and aware, informed and health conscious, striving to improve their quality of life with justified use of their rights. They can curb exploitation in the name of medicine and ensure a decline in quackery.

The empowered can be easily motivated and channelized to enlist support for health programmes and achievement of health goals. Thus health programmes will be a truly people's programme since indifference will cease to exist in health matters. Voluntary participation in health activities will increase.[21]

Dr. Poste and Dr. Everett in their article, "Healthy, wealthy and informed" in *Business Standard* (January 9, 2000) feel that, in new millennium treatment procedures will become more standardized. Equipped with more sophisticated diagnostic information, data about a patient's genetic make up, and access to online guidelines of best clinical practice, the doctor of 2020 will have less excuse to veer from standard procedure. If in doubt, says Dr. Poste, "physician-decision support software" will tell him what to do.[22]

By 2020, people will probably store their personal health records on electronic swipe cards or subcutaneous chips, obviating the need to perform the same tests over and over again.

Monitoring will also become electronic. For example, a patient with hypertension could be fitted with a chip to measure blood pressure. If the reading moves outside a determined level, an alarm would sound—a more effective early-warning system than a fainting spell or a heart attack.

But as we rush towards this future of technologically enhanced health care, one very old question will remain: who is going to pay for it all?

It seems certain that the health gap between the developing world and industrialized nations will widen in the century to come, after vaccines and antibiotics did so much to narrow the disparity in the century just elapsed. Even in the west, patients are unlikely to have equal access to new technologies.

Perhaps a day will come when it will indeed be considered a right to live to 120 with constantly rejuvenated organs, muscles, bone and brain. But for as long as these techniques are new and expensive, many of them will remain a privilege of the rich.[23]

District Hospitals need improvement to serve as a referral system in all aspects mentioned done.

Notes and References

1. WHO, Technical Report Series, 1968, 195, p. 6.
2. Final Report of The Task Force on Health and Family Welfare, Government of Karnataka, April 2007, pp. 31-32.
3. *Ibid.*, p. 32.
4. UN: 'Inter-regional Seminar on Administration of Management Improvement Services', Vol. 1, Copenhagen, Denmark, October 1970, p. 24.
5. UN: "United Nations Programme in the Public Administration" (E/4296-ST/TAO/M/38), pp. 11-12.
6. U.C. Agarwal, Good Governance cutting Edge of Administration, in *IJPA*, July-September, 1998, p. 436.
7. *Ibid.*, p. 33.
8. *Ibid.*, pp. 35-36.
9. *Ibid.*, p. 447.
10 UN: Inter-Regional Seminar on Administration of Management Improvement Services, (Vol. I), Copenhagen, Denmark, 28 September-6 October 1970, 1971, pp. 6-7 (ST/TAO/M/56).
11. M.L. Mishra: Contemporary Management Thinkers, Associated Publishing House, New Delhi, 1980, pp. 120-29.
12. Swami Parmananda, Secret of Right Activity, Madras, Ramakrishna Math, Year Not mentioned.
13. *Ibid.*, p. 51.
14. *Ibid.*, p. 62.
15. *Ibid.*, p. 278.
16. A. Rai and S.P. Singh, Current Ideas and Issues in Indian Administration, New Delhi, Uppal, 1979, p. 209.
17. C.N. Bhalerao (Ed), Administration, Politics and Development in India, *op. cit.*, pp. 227-28.
18. Final Report of The Task Force on Health and Family Welfare, Government of Karnataka, April 2007, p. 292.
19. Khali Gibran, Between Night and Morn, The Philosophical Library, New York, 1972, pp. 8-9.
20. Final Report of The Task Force on Health and Family Welfare, Government of Karnataka, April 2007, p. 353.
21. N.K. Kulshrestha, "Management in Public Administration, the Decision Anatomy X-rayed," in *IJPA*, January-March, 1994, p. 45.
22. Dr. Poste and Dr. Everett, Healthy, Wealthy and Informed, *Business Standard*, New Delhi, January 9, 2000.
23. Vijay Thawani and Kunda Gharpure, Improving Patient in Regional Health Forum, WHO, South-East Asia, New Delhi, Vol. 2, No. 1, 1997, pp. 1851-53.

ANNEXURE 5.1

Percent of Health Care Establishments having Specific Infrastructure Facilities in India, Facility Survey: 2003

Sl. No.	*Infrastructure Facility*	*District Hospitals*	*FRU*	*CHC*
1.	Own Building	97.0	94.7	91.0
2.	Maintenance at least once in three years	40.1	39.9	37.7
3.	Sources of Water—Water Pipe	58.7	49.1	43.9
4.	Water-well (including tube well) water-Pipe	41.2	50.9	56.1
5.	Over head tank	90.5	80.8	70.0
6.	Electricity in all part of the hospital	96.7	91.3	91.8
7.	Operation Theatre	99.5	93.7	87.6
8.	Separate asceptic labour room	44.4	33.3	31.0
9.	Generator functional	91.7	86.9	84.3
10.	Telephone Facility	96.7	74.8	62.2
11.	Vehicles on Road	89.9	56.8	57.4
12.	OPD Facility for RTI/STI	56.4	24.9	16.0
13.	Gynaecology/Obstetric OPD facility	73.7	50.8	36.0
14.	Nameplates to guice clients to Gynaec OPD	83.8	76.8	67.5
15.	Privacy during examination	92.6	89.3	85.8
16.	Facility for counselling	76.7	03.1	03.9
17.	Separate toilet with running water	67.3	62.6	55.0
18.	Facility for sterilizing instruments	87.5	82.9	80.0
19.	Linkage with district blood bank	67.5	27.2	15.8
20.	Regular blooc supply	60.5	27.7	10.5
21.	Quarters for obstetrician/gyaecologist	40.1	28.5	21.0
22.	Quarters for RMD (Residential Medical Officer)	47.1	42.2	44.0
23.	Quarters for Nurse	67.5	66.8	71.0
24.	Personal computer	47.7	14.7	2.0
	Total Surveyed	370	1882	1625

Source: Facility Survey, Phase-II, 2003, Ministry of Health and Family Welfare/IIPS, Mumbai.

APPENDIX FIGURE 5.1

Infrastructure Facilities Available in District Hospitals, India

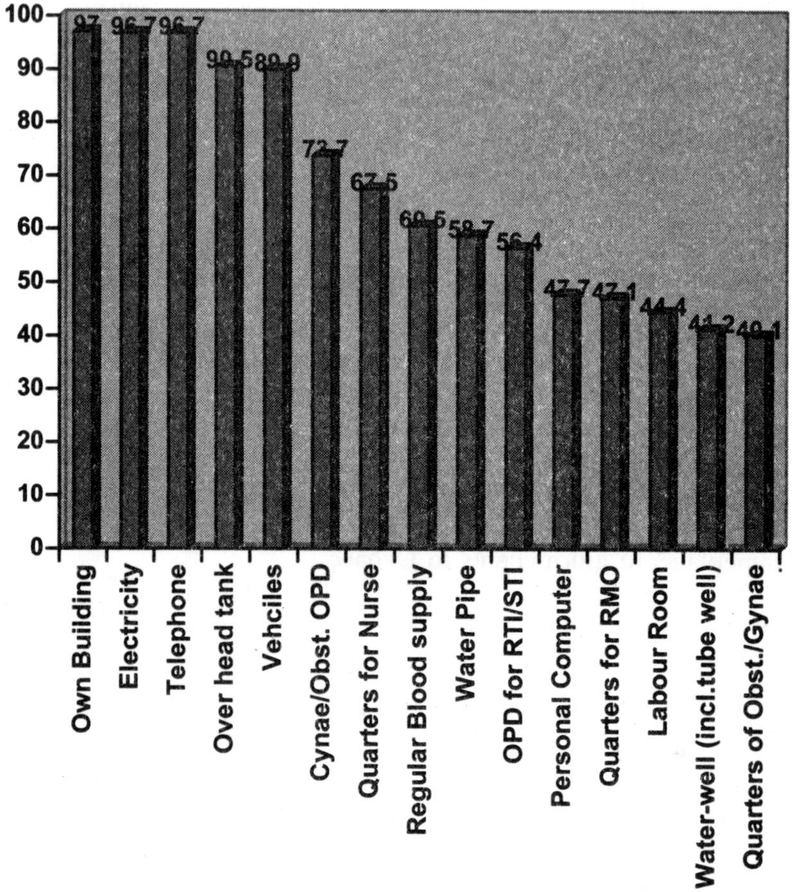

Source: Ministry of Health and Family Welfare, Family Welfare Statistics in India, 2006, p. 86.

APPENDIX FIGURE 5.2

Infrastructure Facilities Available in FRU, India

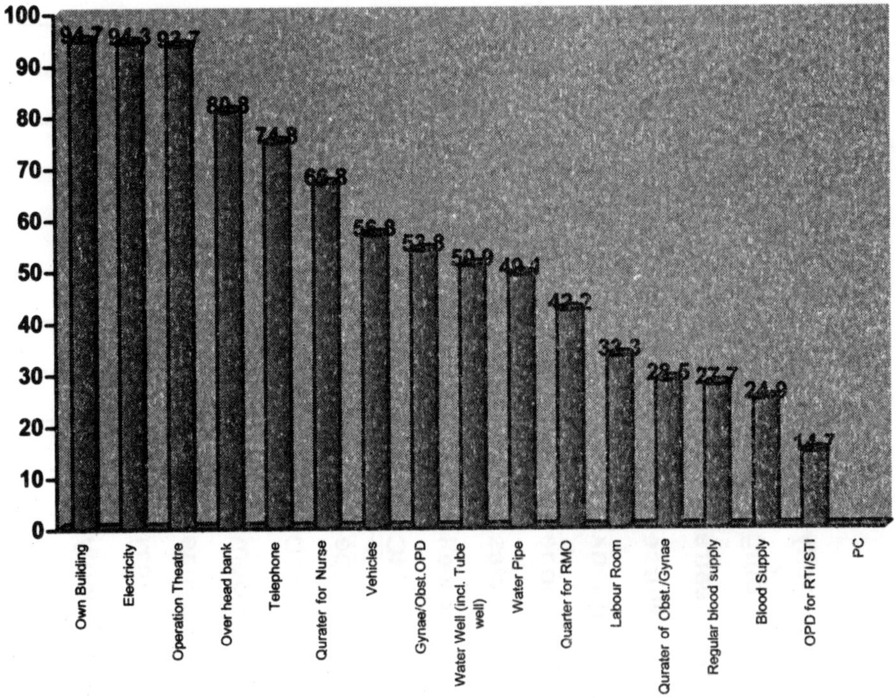

Source: Ministry of Health and Family Welfare, Family Welfare Statistics in India, 2006, p. 86.

APPENDIX FIGURE 5.3

Infrastructure Facilities Available in CHC, India

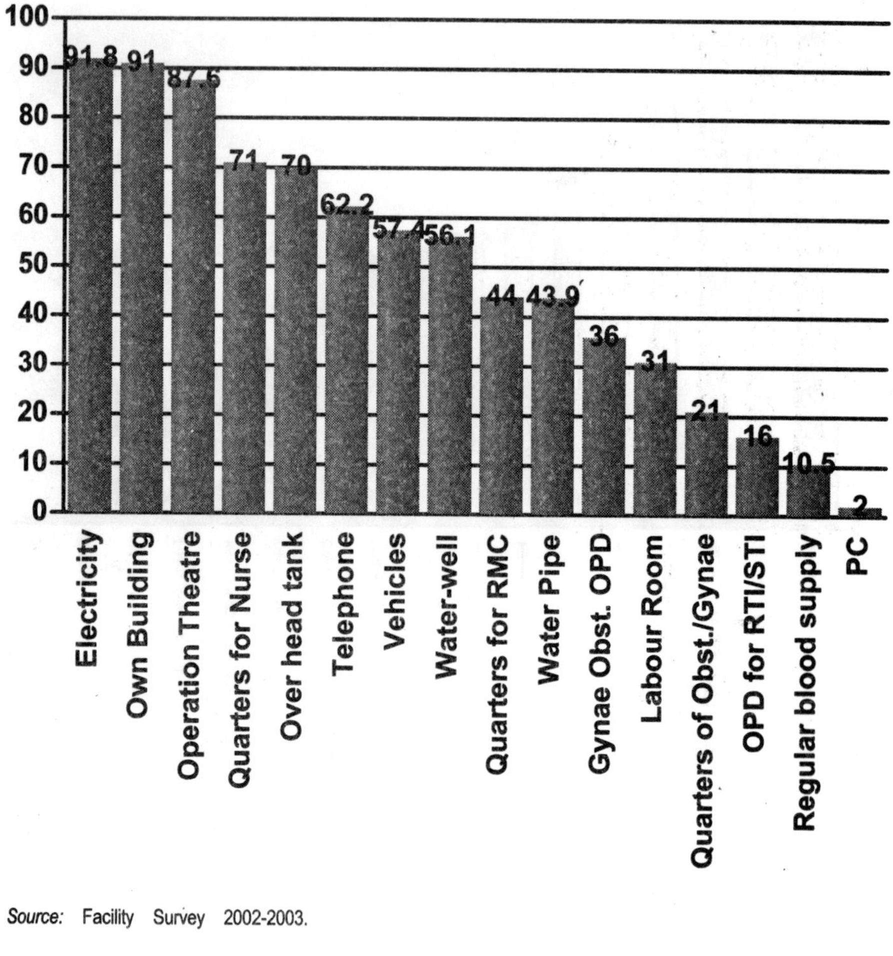

Source: Facility Survey 2002-2003.

APPENDIX FIGURE 5.4

Staff Available in District Hospitals, India

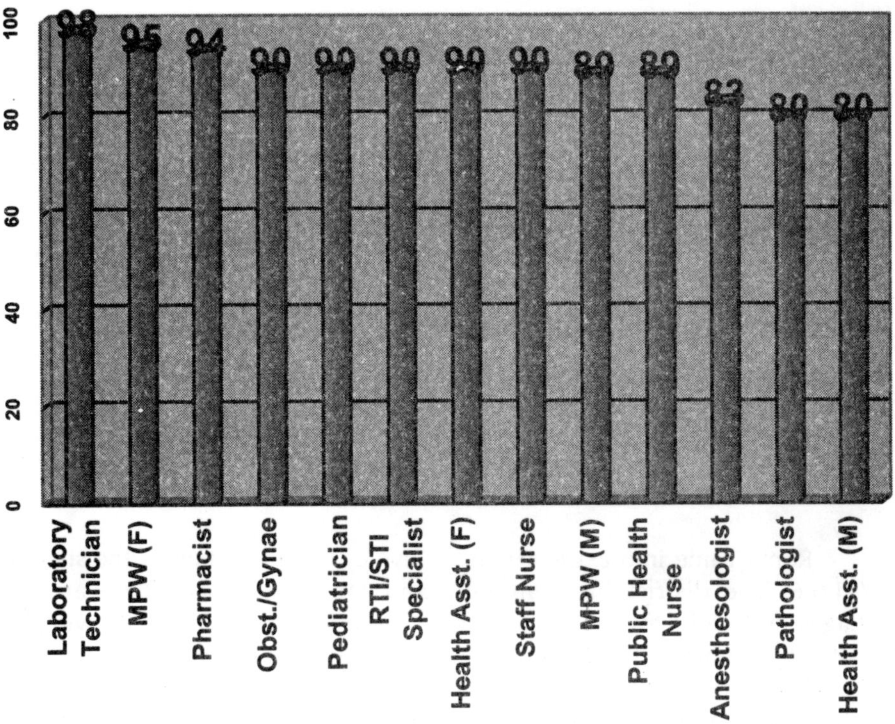

Source: Facility Survey, 2002-03.

6

CHAPTER

Secondary Health Care Administration

A Case Study of Ropar (Rupnagar) District in Punjab

DEMOGRAPHIC PROFILE OF DISTRICT ROPAR

Ropar came into existence on the eve of reorganisation of the state on 1/11/66. The district has semi-hilly and far-flung areas. There are 894 villages and eight towns. According to the information available with the health department, the population of the district is 10, 99,906.

It is spread over an area of 2117 sq. miles. Ropar is placed adjoining to the state capital, i.e. Chandigarh which is on its east. On its west is district of Nawanshahar and on its north are situated Una and Bilaspur district's of Himachal Pradesh while on south is bounded by districts Patiala and Fatehgarh Sahib.

The density of the population on the average is 509 per sq. mile, which is comparatively less than that of the state of Punjab. Agriculture is the most important activity of the people of the district.

Demographic Indicators	*Ropar*	*Punjab*	*India*
Population	11,10,000	2,42,89,296	1,02,70,15,247
Rural	68%	66%	72%
Urban	32%	34%	28%
Birth Rate	19.6	21.5	23.8 (2005)
Death Rate	6.19	7.4	7.6 (2005)
Literacy Rate	100%		64.80
Sex Ratio	870/1000	886	933
IMR	23.5		58 (2005)

MAP I

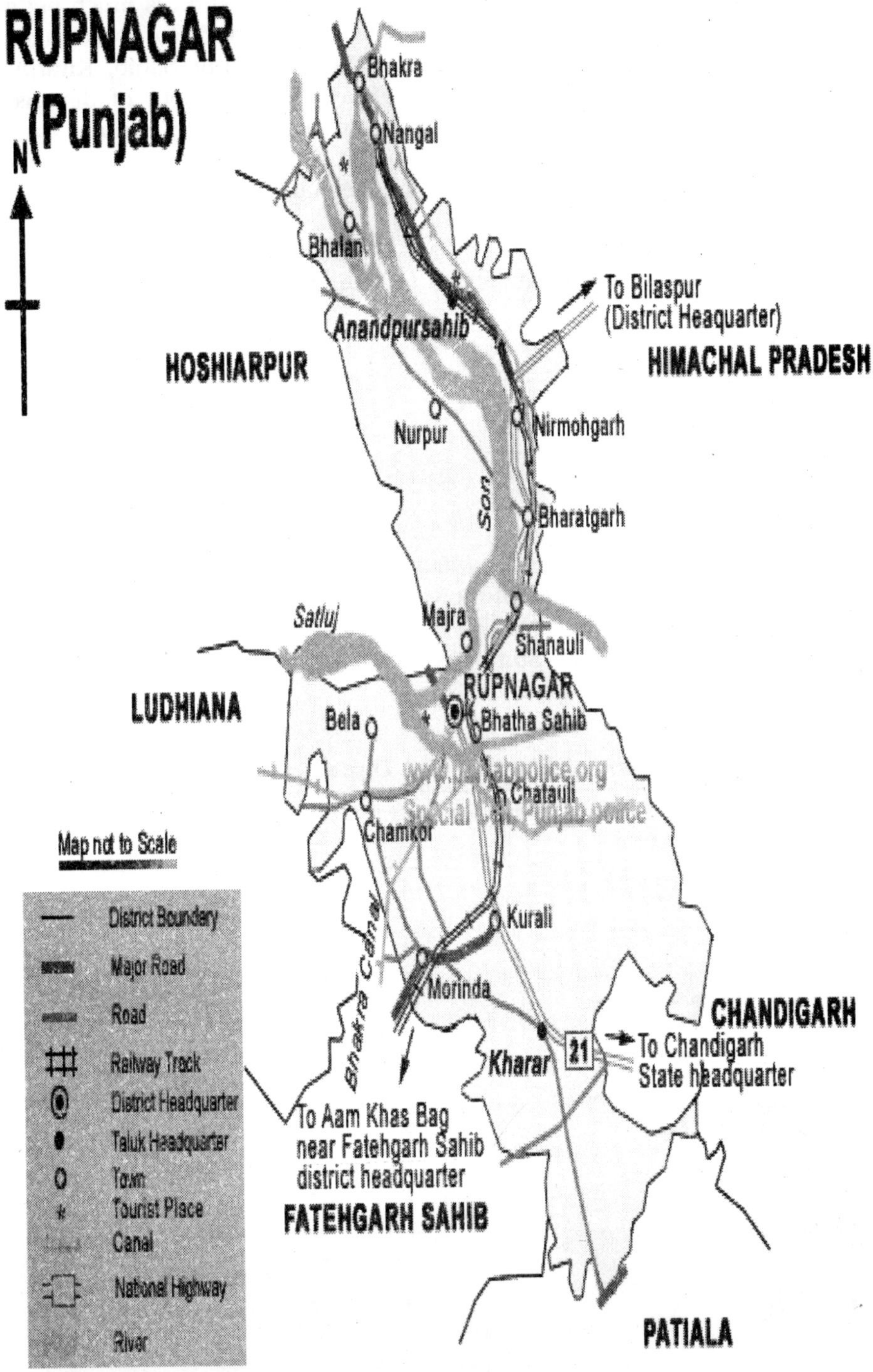
RUPNAGAR
(Punjab)
N
Bhakra
Nangal
Bhalan
Anandpursahib
To Bilaspur
(District Heaquarter)
HOSHIARPUR
HIMACHAL PRADESH
Nurpur
Nirmohgarh
Son
Bharatgarh
Satluj
Majra
Shanauli
RUPNAGAR
LUDHIANA
Bela
Bhatha Sahib
www.punjabpolice.org
Chatauli
Special Cell, Punjab police
Chamkor
Map not to Scale
District Boundary
Major Road
Road
Railway Track
District Headquarter
Taluk Headquarter
Town
Tourist Place
Canal
National Highway
River
Bhakra Canal
Kurali
Morinda
CHANDIGARH
21
Kharar
To Chandigarh
State headquarter
To Aam Khas Bag
near Fatehgarh Sahib
district headquarter
FATEHGARH SAHIB
PATIALA

One of the major rivers of the state Satluj flows through the upper part of the district and lower down it forms its west boundary. Area being sub-mountainous is quite flood prone, though the situation is much better than earlier times because of Bhakhra Dam, Nangal and Ropar barrages.

A number of religious places exp. Sri Anandpur Sahib, Kiratpur Sahib, Naina Devi and a no. of deras attract large number of devotees sometimes running in tens of thousands and brings along various water borne communicable diseases and so also for accidents especially because of fast moving traffic on the highway to the state capital.

Health Infrastructure

District Ropar comprises of the following 6 Blocks:

- Ropar
- Chamkaur Sahib
- Anandpur Sahib
- Nurpur Bedi
- Kharar
- Majri

Each block consists of hospitals, health centres and dispensaries. There are about 244 health institutions in District Ropar. The management of a few health institutions is with PHSC, some fall under DHS and others in the voluntary sector. Summary statement of the hospitals and dispensaries in district Ropar.

Summary Statement of Hospital and Dispensaries in District Ropar

Block	*Ropar*	*Chamkaur Sahib*	*Anandpur Sahib*	*Nurpur Bedi*	*Kharar*	*Majri*	*Total*
Punjab Health Systems Corporation							
District Hospital	1	—	—	—	—	—	**1**
Sub-Div. Hospital	—	—	1	—	1	—	**2**
Area Hospital	—	—	—	—	1	—	**1**
Community Health Centre	—	1	—	1	—	1	**3**
Director Health Services							
Rural Hospital	1	1	1	—	—	—	**3**
Primary Health Care	3	—	—	3	—	1	**7**
Subsidiary Health Care	8	7	7	9	18	15	**64**
Urban Slum Area							
Dispensary	2	—	7	—	2	—	**11**
Civil Dispensary	—	—	—	—	3	—	**3**
Police Line Dispensary	1	—	—	—	—	—	**1**
T.B. Centres	1	—	—	—	—	—	**1**
Sub-Centres	25	17	24	17	25	19	**127**

Hospital and Dispensaries under Director (SI)							
ESI Hospital	—	—	—	—	1	—	1
ESI Dispensary	3	—	—	—	3	—	6
BBMB Hospital	—	—	1	—	—	—	1
Hospitals and Dispensaries under other Management							
BBMB TB Hospital	—	—	1	—	—	—	1
BBMB Dispensary	—	—	3	—	—	—	3
First Aid Posts	—	—	1	—	—	—	1

Source: Punjab Health System Corporation.

District Hospital Ropar

Civil Hospital, Ropar, a 100 bedded district hospital was ranked vary poorly, with hardly any clinical work worth the name, five years ago. On the other hand it is today ranked the best district level hospital in the state of Punjab. This has been possible only with the inputs project. The hospital can boast of having successfully implemented all the health systems, for which it came into existence. The hospital is now well equipped to deal with most of patient's problems as a secondary level hospital. Excepting CT scan almost all tests are being conducted as per norms for a secondary level hospital. Computerization, a Pilot project for district level hospitals, having been successfully implemented, has helped in proper up keep of hospital data apart from centralized collection of user charges. The user charges collected in a month these days may be more than those collected in a year say five years ago. New OT-*cum*-PP Unit block has come up in a place adjoining to the west of B block, linking it with all the floors. It is also linked through a new corridor to old PP Unit and also to Trauma Unit. New Canteen has been built with a wide range of facilities for the patients.

Manpower Position

Sr. No.	*Name of Post*	*Norms Post*	*Sanctioned*	*Available*
Specialist Post				
1.	General Medicine	1	1	1
2.	General Surgery	1	1	1
3.	Obstetrics and Gynaecology	—	—	—
4.	Psychiatry	—	—	—
5.	Paediatric	1	1	1
6.	Pathology/Bio-Chemistry/Microbiology	1	1	
7.	Tuberculosis	—	—	—
8.	Anaesthetics	1	1	1
9.	Radiology	1	1	1
10.	Skin and V.D.	—	—	—
11.	Blood Transfusion Officer	1	1	1
12.	Orthopaedics	—	-	—
13.	Ophthalmology	1	1	1

14.	Incharge CMO/SMO	1	1	1
15.	MO	7	7	7
16.	Casualty Mo	4	4	4
17.	Dental Surgeon	1	1	1
18.	Social Scientist	—	—	—
19.	House Surgeon	5	5	5
Para-Medical Staff				
1.	Matron	1	1	—
2.	Asst. Matron	—	—	—
3.	Statistical Assistant	1	1	—
4.	Computer	1	1	1
5.	Sr. Lab. Technician	1	1	1
6.	Stenographer	—	—	—
7.	FPFW	—	—	—
8.	Nursing Sister	3	3	3
9.	LHV	—	—	—
10.	ANM	—	—	—
11.	O.T. Attendant	—	—	—
12.	Pharmacist	5	5	2
13.	Lab. Tech. Grade I and II	5	5	5
14.	Steno Typist	—	—	—
15.	Lab. Attendant	2	2	2
16.	Radiographer	1	1	—
17.	Physiotherapist	—	—	—
18.	Operation Room Attendant	2	2	2
19.	Cashier	1	1	1
20.	Head Clerk	—	—	—
21.	Dental Mechanic/Elect.	1	1	1
22.	Dietician	—	—	—
23.	AAO/Accountant	1	1	1
24.	Clerk	7	7	7
25.	Typist-*cum*-Clerk	—	—	—
26.	Head Cook	—	—	—
27.	Electrician	1	1	1
28.	Carpenter	1	1	1
29.	Plumber	—	—	—
30.	Driver	1	1	1
31.	Cook	—	—	—
32.	Helpers to Cook	—	—	—
33.	Caretaker	—	—	—
34.	Dhobi	—	—	—
35.	Class-IV	48	48	48
36.	Mali	1	1	Nil
37.	Chowkidar	3	3	3
38.	Storekeeper/Sweeper	11	11	2
39.	Superintendent	1	1	1
40.	Dental Hygienist	1	1	—
41.	Dark Room Asstt.	1	1	1

Note: Nine Posts of Sweepers adjusted in the District Hospitals/Dispensaries for temporary basis.

Equipment Status

Equipment	Norms	Quantity				*Remarks
		On Hand	Usable	Needs Repair	Not Usable	
I. Imaging Equipment						
1. 500mA X-Ray	1	-	-	-	-	Awaited
2. 300mA X-Ray	0	2	1	1	-	Funds not available
3. 100mA X-Ray	1	1	-	1	-	-do-
4. 60mA X-Ray (mobile)	1	1	1	-	-	
5. Dental X-Ray	1	1	1	-	-	
6. Ultra Sound Scanner (Linear)	1	1	-	1	-	Company discontinue
7. Ultra Sound Scanner (Linear Sector) with upgradability	0				-	
8. Ultra Sound Scanner (Linear Sector) with upgradability	1	-	-	-	-	
II. Electro Medical Equipment						
1. E.C.G.	3	2	-	2	-	
2. Cardiac Monitors	2	4	-	4	-	
3. Defibrilators	2	3	3	-	-	
4. Audiometers	1	-	-	-	-	
5. Baby Incubators	4	2	-	2	-	
6. Phototherapy Unit	2	1	1	-	-	
7. Endoscipe Fibre Optic	1	-	-	-	-	
8. Operating Microscopes	2	1	-	1	-	
9. Cyro Surgery (Deluxe)	1	-	-	-	-	
10. Foetal Monitor	3	2	-	2	-	
11. Short wave Diathermy	1	2	-	2	-	
12. Ventilators	2	2	-	2	-	
13. Boyles Apparatus with circle absorber	2	5	1	4		
14. Boyles, Apparatus without flout	2	1	-	1	-	
15. Opthaamoscope	3	2	2	-	-	
16. Slit Lamp	1	1	2	-	-	
17. Retino Scope	1	1	1	-	-	
18. Perimeter	0	1	1	-	-	
19. Emergency Resuscitation Kit	3	-	-	-	-	
20. Sigmoid Scope	1	-	-	-	-	
21. Head Light	1	3	2	1	-	
22. Plus Air Tonometer	1	1	1		-	
23. AMC Equipment (2 Monitor, 1 Ventilator, 1 Defibrillator, A/c	1	-	-	-	-	
24. Holter Monitor	1	-	-	-	-	
25. Endoscope with Lapro catorand and Accessories	1	-	-	-	-	
26. Radiant Heater (4KW)	1	1	1	-	-	
27. Cryo surgery (Basic)	1	-	-	-	-	
28. Pulse Oxymeter	1	-	-	-	-	
29. Blood Gas Analyzer	1	-	-	-	-	

III. Pneumatic, Hydraulic and Sterilization Equipment				
1. Dental Unit	1			
2. Dental Chair	1	3	2	1
3. Air rotor	1	1	1	-
4. Ultrasonic Scalar	1	-	-	-
5. Operation Table	3	4	4	-
6. Operation Table (Hydraulic)	3	2	2	-
7. Autoclave HP (Horizontal)	3	-	-	-
8. Autoclave HP (Vertical)	2	2	2	-
9. Autoclave with Burners 2 bin	0			-
10. Shadowless lamp (mobile)	4	3	1	2
11. O.T. Lights (Shadowless)	3	2	1	1
12. Focussing Lights (Mobile)	2	1	1	-
13. Suction Apparatus (High Vacuum MTPL)	4	3	2	1
14. Suction Apparatus (High Vacuum MTPL)	15	10	8	2
15. Foot Suction Apparatus	2	6	5	1
16. Vacuum Extractor	2	1	1	-
17. Instrument Sterilizer	2	20	18	2
18. Diathermy Machine	25	-	-	-
19. Gynaec electric cautery	2	1	1	-
20. Automist	3	-	-	-
21. Dental Lab (Bath, Motor, Lathe)	0	-	-	-
IV. Laboratory Equipment				
1. Microscopes (Binocular)	5	2	2	-
2. Chemical Balances	1	1	1	-
3. Simple Balances	1	1	1	-
4. Photo Electric Calorimeter	2	5	1	4
5. Flame Cell Photometer	1	-	-	-
6. Spector Photometer	1	-	-	-
7. Auto Analyzer		1	-	1
8. Micro Pipettes	1	4	4	-
9. Electrophoresis	-	-	-	-
10. Water Bath	2	2	2	-
11. Hot Air Oven	1	1	1	-
12. Incubators	1	1	1	-
13. Distilled Water	1	-	-	-
14. Centrifuges	3	6	1	5
15. Centrifuge (Haematocrit)	2	2	-	2
16. Hot Plates	1	2	1	1
17. Rotor/Shaker	1	-	-	-
18. Counting Chamber	3	2	2	-
19. PH meter	1	1	1	-
20. Glucometer	2	4	-	4
21. Hemoglobin Meter	3	8	6	2
22. Microtom	1	-	-	-
23. Oven (Wax embedding)	1	-	-	-
24. Tissue Processor	1	-	-	-
25. Timer stop watch	2	1	1	-
26. Alarm clock	2	-	-	-
V. Refrigerator and Air-Conditioning				
1. Refrigerator 165 Ltrs.	8	12	8	4
2. Refrigerator 300 Ltrs.	2	3	2	1

3.	A/C Machine with Stabilizer	8	8	3	5	
4.	Water Coolers	3	2	1	1	
5.	Two body Mortuary (Cold Storage)	3	-	-	-	
VI.	**Hospital Plants**					
1.	Generator 5 KVA	0			-	
2.	Generator 15 KVA	0	2	2	-	
3.	Generator 50 KVA	0	-	-	-	
4.	Generator 62.5 KVA	1	1	1	-	
5.	Hot water system (solar unit)	3	1	1	-	
6.	Incinerator 3 KW	-			-	
7.	Incinerator 5 KW	-			-	
VII.	**Administration**					
1.	Typewriters	4	1	1	-	
2.	Photocopier	1	1	1	-	
3.	Cyclostyling Machine	1	-	-	-	
4.	Intercoms (40 lines)	1	-	-	-	
5.	Intercoms (10 lines)		1	-	1	
6.	Fax Machine	1	-	-	-	
7.	Telephone (external lines)	12	3	3	-	
8.	Library (Facility)	1	-	-	-	
VIII.	**Transport**					
1.	Ambulance	2	2	-		
2.	Pick-up	-	-	-		
IX.	**Surgical Instrument Packs**					
1.	D.D. and C.	3	4	4	-	
2.	M.T.P.	3	4	4	-	
3.	Cervical Biop	4	2	2	-	
4.	Evacuation	3	2	2	-	
5.	Delivery	3	4	4	-	
6.	P.N. Sterilization	6	-	-	-	
7.	Epiosotomy	3	2	2	-	
8.	Venisection	4	4	4	-	
9.	Copper T	4	6	6	-	
10.	Caserean Section	3	8	8	-	
11.	Incision and Drainage	4	4	4	-	
12.	Vaginal Hysterectomy	2	4	4	-	
13.	Abdominal Hysterectomy	2	4	4	-	
14.	Vagotomy	1	2	2	-	
15.	Appedectomy	2	2	2	-	
16.	Hydrocele	2	2	2	-	
17.	Gastro Jejunostomy	2	2	2	-	
18.	Hemorthoidectomy	2	2	2	-	
19.	Suture Removal	4	1	1	-	
20.	Suturing Tray	4	2	2	-	
21.	L.P. Tray	2	10	10	-	
22.	Cholecystectomy	1	2	2	-	
23.	Thyroid	1	1	1	-	
24.	Chaterization Tray	3	2	2	-	
25.	I.M. Nailing	1	-	-	-	
26.	S.P. Nailing	1	-	-	-	
27.	Dynamic Comeression Plating	1	-	-	-	-
28.	A.M. Prosthesis	1	-	-	-	-

29. Dynamic Hip Screw Fixation	5	-	-	-	-
30. Fixation of Radius and Ultra	1	-	-	-	-
31. Cataract operation	2	4	4	-	-
32. Needing and Cataract Evacuation	2	2	2	-	-
33. Tridectomy	2	2	2	-	-
34. Irindenculisis	2	2	2	-	-
35. Extra Capsular Operation	2	4	4	-	-
36. Chalazon	3	4	4	-	-
37. Tarsorraphy	3	2	2	-	-
38. Enucleation	1	2	2	-	-
39. Probing of Lachrymal Passage	2	2	2	-	-
40. D.C.R.	1	1	1	-	-
41. Lachrymal Sac Extension	1	1	1	-	-
42. Trabeculectomy	1	1	1	-	-
43. Pterygium Excision	1	1	1	-	-
44. Entropion Correction	1	1	1	-	-
45. Foreign Body Corenea	2		1	-	-
46. Foreign Body in AC	2	1	1	-	-
47. Conjectval Cyst Excision	2	2	2	-	-
48. Ear Examination	2	2	2	-	-
49. Mastectomy	2	1	1	-	-
50. Macro ear set Myringo, Tympano, Stepedo Plasty	1	-	-	-	-
51. Nasal set SMR Stetoplasty	1	1	1	-	-
52. D.N.S.	1	1	1	-	-
53. Rhinoplasty	1	1	1	-	-
54. Adeno Tonsillectomy	2	1	1	-	-
55. Tracheostomy	3	2	2	-	-
56. Endo Laryngea Micro Surgery	1	-	-	-	-
57. ENT. General	1	1		-	-
58. Anesthesia Kit	1	-	1	-	-
59. General Orthopaedic Kit	1	1		-	-
60. Dental Kit	1	1		-	-
X. Minor Equipment					
1. X-Ray Viewing Box	10	20	2	18	-
2. Developing tanks (X-ray)	3	2	2	-	-
3. Safe Light X-ray Dark Room	3	1	1	-	-
4. Cassettes X-ray	32	10	6	4	-
5. Intensifying Screen (various)	32	15	3	12	-
6. Lead aprons	4	1	1	-	-
7. Lead Protection Screen	2	1	1	-	-
8. Chest Stands X-ray	2	1	1	-	-
9. B.P. Apparatus	24	48	6	42	-
10. Weighing machine Adult	1	10	8	2	-
11. Weighing machine Infant	4	4	4	-	-
12. Infra-red Lamps	6	2	2	-	-
13. Oxygen cylinders	40	33	18	15	-
14. Nitrogen cylinders	20	12	12	-	-
15. Regular Flowmeter for medical Gas	16	12	8	4	-
16. Ambu Bags	16	12	4	8	-
17. Angle Poise Lamp	4	2	1	1	-
18. Hot plate Domestic	6	4	2	2	-
19. Emergency Lamp	16	32	-	32	-
20. Sewing Machine	2	1	1	-	-
21. Fire Extinguishers	6	-	-	-	-

22.	Laryngoscope	4	6	6	-	-
23.	Otoscope	2	2	2	-	-
24.	Universal Bone Drill	2	1	1	-	-
XI.	**Furniture and other Equipment**					
1.	Examination Table	30	12	12	-	-
2.	Delivery Table	60	2	2	-	-
3.	Foot Steps	30	6	6	-	-
4.	Bedside Screen	40	12	4	8	-
5.	Revolving Stool	40	20	5	15	-
6.	Arm Board Adult and Child	60	50	15	35	-
7.	Saline Stand	50	12	8	4	-
8.	Wheel Chair	12	5	1	4	-
9.	Emergency recovery Trolley	4	6	1	5	-
10.	Stretcher on Trolley	12	4	1	3	-
11.	Oxygen Trolley	16	6	1	5	-
12.	Height Measuring stand	4	2	2	-	-
13.	Fowler Bed	4	-	2	-	-
14.	Iron Cot	110	120	80	40	-
15.	Baby Cot	12	24	6	18	-
16.	Beside Locker	110	150	50	100	-
17.	Dressing Trolley	12	6	1	5	-
18.	Mayo's trolley	4	-	-	-	-
19.	Instrument Cabinet	8	3	-	3	-
20.	Instrument trolley	8	4	4	-	-
21.	Linen trolley	8	-	-	-	-
22.	Kick Bucket	16	4	1	3	-
23.	Attendant Stool	100	100	60	40	-
24.	Traction Systems	8	-	-	-	-
25.	Postmortem Table	1	-	-	-	-
26.	Wash Basin	40	40	10	30	-
27.	Instrument Tray	24	10	8	2	-
28.	Chairs	50	100	50	50	-
29.	Wooden Tables	40	4	-	4	-
30.	Steel Cabinet	36	30	28	2	-
31.	Swab Rack	4	16	16	-	-
32.	Table (Fracture)	2	2	2	-	-
33.	Blood Donor Table Wooden	4	2	2	-	-
34.	Matteress	110	250	250	-	-
35.	Pillows	110	50	50	-	-
36.	Wooden Benches	100	-	-	-	-
37.	Cheatle Forceps Jar	20	10	10	-	-
38.	Patella Hammer	8	6	6	-	-
39.	Tongue Depressor	20	10	10	-	-
40.	Oxygen Mask	8	500	500	-	-
41.	Torch light	12	10	2	8	-
42.	Medicine Cabinet	10	2	2	-	-
43.	Side Rals	10	24	24	-	-
44.	Bucket Galvanised	20	-	-	-	-
45.	Beds Pans and Urinals	20	60	60	-	-
46.	Bowls	100	15	15	-	-
47.	Kidney Tray	40	6	6	-	-
48.	Racks	48	3	3	-	-
49.	Patient's Attendant Cots	50	-	-	-	-
50.	Wooden Tables	50	-	-	-	-
51.	Wooden Chairs	50	6	-	6	-

Source: Ibid.

Hospital Layout

Civil Hospital Ropar is a 100 bedded hospital. It is located in the heart of city. The present complex was built in 1972. Apart from the hospital in form of various blocks, the complex also houses the office of the Civil Surgeon and the District T.B. Centre. The residential area of the hospital has old block for D category Staff and new blocks for A, B, C, category Staff. It consists of various distinct units, i.e.

A Block

Ground Floor:

Various OPD's
Computerized Registration Room,
Physio-therapy Unit
ECG room and
School Health Clinic

First Floor:

Medical and Eye and ENT Ward,
Medical Store and CSSD

Second Floor:

Audiometer Room
Private Wards
General Store and
Electrical workshop

B-Block

Ground Floor:

Offices of Deputy Medical Commissioner/Ropar and
Senior Medical Officer I/C
X-Ray Department
Clinical Laboratory and
Medical Record Room

First Floor:

Gynae
Antenatal
Postnatal
Neonatal and
Female Orthopedic Wards

Second Floor:

Surgical Wards
New OT Block

Ground Floor:

PP Unit including Immunization and
Antenatal Clinics

First Floor:

Labour Room, Gynae OT Theatre

Second Floor:

Surgical and Eye OT's

Trauma Unit

A ten bed trauma unit is attached to take care of emergency services. A two bed ICU is also working for care of Cardiac patients. It is linked through a new corridor to old PP Unit and A and B blocks for patient convenience.

Blood Banks:

A very busy and progressing blood bank is housed in Trauma Unit.

T.B. Clinic:

It houses the TB Clinic, which has been attached to the Civil Hospital recently.

New Canteen:

A beautiful independent complex of canteen for hospital come up adjoining to the A and B Blocks. It has four components, i.e. waiting area for patient attendants, Dining Hall, Kitchen and STD-*cum*-Tuck Shop for toiletries, etc.

Impact of PHSC Health Systems:

Referral

CH Ropar was selected as a pilot district for referral system, for which following steps have been taken, which has resulted in establishing a good referral systems, i.e.

Training

All the staff has been trained in referral systems and it has helped in its proper and successful implementation. Care is taken to guide and train in referral system, any new staff of any category joining the hospital on transfer from outside.

Mismatch

With the effective control of mismatching, which was quite prevalent in the past, the improved results and quality of services have been achieved. At present through there is shortage of staff but there is hardly any mismatch in the institution.

Equipment

Before the start of PHSC, a lot of equipment and machinery was lying idle because of want of repair, some of them very minor ones. Due to PHSC all the repairable equipment was got repaired, which brought the hospital back on rails, till the new equipment started coming to all the departments as per referral norms. The rest is being condemned from time to time.

Apart from mattresses, bed sheets and other linen, a lot of major equipments have been provided. To name a few are as under:

(a) Cardiac Monitors and Defibrillators;
(b) Semi Auto Analyzer
(c) Boyles Apparatuses;
(d) Photo Therapy Units;
(e) Electro Surgical Cautery;
(f) Hydraulic OT Tables
(g) Audio Meter
(h) Horizontal Autoclaves;
(i) Operating Autoclaves
(j) Operating Eye Microscope;
(k) Operating ENT Microscope;
(l) Audio Meter.

Waste Management

Again Civil Hospital, Ropar was selected for pilot project for hospital waste management. Scientific disposal of biomedical waste after proper treatment is now mandatory under the law, to avoid the spread of dreaded diseases. Various steps have been taken by PHSC in this regard.

They are:

- All the staff of the hospital including the waste handlers has been trained in waste management.
- Various steps in the management of the hospital waste have been successfully implemented.
- Pits have been prepared as per guidelines for proper disposal of various segments of segregated hospital waste after rendering it non-infective.

Most important point this regard is the segregation at generation of the hospital waste.

Segregation at generation

Various color coded bins have been provided at various pint of generation.

Red – Septic Waste
Yellow – Human anatomical waste

White	–	Sharps and Needles
Green	–	For ordinary wastes

Transportation

In segregated form, the septic waste (Red) is weighed and collected and taken to treatment room for over night treatment with one percent hypo chloride or 10 gem/liter of bleaching powder solution. The fluid is then drained after neutoralizing it with HCL to bring its ph to between 5 to 9.

The waste is paced in polythene bags and disposed along general waste.

The human anatomical waste (Yellow) is dumped into specially made pits using bleaching powder and earth on top of it. Sharp (White), which include glass ampoules, blades and needles (with the tips burnt with the use of needle cutter) are dumped in specially made pits after treating with hypo-chloride or bleaching powder solution. The general waste (Green) is collected as such and sent as municipal waste. The waste handlers use protective measures, e.g. gumboots, masks, gloves and aprons to protect themselves from dreaded disease like Hepatitis and AIDS.

Privatization of Sanitation

On contractual basis, sanitation of Civil Hospital, Ropar has been privatized. Again this hospital was selected as one of the first few to implement it. Initially 15 safai sewaks were permitted. But after the up coming of new OT Blocks canteen and new corridor, leading to increase in covered area there strength has been increase to 20 with the privatization of sanitations services the level of cleanliness has improved a lot. The contractors employs the desired number of safai sewaks, provides the cleaning materials and proactive gears.

Quality Assurance

Training in Clinical Skills:

- Updating of clinical skills and knowledge, of various categories of a large number of employees, resulted in their better working.
- Each category of staff has been sent for training at the best possible institutions, i.e.
  SMO-Hospital Management—at AIIMS, New Delhi
  - o IIHMR, Jaipur
  - o ASCI, Hyderabad
- Doctors and paramedical—Clinical Skills—PGIMER, CHD.
- Surgeon-laparoscopic surgery—CMC Ludhiana

Quality Control

- o To ensure proper quality control in clinical laboratories, we are having internal and external quality control systems. For the latter our laboratories get sample sera from CMC, Vellore.

- o Swab Test for various operation theatres is being done from time to time.
- o Quality assurance group meeting is held on 25th of every month in which various QA measures are discussed.
- o Utmost care is being given to cleanliness of the hospital.

Medical Audit

- o Peer group review meetings for proper case files, death case files are being held on regular basis. On 25th of every month quality assurance group meeting is held to review various quality controls measured for proper health care management of patients.
- o Training on medical audit is being imparted at ASCI, Hyderabad, IIHMR, and Jaipur and at State Training Institute, Kharar.
- o Compterization has been started in February 2002 as part of medical audit.
- o International code of diseases is being followed for the purpose of proper statistical data.
- o Double purchee systems have already been introduced.

Surveillance

The entire doctors and staff member have been trained to watch for the diseases under surveillance, i.e. Gastroenteritis, cholera, hepatitis and Japanese encephalitis. AFP (Acute Flaccid Paralysis) even nil reporting is being given on regular weekly basis, since no polio case has been reported from the hospital from quite some time. Recently survey of all the workers working in all the factories in the district has been done by the specialists of the hospital, for communicable diseases, i.e. Tuberculosis (TB), leprosy and other skin problems. For the control of any epidemic of water borne diseases during floods or rainy season, advance preparation in the form of teams building and purchase of necessary medicines and equipment is done well in advance. Fortunately, there had been no such situation during the last three years.

Some other important areas of the hospital

User Money

With the decision to retain the user charges collected by the institution for day-to-day use in patient care, the PHSC (World Bank Project) has infused life into limping health services of government hospitals.

Necessary guidelines are being issued for the judicious and proper use of collected money for the patient welfare, which is being done as per the guidelines of PHSC.

This step has been very effective in proper upkeep of the equipments and smooth running of the hospital.

Free Service and Poor Patients:

New Policy for poor deserving patients:

To facilitate treatment for poor patients free of cost a very comprehensive procedure has been devised by the PHSC which permits equivalent of 2.5% of the user charges collected can be allowed by joint approval of SMO and the treating physician.

Otherwise all other categories continue to enjoy the earlier facilities as per government guidelines.

- o All government employees, retiree, freedom fighters are given free services.
- o To the people below the poverty line who are holding valid yellow cards are also entitled to all the free services of the hospital.
- o Unattended accidental cases and mass casualty cases are also given all types of service (Treatment, X-Ray and lab investigations) free of cost, even the purchee fee is not taken from them.
- o In the OPD, certain range of medicines is available free to all the patients.
- o Free Ambulance services are also provided to accidental unattended cases, mass casualty cases, and yellow card holder poor patients.

IEC Activities

- o Doctors and Paramedical Staff is being given clinical skill training to improve their skills, from time to time at the best institutions identified by PHSC from time to time.
- o Library facilities have been provided.
- o For patients ICE activities wall posters, arrow marking of equipments, etc. has been done.
- o CME participation of doctors for different type of specialties as and when they are held in PGI, GMCH, 32 hospitals and other institutions. CMEs are also held in the hospital on an average once a month.

Functioning of various units:

Medical Unit

The quality care has improved because of following factors in the department:

- o Prevision of a two bed ICU in trauma ward with care monitor.
- o Holter monitor
- o Round the clock availability of fully equipped facilities.

Surgical Scope

It has been provided with:

New operation theater, with new equipments like electrocute, etc.
Sigmoid scope
Proctoscope

All resulted in better quality operations and care of the patients and more.

TOR (Turn over rate).

Orthopedic Unit

Provision of new equipment and instruments has resulted in better quality of operation some of the new equipment's provided are:

Shortwave diathermy

Electronic traction set

Spica table

Ortho

Instruments pack consisting of 180 instruments quality surgery is being done. Under the project of National Programs for Physically Disabled, corrective surgeries are being done for handicapped people. Survey camps are necessary certificates/I Card, for which both the orthopedic surgeons have been honored with commendation certificates at the district level function on Independence Day this year.

Gynae and OBS Unit

Provision of—

- o Foetal monitor
- o New labor room
- o Separate operation theatre
- o And proper wards at the same floor

has helped in better results of the department. Patients are on record where they preferred their second delivery in the hospital than in the nursing home where the first delivery was conducted and they went satisfied.

Paediatrics:

The department has been provided with—

- o Baby incubator
- o Photo-therapy unit and other equipments
- o Independent wards ensuring better care of the new born and other children.

Eye Unit:

- o Latest operating eye microscope
- o Large number of eye camps are arranged in the hospital with the help of various voluntary agencies from September onward to March next year. Other equipments helped in reducing operating completions and in the proper IOL and other operations.

ENT Unit:

It has been equipped with—

- o Latest operating microscope for middle ear operations. A large number of operations are being done with it, which were hitherto not possible.

Dental Department:

It is well equipped with Dental Chair, Dental X-Ray machine and other equipments to be able to handle all types of cases.

PP Unit:

It has been recently attached to the Civil Hospital for better care and management of the patients attending the PP Unit.

TB Clinic:

Again like PP Unit has been attached to the Civil Hospital for better care of the patients and proper running of the clinic as regards to its upkeep and medicine supplied.

Skin Unit:

With the posting of skin specialist in the hospital, a long standing demand of the area was fulfiled. It is one of busy OPD.

Trauma Unit:

A ten bed trauma unit has two beds ICU also. It is one of the busy and volatile areas of the hospital and as usual a source of good, bad and ugly. But invariably it has come out of many testing times with flying colors. It is well equipped to handle all types of emergencies.

OT and Anesthesia Department:

Operation Theatres are well equipped with OT lights, OT Table, and other gadgets. Availability of Boyles Apparatus, Bains Circuit, etc. enables surgery under any kind of Anesthesia.

Radiology:

New 500mA (Siemens), 300mA and Portable X-Ray Plants, new Ultrasound Machine has helped in availability of all invasive and non-invasive tests in the hospital.

Blood Banks:

The turn over of the blood bank has grown a lot in the recent past. All equipments required for full and proper functioning of the blood bank have been provided. Privatization of services has helped in running round the clock, with the help of contractual employees.

Pilot Projects conducted successfully:

The hospital has been given various pilot projects by the PHSC from time to time. The staff can certainly boast of having been a part of these for the effort they put in to successfully implement it at a district level. Some of these are:

- o Waste Management
- o Referral Systems
- o Computerization at District Level Hospital
- o Privatization of Sanitation Services

TABLE 6.1

Hospital Performance Indicators

(Rs. in lakhs)

	Year						
	1998	*1999*	*2000*	*2001*	*2002*	*2003*	*2004*
OPD	63218	90672	63490	114159	146595	160671	161526
IPD	6435	7607	7147	7257	8066	8919	8210
Delivery	672	773	999	1029	117[	1154	706
X-ray	5145	5807	*5789*	9478	10611	13079	15383
Lab. Test	24101	28550	31481	49409	53660	55933	61505
User Charges	7.79	11.06	18.26	25.15	33.05	35.54	40.08

There has been a great increase in all the areas from 1998-2004.

Critical Appraisal (Civil Hospital, Ropar)

Working of District Hospital, Ropar—We have already discussed the organisation structure of District Hospital, Ropar with Senior Medical Officer as In-charge of the Hospital. It was quite hearteoung to see that

District Hospital, Ropar, a 100 bedded hospital has been provided all the infrastructure facilities through Punjab Health System Corporation. However, inspite of the existence of all sorts of facilities, the working has not been as good as expected. Let us discuss some facts and suggestions.

1. SMO In-charge Hospital Lack Administrative Capability by and Capacity to manage the hospital efficiently and effectively

It has been found by personal visit that senior health persons lack administrative skill which impede the functioning of hospital efficiently. Administration is a basic operative force in all-complex and purposive organisations. Management is the process and agency which guides the operations of an organisation in the realization of established goals. In simple works, management is the handling of tools and techniques to achieve a desired goal. In other words, management embraces planning, organizing and controlling of human and other resources to achieve the specified goals. MC-Namara, former World Bank President has rightly said that Management is the heart of development.

There is a need of giving intensive training to Senior Persons in a hospital to make them dynamic and make use of resources efficiently.

2. Dichotomy between people and medical personnel affecting the quality of health services

Public relations is the establishment of climate of understanding. It means interpreting the programme of an health organisation to the public and *vice versa*. The purpose of public relations is not only to supply information, but also to encourage understanding and co-operation between the citizens and the public servants. It is the duty of every member of the organisation to maintain public relations.

At present, we find a great deal of alienation between the people and the health organisation. This has undermined the legitimacy, effectiveness and credibility of the public administration in our country. We need to promote harmony and mutual trust among the people and public administration. The objectives of public relations should be to increase prestige and goodwill and protect the life of the District Hospital by safeguarding it against unwarranted attacks as well as to remove the genuine complaints and grievances of the people.

To improve understanding between the citizens and the personnel, public relations need to be developed in an effective manner to create favourable community opinion towards public services. This would create confidence in the minds of the people towards the competence, fairness, honesty, impartially and sincerity of the public services.

We must give power to the people to make them feel important. P.K. Bajpai in his Article, "People's Participation in Development" in *IJPA*, October-December 1998 has rightly suggested that Government must understand that conscientisation of the people and their active participation in the development process on the one hand and asserting their right on the other, does not weaken democracy. It rather strengthens democracy.

3. Lack of Administrative Reforms

Medical personal and their administrative staff follow the outdated practices. There is a need to change to make the people understand and participate.

Administrative reforms are not only to be planned but implemented as well, with sincerity at all levels, to achieve the desired results. There has to be a genuine desire to ensure just and impartial administration. Making improvements in procedures and practices, form and techniques of administration are only partial remedies. These alone may not give the desired results unless the human elements in-charge of running the administrative machinery show genuine commitment to bring about good governance. Unfortunately, the deteriorating quality of leadership has adversely affected the quality of administrative machinery as well. For, unless the top is clean and truly dedicated to the well being of the people, other layers of administration are unlikely to behave any better. The lower ones generally follow the footsteps of the higher ones.[1]

Substantial change can be introduced either piecemeal or as one comprehensive innovation. Piecemeal change may offer the advantage of minimizing stress and may be the only form available if the change manager is constrained by overall rules and practices. On the other hand, there are certainly cases where piecemeal change produces confusion, destroying established patterns of communication and co-oridnation and carrying a heavy cost. These behavioural concepts of change management have received much research attention in recent years and offer improvement methods to those responsible for changing organisations.

4. Lack of morale and motivation among the members of District Hospital

The Hospital Leadership should encourage their subordinate to achieve results. The most important task of an organisation must be to give abundant and constant evidence of its belief that personnel in an organisation are key to development. This requires proper motivation of the employees. Motivation is of utmost importance, as it constitutes the base for the management functions of planning and organizing. The personnel of a department must devote considerable time and effort in planning for and achieving high levels of motivation and morale. It has been noticed that the performance of the personnel, either as individuals or as members of a group, is less as compared to their capabilities in terms of skills, abilities and capacities. Finer, for example, states that demonstrated performance generally never exceeds more than fifty per cent of the individuals to perform.[2] Most individuals tend to balance their efforts around an assessment of relative costs (time and energy) and benefits.[3]

5. Lack of Teamwork

There is a need to practise 'Management by Objectives' to ensure fruitful participation. Management by Objectives shifts the focus to goals, to the purpose of the activity rather than the activity itself. It is a process whereby the superior and subordinate personnel of an organisation jointly identify its common goals and ensure performance.[4]

The trend of management today should be to make use of authority in collaboration with colleagues developing teamwork. Teamwork is a plan which makes possible utilization of all levels of personnel to achieve maximum output. Personnel in an organisation form a team in each organisation. Of necessity, each team is made up of varied elements, but each official should be committed to bend all his efforts towards creating a homogenous working group.[5]

6. *Poor maintenance of wards*

Though 100-bedded hospitals have been set-up. However, the occupancy is less as most of the specialists do not stay at Ropar inspite of good accommodations for them.

Robert M. Hutchins states (quoted in M.R. Pinto, "Values in Public Services", *IJPA*, January-March 1989). "Thus, all organisations can function and achieve excellence provided all its members strive to purse the goals of the organisation earnestly, sincerely, whole-heartedly and with dedication."

Our thought is the seed which determines the fruit of our action. If the seed is good, then the flowers and fruit which come from the seed must be good and must prove beneficial to ourselves and others. But if we plant in our hearts a poisonous seed, it will harm not only ourselves but all who come in contact with us. Human life is a great responsibility. Only a thoughtless man will say: I cannot help what happens, I am not responsible. We are constantly influencing ourselves and our fellow-beings by what we think, because our thought shapes our inner nature and we radiate consciously or unconsciously what we are. Let us be wakeful then. Let us be thoughtful in whatever we do. Let us be faithful to our true self; for all blessings must come to us, if we prove ourselves true to our higher nature.

7. *Lack of decision-making of right quality at night*

Nothing is more difficult and therefore more precious than to be able to decide. According to Manley H. Hones: "Broadly, decision-making involves making organisation committed to adoption of a specific course of action and use of resources in a particular manner."

New problems demand new solutions and the Chief Executives who can come out from the routine are highly prized. This requires creativity in the sphere of decision-making. Newmann has indicated five distinct stages which can help the Chief Executive in this process.[6]

1. *Saturation*: to be familiar with the problem;
2. *Deliberation*: to consider alternative solutions and to rearrange them.
3. *Incubation*: to let the sub-consicous mind work on the problem.

4. *Illustration*: to get a new ideas and sensing that it may work.
5. *Accommodation*: to work out the new ideas so that it is a practical solution to the problem.

Hicks[7] gives the following types of creativity in sound decision-making:

1. *Innovative*: Creativity to think totally new ideas.
2. *Synthesis*: Creativity to absorb, combine and use ideas from different sources and making it new.
3. *Extension*: Creativity to use old or new ideas.
4. *Duplication*: Creativity to use the other's successful ideas.

According to W. Brooke Grove, "Decision-making is the selection from two or more reasonable possibilities of a course that will, at the time and under circumstances, provide the most suitable solution of the problem at hand."[8]

8. *Most of the Equipment not functional.*

9. *Referral system not functioning as desired.*

10. *No cleanliness of hospital premises.*

11. *Patients are not treated as dignified citizens.*

12. *Corrupt practices.*

13. *Wards are a machinery of medical administration.*

Notes and References

1. U.C. Agarwal, Good Governance Cutting Edge of Administration, in *IJPA*, July-September 1998, p. 436.
2. H. Finer: Theory and Practice of Modern Government, p. 106.
3. Eli Ginzber: "Perspectives on Work Motivation", *Personnel*, Vol. 31, (July) 1959, pp. 48-49.
4. George S. Odoirne: Management by Objectives, New York, Pitman, 1965, p. 55.
5. W.J. Reddin, Effective/Management by Objectives, New York, McGraw Hill, 1970.
6. Newmann William, H. and others: Process of Management (Englewood Cliffs, N.J., Prentice Hall, 1967), pp. 338-45.
7. Hicks, Herbert G., "The Management of Organisations" (New York, McGraw Hill, 1967), pp. 169-71.
8. W. Brooke Groves: Public Administration in a Democratic Society, Boston, 1950, p. 434.

7

CHAPTER

Secondary Health Care Administration

A Case Study of Kharar Civil Hospital

It came into existence as Civil dispensary with two posts of Medical Officers and was upgraded to PHC with the addition of CHC Component in the year 1982. Later on it was upgraded to 30-bedded CH and Trauma Unit was added to it and PHC component was shifted to village Gharuan. The hospital was taken over by Punjab Health Systems Corporation in October 1996 under the World Bank Project and was upgraded to 50-bedded hospital to provide better quality of professional services to people at secondary level health care.

Kharar is one of the fast upcoming satellite townships and is gateway of Punjab to Chandigarh. The vehicle traffic is enormous and makes it an accident-prone area. The situation of Civil Hospital Kharar is at a very strategic point.

Manpower Position

Sl. No.	*Name of Post*	*Norms*	*Sanctioned Post*	*Available*
Specialist Post				
1.	General Medicine	1	1	—
2.	General Surgery	1	1	1
3.	Obstetrics and Gynaecology	—	—	2
4.	Psychiatry	—	—	—
5.	Paediatric	1	1	1
6.	Pathology/Bio Chemistry/Microbiology	1	1	1
7.	Tuberculosis	—	—	—
8.	Anaesthetics	1	1	—

9. Radiology	1	1	—
10. Skin and V.D.	—	—	—
11. Blood Transfusion Officer	1	1	—
12. Orthopaedics	—	-	—
13. Ophthalmology	1	1	1
14. Incharge CMO/SMO	1	1	1
15. MO	7	7	1
16. Casualty MO	4	4	4
17. Dental Surgeon	1	1	1
18. Social Scientist	—	—	—
19. House Surgeon	5	5	—
Para-Medical Staff			
1. Matron	1	1	—
2. Asst. Matron	—	—	—
3. Statistical Assistant	1	1	—
4. Computer	1	1	—
5. Sr. Lab. Technician	1	1	1
6. Stenographer	—	—	—
7. FPFW	—	—	—
8. Nursing Sister	3	3	1
9. LHV	—	—	1
10. ANM	—	—	—
11. O.T. Attendant	—	—	—
12. Pharmacist	5	5	3
13. Lab. Tech. Grade I and II	5	5	2
14. Steno Typist	—	—	—
15. Lab. Attendant	2	2	2
16. Radiographer	1	1	1
17. Physiotherapist	—	—	—
18. Operation Room Attendant	2	2	1
19. Cashier	1	1	—
20. Head Clerk	—	—	—
21. Dental Mechanic/Elect.	1	1	—
22. Dietician	—	—	—
23. AAO/Accountant	1	1	—
24. Clerk	7	7	2
25. Typist-*cum*-Clerk	—	—	—
26. Head Cook	—	—	—
27. Electrician	1	1	—
28. Carpenter	1	1	—
29. Plumber	—	—	—
30. Driver	1	1	2
31. Cook	—	—	1
32. Helpers to Cook	—	—	—

33. Caretaker	—	—	—
34. Dhobi	—	—	1
35. Class-IV	48	48	48
36. Mali	1	1	Nil
37. Chowkidar	3	3	—
38. Storekeeper/Sweeper	11	11	2
39. Superintendent	1	1	—
40. Dental Hygienist	1	1	—
41. Dark Room Asstt.	1	1	—

Note: Nine Posts of Sweepers adjusted in the District Hospitals/Dispensaries for temporary basis.
Source: Punjab Health System Corporation.

Equipment Status

	Norms	*Quantity*				*Remarks**
		On Hand	*Usable*	*Needs Repair*	*Not Usable*	
	1	*2*	*3*	*4*	*5*	*6*
I. Imaging Equipment						
1. 500mA X-Ray	0	-	-	-	-	Awaited
2. 300mA X-Ray	1	2	1	-	-	Funds not available
3. 100mA X-Ray	0	1	-	1	-	
4. 60mA X-Ray (mobile)	1	1	1	-	-	
5. Dental X-Ray	1	1	1	-	-	
6. Ultra Sound Scanner (Linear)	0	1	-	1	-	Company discontinue
7. Ultra Sound Scanner (Linear Sector) with upgradability	1				-	
8. Ultra Sound Scanner (Linear Sector) with upgradability	0	-	-	-	-	
II. Electro Medical Equipment						
1. E.C.G.	2	3	-	2	-	
2. Cardiac Monitors	1	1	-	4	-	
3. Defibrilators	1	1	3	-	-	
4. Audiometers	0	1	-	-	-	
5. Baby Incubators	2	1	-	2	-	
6. Phototherapy Unit	1	1	1	-	-	
7. Endoscipe Fibre Optic	0	-	-	-	-	
8. Operating Microscopes	0	1	-	1	-	
9. Cyro Surgery (Deluxe)	1	-	-	-	-	

10. Foetal Monitor	2	1	-	2	-
11. Short wave Diathermy	1	1	-	2	-
12. Ventilators	1	-	-	2	-
13. Boyles Apparatus with circle absorber	1	3	1	4	-
14. Boyles Apparatus without flout	1	-	-	1	-
15. Opthaamoscope	1	1	2	-	-
16. Slit Lamp	1	1	1	-	-
17. Retino Scope	1	-	1	-	-
18. Perimeter	0	1	1	-	-
19. Emergency Resuscitation Kit	2	1	-	-	-
20. Sigmoid Scope	1	-	-	-	-
21. Head Light	1	1	2	1	-
22. Plus Air Tonometer	1	-	1		-
23. AMC Equipment (2 Monitor, 1 Ventilator, 1 Defibrillator, A/c	1	-	-	-	-
24. Holter Monitor	1	1	-	-	-
25. Endoscope with Lapro catorand and Accessories	1	-	-	-	-
26. Radiant Heater (4KW)	1	-	1	-	-
27. Cryo surgery (Basic)	0	-	-	-	-
28. Pulse Oxymeter	1	1	-	-	-
29. Blood Gas Analyzer	0	-	-	-	-

III. Pneumatic, Hydraulic and Sterilization Equipment

1. Dental Unit	1	1
2. Dental Chair	1	1
3. Air rotor	1	1
4. Ultrasonic Scalar	1	-
5. Operation Table	2	2
6. Operation Table (Hydraulic)	2	4
7. Autoclave HP (Horizontal)	2	1
8. Autoclave HP (Vertical)	1	1
9. Autoclave with Burners 2 bin	1	2
10. Shadowless lamp (mobile)	3	2
11. O.T. Lights (Shadowless)	2	2
12. Focussing Lights (Mobile)	2	2
13. Suction Apparatus (High Vacuum MTPL)	2	-
14. Suction Apparatus (High Vacuum MTPL)	2	10
15. Foot Suction Apparatus	1	4
16. Vacuum Extractor	1	-
17. Instrument Sterilizer	10	10
18. Diathermy Machine	1	1
19. Gynaec electric cautery	2	-

20. Automist	2	-
21. Dental Lab (Bath, Motor, Lathe)	0	-
IV. Laboratory Equipment		
1. Microscopes (Binocular)	3	4
2. Chemical Balances	1	-
3. Simple Balances	1	2
4. Photo Electric Calorimeter	1	1
5. Flame Cell Photometer	1	-
6. Spector Photometer	0	-
7. Auto Analyzer	1	1
8. Micro Pipettes	1	4
9. Electrophoresis	0	1
10. Water Bath	1	1
11. Hot Air Oven	1	1
12. Incubators	1	1
13. Distilled Water	1	-
14. Centrifuges	2	1
15. Centrifuge (Haematocrit)	1	-
16. Hot Plates	1	1
17. Rotor/Shaker	1	-
18. Counting Chamber	2	2
19. PH meter	1	1
20. Glucometer	1	1
21. Hemoglobin Meter	2	4
22. Microtom	0	-
23. Oven (Wax embedding)	0	-
24. Tissue Processor	0	-
25. Timer stop watch	1	1
26. Alarm clock	1	1
V. Refrigerator and Air-Conditioning		
1. Refrigerator 165 Ltrs.	5	3
2. Refrigerator 300 Ltrs.	1	2
3. A/C Machine with Stablizer	5	10
4. Water Coolers	2	2
5. Two body Mortuary (Cold Storage)	2	1
VI. Hospital Plants		
1. Generator 5 KVA	0	-
2. Generator 15 KVA	0	-
3. Generator 50 KVA	1	1
4. Generator 62.5 KVA	0	-
5. Hot water system (solar unit)	1	1
6. Incinerator 3 KW	-	-

7. Incinerator 5 KW	-	-			
VII. Administration					
1. Typewriters	3	1			
2. Photocopier	0	1			
3. Cyclostyling Machine	0	-			
4. Intercoms (40 lines)	0	-			
5. Intercoms (10 lines)	1	1			
6. Fax Machine	0	-			
7. Telephone (external lines)	6	2			
8. Library (Facility)	6	1			
VIII. Transport					
1. Ambulance	-	1			
2. Pick-up	-	-			
IX. Surgical Instrument Packs					
1. D.D and C	2	4	-	-	
2. M.T.P.	2	2	-	-	
3. Cervical Biop	4	1	2	1	
4. Evacuation	2	1	2	-	
5. Delivery	2	4	4	-	
6. P.N. Sterilization	1	-	-	-	
7. Epiosotomy	2	2	2	-	
8. Venisection	2	4	4	-	
9. Copper T	2	6	6	-	
10. Caserean Section	2	8	8	-	
11. Incision and Drainage	2	4	4	-	
12. Vaginal Hysterectomy	2	4	4	-	
13. Abdominal Hysterectomy	1	4	4	-	
14. Vagotomy	1	2	2	-	
15. Appedectomy	0	2	2	-	
16. Hydrocele	2	2	2	-	
17. Gastro Jejunostomy	2	2	2	-	
18. Hemorthoidectomy	2	2	2	-	
19. Suture Removal	0	1	1	-	
20. Suturing Tray	2	2	2	-	
21. L.P. Tray	2	10	10	-	
22. Cholecystectomy	1	2	2	-	
23. Thyroid	1	1	1	-	
24. Chaterization Tray	2	2	2	-	
25. I.M. Nailing	2	-	-	-	
26. S.P. Nailing	0	-	-	-	
27. Dynamic Comeression Plating	0	-	-	-	-
28. A.M. Prosthesis	0	-	-	-	-

29. Dynamic Hip Screw Fixation	0	-	-	-	-
30. Fixation of Radius and Ultra	0	-	-	-	-
31. Cataract operation	1	4	4	-	-
32. Needing and Cataract Evacuation	1	2	2	-	-
33. Tridectomy	1	2	2	-	-
34. Irindenculisis	1	2	2	-	-
35. Extra Capsular Operation	1	4	4	-	-
36. Chalazon	2	4	4	-	-
37. Tarsorraphy	2	2	2	-	-
38. Enucleation	1	2	2	-	-
39. Probing of Lachrymal Passage	1	2	2	-	-
40. D.C.R.	0	1	1	-	-
41. Lachrymal Sac Extension	0	1	1	-	-
42. Trabeculectomy	1	1	1	-	-
43. Pterygium Excision	1	1	1	-	-
44. Entropion Correction	1	1	1	-	-
45. Foreign Body Corenea	1		1	-	-
46. Foreign Body in AC	1	1	1	-	-
47. Conjectval Cyst Excision	1	2	2	-	-
48. Ear Examination	1	2	2	-	-
49. Mastectomy	1	1	1	-	-
50. Macro ear set Myringo, Tympano, Stepedo Plasty	0	-	-	–	
51. Nasal set SMR Stetoplasty	0	1	1	-	-
52. D.N.S.	0	1	1	-	-
53. Rhinoplasty	0	1	1	-	-
54. Adeno Tonsillectomy	0	1	1	-	-
55. Tracheostomy	3	2	2	-	-
56. Endo Laryngea Micro Surgery	1	-		-	-
57. ENT. General	0	1		-	-
58. Anesthesia Kit	1	-	1	-	-
59. General Orthopaedic Kit	0	1		-	-
60. Dental Kit	1	1		-	-

X. Minor Equipment

1. X-Ray Viewing Box	6	1	2	18	-
2. Developing tanks (X-ray)	2	2	2	-	-
3. Safe Light X-ray Dark Room	2	1	1	-	-
4. Cassettes X-ray	12	4	6	4	-
5. Intensifying Screen (various)	12	10	3	12	-
6. Lead aprons	2	2	1	-	-
7. Lead Protection Screen	1	1	1	-	-
8. Chest Stands X-ray	1	2	1	-	-
9. B.P. Apparatus	12	30	6	42	-
10. Weighing machine Adult	4	1	8	2	-

11.	Weighing machine Infant	2	2	4	-	-
12.	Infra-red Lamps	4	1	2	-	-
13.	Oxygen Cylinders	20	30	18	15	-
14.	Nitrogen cylinders	10	10	12	-	-
15.	Regular Flowmeter for medical Gas	8	4	8	4	-
16.	Ambu Bags	8	6	4	8	-
17.	Angle Poise Lamp	2	-	1	1	-
18.	Hot plate Domestic	3	-	2	2	-
19.	Emergency Lamp	8	10	-	32	-
20.	Sewing Machine	0	1	1	-	-
21.	Fire Extinguishers	4	1	-	-	-
22.	Laryngoscope	2	1	6	-	-
23.	Otoscope	1	-	2	-	-
24.	Universal Bone Drill	1	1	1	-	-
XI.	**Furniture and other Equipment**					
1.	Examination Table	15	10	12	-	-
2.	Delivery Table	4	2	2	-	-
3.	Foot Steps	15	10	6	-	-
4.	Bedside Screen	20	10	4	8	-
5.	Revolving Stool	20	35	5	15	-
6.	Arm Board Adult and Child	40	30	15	35	-
7.	Saline Stand	25	15	8	4	-
8.	Wheel Chair	4	4	1	4	-
9.	Emergency recovery Trolley	2	4	1	5	-
10.	Stretcher on Trolley	4	4	1	3	-
11.	Oxygen Trolley	8	10	1	5	-
12.	Height Measuring stand	2	-	2	-	-
13.	Fowler Bed	2	1	-	-	-
14.	Iron Cot	55	50	80	40	-
15.	Baby Cot	6	10	6	18	-
16.	Beside Locker	55	50	50	100	-
17.	Dressing Trolley	4	4	1	5	-
18.	Mayo's trolley	2	2	-	-	-
19.	Instrument Cabinet	4	6	-	3	-
20.	Instrument trolley	4	4	4	-	-
21.	Linen trolley	4	2	-	-	-
22.	Kick Bucket	8	2	1	3	-
23.	Attendant Stool	20	50	60	40	-
24.	Traction Systems	4	1	-	-	-
25.	Postmortem Table	1	2	-	-	-
26.	Wash Basin	20	4	10	30	-
27.	Instrument Tray	12	10	8	2	-
28.	Chairs	24	10	50	50	-
29.	Wooden Tables	20	15	-	4	-

30. Steel Cabinet	12	12	28	2	-
31. Swab Rack	2	-	16	-	-
32. Table (Fracture)	1	1	2	-	-
33. Blood Donor Table Wooden	2	2	2	-	-
34. Matteress	55	50	250	-	-
35. Pillows	55	50	50	-	-
36. Wooden Benches	40	15	-	-	-
37. Cheatle Forceps Jar	10	-	10	-	-
38. Patella Hammer	40	10	6	-	-
39. Tongue Depressor	12	15	10	-	-
40. Oxygen Mask	4	10	500	-	-
41. Torch light	8	4	2	8	-
42. Medicine Cabinet	4	2	2	-	-
43. Side Rals	4	-	24	-	-
44. Bucket Galvanised	8	-	-	-	-
45. Beds Pans and Urinals	8	30	60	-	-
46. Bowls	48	40	15	-	-
47. Kidney Tray	20	15	6	-	-
48. Racks	24	10	3	-	-
49. Patient's Attendant Cots	20	-	-		-
50. Wooden Tables	20	4	-	-	-
51. Wooden Chairs	20	50	-	6	-

Source: Ibid.

Utility

- Sub-Divisional Hospital providing services to the population of Kharar Town and Khanpur (>32696) and about 100 villages located around the town catering to medical needs of about 1.5 lakh people.
- Situated on the Morinda bye Pass near Ludhiana-Ropar Intersection and Caters to road-side feeding area.
- In addition to OPD, Indoor Services runs round the clock emergency and RCH services for the feeding area.
- Receives referred cases from Kurali, Morinda, PHC Gharuan and its subsidiary health centres and also caters to the referred back from PGIMER and Government Medical College, Chandigarh/General Hospital, Chandigarh.

Renovation and Expansion after Inception of PHSC

Renovation

After the hospital was taken over by PHSC a sum of Rs. 15.00 lakh approximately was earmarked in the year 1997-98 for repair, renovation, facelift and landscaping of hospital in the 1st phase and roofing of OPD complex was also done. In addition, following activities were also undertaken.

- Complete replacing of Electrical Wiring and Fittings
- Flooring
- New Parking Space
- Pointing (Teep)

Expansion

Then a sum of Rs. 70.0 lakh was earmarked for future expansion of hospital. This was started in December 1999 and completed in January 2001. In this phase, 2 Operation Theatres, 4 Wards were constructed and existing structure of OPD and Trauma Unit was interconnected. Now the hospital has following separate wings:

- OPD Complex
- Maternity and Female Ward with Labour Room
- Male Ward
- Trauma Unit
- Two Modern Operation Theatre
- Laboratory and Blood Bank
- Dental Unit
- Post Partum Unit

Prior to the Inception of PHSC. This Hospital was mainly concentrating on:

- Curative Services
- Preventive Services
- All the National Health Programmes

After this hospital was taken-over by the PHSC, in addition to the above activities special emphasis is being given to the following:

- Biomedical/Hospital Waste Management Programme
- Referral System
- Quality Assurance

Waste Management Programme

PHSC selected Ropar and Bathinda Districts for a special hospital waste management programme. Before this, there was no clear cut policy or disposal of solid and biological waste.

After this programme, the first step was imparting training to all categories of staff. This training programme laid emphasis on scientific disposal of different types of wastes.

Presently, in this hospital, following measures have been undertaken:

- Provision of deep burial pits for biological waste and sharp pointed objects.
- Provision of a microwave-oven for sterilization of sharp and pointed objects and body fluids, before disposal.
- Provision of protective devices like glasses, apron, masks, gum boots, gloves and wheel burrows to safai karamcharis.

Segregation of Different Types of Waste

In this regard, different coloured buckets have been provided at various points of generation of waste like; Emergency, OT, Wards, Labour Room, PP Unit, etc. the staff has been trained to segregate the waste. Yellow, Red, White and Green Buckets are being used for different types of wastes.

Waste is segregated at all the points of generation in the colour coded buckets. Shredders are used for destroying needless and syringes. Then the waste collected by Safai Karamcharis is taken directly to the pit specially prepared for the purpose. Sharp pointed and all the waste collected in the red bucket is sterilized in the Microwave and then sharp pointed objects are thrown into the pit specially prepared for this purpose. Plastic objects, syringes, etc. are further segregated and disposed as plastic. Other infected waste like Cotton, Gauges, etc. is disposed in the general waste after micro-waving to be taken away by the Municipal Council Staff.

Specification of this pits:

- For Pointed Sharps 2′ × 2′ × 4′
- For Human Anatomical Waste 4′ × 4′ × 6′

Referral System

There was no Referral System under operations in the hospitals of Punjab. PHSC introduced Referral System in the hospitals to strengthen and improve the hospital services. Under this system, the services will be improved by following measures. Renovating and upgrading hospital buildings to provide appropriate space for services. Upgrading and updating clinical skills of Medical Officers and Staff Nurses through an effective training programme. Providing Ambulances for Transporting critical patients. Financial powers to SMO In-charge of the hospitals to accord necessary single sanction up to Rs. 10000 (Rs. Ten Thousand Only). The user charges are to be retained at the facility level. These are to be sued by the SMO In-charge of the hospital as per guidelines. The doctors were given training for 3 days in Referral System. Similarly, Paramedical Staff was also trained.

Quality Assurance

For improvement and quality, following things are needed:

(i) Positive Attitude
(ii) Updating Knowledge
(iii) Better Organisation
(iv) Better Work Culture
(v) Better Results.

Prior to inception of PHSC reputation of Government Hospitals was getting bad to worse because of so many factors, i.e. non-availability of sufficient budgetary provisions and negative attitude of the staff, etc. after taking over of 156 hospitals by the PHSC tremendous improvement in quality and performance has taken place because of availability of adequate finances, improvement in infrastructure, delegation of financial powers to SMOs and change in the attitude of the staff itself. In C.H. Kharar now quality is visible and is being appreciated by public because of the following factors.

Adequate Space

- Adequate space for OPD patients with facility like; cold drinking water, proper sitting arrangement with shell type chairs and electric fans, etc. two rooms were also constructed in the OPD complex.
- To modern well equipped AC Operation Theaters.
- Well spaced and well equipped Indoor Female Ward, Male Ward, Emergency Wing.
- All other wings like Dental Unit, Lab. Blood Bank, PP Unit, Labour Room are adequately spaced.

Equipments

In addition to the iron beds, mattresses, bed-sheets, almiras, chairs, revolving chairs for doctors, tables and other major equipment provided by PHSC in the recent time is as follow:

- ***Computerization:*** Kharar hospital is the first to start computerization of OPD Department. With this lot of. improvement in working out statistics has taken place and there is significant reduction in waiting period for patients.
- ***30KVA Genset:*** It has stared working and can take the load of the whole of the hospital. With this there is definite improvement dealing with emergencies and delivery cases specially at night.
- ***Mechanized Laundry Plant:*** It has started working with its installation there is definite improvement in the quality of washing, saving in material, saving labour and increase in the life of the linen.
- ***Microwave Oven:*** Microwave Oven of 6L capacity has been installed for disinfection of infected waste. This hospital is the

first to get this facility in entire Punjab. With its installation there is definite improvement in disinfection of the infected waste and its disposal.

- Two Air Conditioners have been provided for the newly constructed Operation Theatre.
- New Ambulance for shifting the patients under Referral System has been provided at confessional rates.
- Portable X-ray Machine, Computerized ECG Machine, 30mA X-ray Machine, Ultrasound Machine, Water Cooler for patients, New Dental Unit, Cardain Monitor, Defibrillator, Computerized Feato Meter, Photo Therapy Unit, Semi-Auto Analyzer, Computerized Traction Set, O.T. Lights with Inverter, Opthalmic Instruments like; Ascan, Keratometres, Slit Lamp and Operating Microscope for Contract Surgery has also been provided to this hospital.
- Blood Bank became operational in October 2002.
- The Cardiac Department of PGIMER, Chandigarh has decided to set-up an IHD clinic (Ischaemic Heart Disease Clinic).

Medicine

All the vital life saving drugs are available in emergency wing and patients are not asked to bring the drugs.

- In OPD all the basic drugs like Analgesics, Antihistaminic, Antibiotics, Antacids, etc. are available as per guidelines given by the PHSC.
- Performance indicators show that there is definite improvement in the results. After this, hospital was taken over by PHSC, the no. of OPD, indoor patients, emergency patients; no. of operations and no. of deliveries have increased. Though, the hospital is charging for the services rendered still there is increase in the no. of patients every year. This shows that public is accepting, appreciating the services even after payment and this has happened because of improvement in the quality of health care services at the secondary level.

Quality Check-up

To improve and maintain quality both external and internal quality checkup system has been evolved.

(i) For external checkup of quality in the laboratory, the hospital is getting sera from Medical College, Vellor for cross checkup.

(ii) For internal checkup of quality regular cross checks are arranged with the district level laboratory and from the private laboratories. Further quality control sera has been purchased for internal quality control on day-to-day basis.

(iii) To maintain proper check on the disinfection process of the OT, LR, and Microwave, regular swab test are being done.

Services Rendered by the Hospital

1. Medicine
2. Surgery
3. Orthopaedics
4. Gyane
5. Paediatrics
6. Eye
7. ENT
8. Skin and VD
9. Dental
10. Indoor Facility
11. Round the clock Es.
12. Round the clock LR facility
13. Lab. Services
14. Family Operation
15. Ultrasound

Source: *Ibid.*

Free Facility for Patients

The following categories of patients are exempted from payment of any charges:

(i) Yellow cardholders;
(ii) Punjab Government Employees and Pensioners;
(iii) Freedom Fighters;
(iv) Handicapped;
(v) Unknown Patients;
(vi) Roadside Accidents; and
(vii) Critically ill-patients.

Hospital Performance Indicators

	Year						
	1998	*1999*	*2000*	*2001*	*2002*	*2003*	*2004*
OPD	52220	53935	52814	87866	95448	103585	106929
Admission	4773	4884	4701	4779	5315	5311	5670
Delivery	1071	1129	1072	1086	1045	1097	1193
X-ray	1783	1348	1930	3657	4858	4732	4868
Lab. Test	9961	10813	12523	13549	14016	21530	23182
User Charges (Rs. in lakh)	3.34	5.30	6.16	9.56	10.82	14.11	17.21

Source: Ibid.

Deficiencies

The following deficiencies in the hospital requires urgent attention from the Government:

(i) Hotline Facility with independent Transformer should be provided.
(ii) Sarai/Shelter for patients attendants.
(iii) Conference Room.
(iv) Drip Irrigation System for lawns.
(v) Parking space for scooter/car, etc. should be provided with concrete.
(vi) Post of Mali, ANM, Health Worker (Male) should be provided immediately to further improve the working of the hospital.
(vii) Medical Specialist, Paediteision, Skin Specialist, Paediatrician, Ultrasonologist, etc.

Critical Appraisal (Civil Hospital Kharar)

The author visited a number of times Kharar Civil Hospital and through observation and discussion found the following problems which need attention and care—

1. *Specialist and other doctors stay away from Kharar:* Kharar being nearere to Chandigarh, most of the doctors come back to Chandigarh to engage in private practice. The patients for whom they are appointed are deprived of the services.
2. *Wards remain unoccupied:* Since the doctors have to go to Chandigarh, they do not admit any patient which requires their night stay. They use simple method cleverly, i.e. refer them to PGI Chandigarh.
3. *The Specialists are not well read:* Whatever they have learnt during their Education they are using. There is no habit of reading.
4. *A lot of corrupt practices are prevalent.*
5. *The wards are not properly maintained.*
6. *Patients feel suffocated in wards.*
7. *There is no adequate arrangement of food, etc. in wards.*
8. *Most of the diagnostic equipment is out of order.*
9. *Doctors have collisim with Private Laboratories. They asks the patients to get the tests done from outside as their machines are not good. The doctors get 50 per cent commission on these tests and diagnostic tests.*

Suggestions

Imparting Appropriate Knowledge

Research has demonstrated that patients' understanding of their conditions and treatments is positively related to adherence, and that adherence, satisfaction, recall, and understanding are all related to the amount and type of information given. Many studies have shown that patients do not always understand prescription instructions and often forget considerable portions of what health care practitioners tell them. Studies have shown that patients who understand the purpose of the prescription are twice more likely to follow it than those who do not understand the purpose. The physicians can provide effective patient education by: (1) limiting instructions to 3 or 4 major points during each discussion; (2) using simple, everyday language, especially when explaining diagnosis and giving instructions; (3) supplementing oral teaching with written materials; (4) involving the patient's family members and friends; and (5) reinforcing the concepts discussed. This is especially true for millions of citizens with low literacy skills.

Modifying Beliefs and Human Behaviour

It is worthwhile to address patients' beliefs, intentions, and self-efficacy. This is because knowledge alone is not sufficient to enhance adherence in recommendations involving complex behaviour change. Clinicians can optimize behaviour change by ensuring that the patients: (1) perceive themselves to be at risk due to lack of adoption of healthy behaviour (perceived susceptibility), (2) perceive their medical conditions to be serious (perceived severity), (3) believe in the positive effects of the suggested treatment (perceived benefits), (4) have channels to address their fears and concerns (perceived barriers), and (5) perceive themselves as having the requisite skills to perform the healthy behaviour (self-efficacy).

Patient Communication

At least 50% of patients leave their doctors' offices not knowing, what they have been told. Studies have shown that (1) 50% of psychosocial and psychiatric problems are missed by physicians due to lack of proper communication, (2) physicians interrupt patients on an average of 18 seconds into the patients' descriptions of the presenting problems, (3) 54% of patients' problems and 45% of patient concerns are neither elicited by the physician nor disclosed by the patient, and (4) 71% of patients stated poor relationships as a reason for their malpractice claims.

Ask a patient about his feelings and concerns and his views about psychological factors on the adherence, so as to arrive at a common understanding to the nature of the problem. Then provide them with information about all areas that individual finds pertinent, and encourage them to share in decision-making when a plan for management is formulated. Most importantly, successful collaboration requires tailoring strategies to individual patients rather than basing communication on general assumptions. On the same note, communication with the patient's family and the patient's own perception of social support is significantly and positively related to adherence. The family's role becomes all the more important if a patient is suffering from a chronic disabling condition requiring continued support and understanding.

Lifestyle Interventions may be the Key in India

Scientists remind us that an autopsy may show a diseased organ as the 'cause' of death, the proximal cause of the disease may be changes in bodily function producing too much blood sugar or cholesterol. These in turn may be 'cause' by the patient's lifestyle in regard to diet, drinking and exercise. The social environment including education, housing, working conditions, stability of family life, or affordability of food and drink, in turn may cause these. Back off another step and we see that these factors are caused by political and economic factors. Miller says that investigating and throwing attention on these 'deep-spaces', what Diamond would call 'ultimate causes', " . . . . is the stuff of political medicine."

There is still polio, somewhere a child dies every minute of every day from diarrhoea and every 6 minutes a woman dies from pregnancy-related causes. Female foeticide is raging-ironically in wealthier districts, and even in districts where female literacy is the highest. Road traffic accidents in Delhi alone are of epidemic proportions. Tackling these problems does not require more research or the application of more expensive technologies. Each of these deaths is preventable with low-tech technology already well known for decades. We do not need a better polio vaccine or better oral re-hydration salts. So what is 'causing' these problems, and a myrid more that leave countless millions every year disabled, dysfunctional and often dead?

The biggest killer in India today is not the mosquito, not the salmonella, staphylococcus or streptococcus bacteria, not tobacco, and certainly not the polio bacterium despite the disproportionate effort spent on eradicating it, it is corruption.

Effects of Social and Economic Inequality on Health is Profound

The desire for a healthy family, healthy society and a healthy country drives individuals and governments alike. The government is supposed to create settings that will provide equal opportunity for an individual. to fulfil these desires. There is an undisputed association between this social equality, social integration and health. The effect of social and economic inequality on health is profound too. Poverty, which is a result of social and economic inequality in a society, is detrimental to the health of population. The indicators of health (mortality, morbidity and life expectancy) are all directly influenced by the standards of living of any population. Various international studies have documented a strong association between income inequality and excess mortality.

When applied to. Indian context these theories translate into millions of lives that perish due to a lack of socio-economic equality. Since the emergence of free India in 1947, Socialism and government-centered economic policies were favoured over the profit-making private enterprise and capitalism. Though admirable for its motives, these policies led to over-dependence on the bureaucracy and stifled the growth of free enterprise. Slow and unequal social mobilization in various parts of India led to an uneven economic growth. Caste and social polarization, literacy and educational levels, natural resources, levels of corruption and role of political leadership has resulted in some Indian states doing better than others on the economic growth that India has witnessed in the last two decades. Amidst the rising standards of living, lie pockets of terrible poverty and deprivation.

8

CHAPTER

Secondary Health Care Administration in Thailand*

Before we discuss the hospital administration, let us mention briefly the structure and role of Ministry of Public Health in Thailand. The country's administrative structure consists of Bangkok Metropolis area, 73 provinces and 163 municipalities. The Bangkok Metropolis is headed by a governor and his four deputies. Each province is headed by a governor who is appointed by the Ministry of interior. Each Municipality is headed by a mayor who is elected by Municipal Council.[1]

The typical province has a population of about 500,000 and the smallest well over 10,000. Each province is composed of about 3-20 districts (amphoes) depending on population and area. There are 628 district (amphoes) and 82 smaller districts (gingamphoes). Each district is administered by district officer (nai Amphoe), a civil servant appointed by the Interior Ministry who is responsible to the Provincial Governor. Each sub-district is under the supervision of a deputy district officer responsible to the district officer.

There are 5,608 communes (tambons) and 56,286 villages (mubans). Majority of the communes and villages are not legally recognized as part of the administrative system of the country. A commune consists of a group of villages. The tambon head official acts as registrar and as intermediary between the district officer and the village headman. The village is the smallest unit consisting of a cluster of 50 households, having about 200 inhabitants, and is headed by a village headman (puyaiban) elected by the inhabitants of the village.

This is a piece of doctoral Research by Krienkerai Klnoboul, first Secretary, Thais Embassy, under the guidance of the Author who visited Thailand alongwith the students.

The functions of the various Ministries in Thailand are very similar to those of the major sub-division of the executive branch of any modern government. The general pattern of organisation at the ministry level is relatively standardized and long established. The head of each Ministry is its political chief—the Minister—who is responsible to the Cabinet for the proper functionings of his Ministry and its subordinate Departments. The minister may be assisted by one deputy or assistant Minister or more holding a political appointment. Each Minister has attached to him one political secretary or more whose appointment and removal is effected by the Cabinet. In each Ministry, the Secretary, his assistants and staff, form the Office of the Secretary to the Minister.

Ministry of Public Health

The principal governmental agency (but by no means the only one responsible for health services is the Ministry of Public Health.[2] The Ministry of Public Health (MOPH) has undergone several re-organisations since its founding and at present (2000) its responsibilities at the central level are divided among six departments or offices:

1. Office of the Under-Secretary of State for Public Health.
2. Department of Medical Services.
3. Department of Communicable Disease Control.
4. Department of Health.
5. Department of Medical Sciences.
6. Office of Food and Drugs Committees.

The six Departments of Offices of the Central MOPH further organized into 'divisions' with a wide variety of functions.

1. Office of the Under-Secretary of State for Public Health

The office of the Under-Secretary of State, besides its administrative functions and correlation of the work of the various departments, exercises its duties through the Divisions of Medical Registration, International Health, Food and Drug Control, Nursing and also through the Medical Council, the Committee for the Control of Drugs, the Committee for Food Quality Control, the Committee TB Control, the Committee for V.D. Control, the Filariasis Contol Board, the Primary Health Care Board, and Office of National Advisory Board for Disease Prevention and Control. Latest additions to this are the Division of Malaria Eradication, the Division of Filaria, the Division of Vital Statistics and the Health Planning Division.

2. Department of Medical Services

The Department is responsible essentially for the management or supervision of large governmental hospitals. These include, for example, the mental hospitals operated directly by the Central Ministry and the large general hospitals at the provincial level. The National Cancer Institute and the Institute of Pathology, which engage themselves in both patient care and research, are also under this Department. It should be noted, however, that they are numerous smaller district hospitals of the MOPH that are not under the supervision of this Department. Furthermore, there are several hospitals under other ministries of the Government, and also an expanding number of purely private hospitals (both non-profit and for-profit) which are not supervised by the Department of Medical Services.

3. Department of Communicable Disease Control

This Department is responsible for nation-wide campaigns against several selected communicable diseases of relatively high prevalence in Thailand. These include malaria, tuberculosis, filariasis, venereal disease and leprosy. The operation of these disease control programmes are mainly through a "vertical" flow of authority from the Central Government out to the provinces and municipalities. Although, there has been, in recent years, a movement to decentralize health programmes and enlarge the "horizontal" scope of authority at the provincial level, these communicable disease control programmes are still managed essentially from the top of the pyramidal structure of the IMOPH.

4. Department of Health

This Department is responsible for supervision of most of the other preventively-oriented programmes of the Ministry. These include such fields as nutrition, family health, dental health services and environmental sanitation. Highly important has been the delegation to this Department of responsibility for several special innovative programmes in "primary health care." Moreover, since most of the family (maternal and child health and also family planning) health services are delivered through a nation-wide network of facilities for ambulatory service health centres, mid-wifery centres, and also 'medical and health centres' the standards for operation of these facilities are promulgated and supervised by the Department. Most of the medical and health centres are at the district level and contain a small number of beds (10 to 30) for minor illness or emergency cases. These centres have recently come to be designated as "district hospitals." Inspite of the functions of these small hospitals being mainly curative rather than preventive, their technical supervision has remained with the Department of Health.

5. Department of Medical Sciences

This Department has as its main objectives for promotion of research in medical sciences and the provision of modern diagnostic procedures in the treatment of prevention of diseases. It is also responsible for the management of a variety of technical services which are performed mainly at the Central Government level. These include, for example, a Radiation Protection Service Division, an Entomology Division and a Virus Research Institute. The National Health Laboratories Project Division is exceptional in attempting to organize a network of clinical laboratory services throughout the country, as well as operating a major central laboratory in Bangkok.

6. Office of Food and Drugs Committee

Office of Food and Drugs Committee, the newest of the major administrative entities of the MOPH, has responsibility for protecting the population against hazards in the consumption of food or drugs or the use of the cosmetics. As we shall see, the use of drugs in Thailand both those that are medically prescribed and those purchased directly over the counter by patients—absorbs a substantial share of all expenditures for health purposes in the nation. The establishment of this Department signifies an effort by the MOPH to introduce greater controls over this important health problem. Tackling the problems of substances' abuse (drug addiction) is only part of this larger pharmaceutical problem.

Under the general surveillance of the latter Department but operating as a semi-autonomous government enterprise, is the Governmental Pharmaceutical Organisation (GPO). This public entity was started in 1939, originally under the Ministry of Economics to prepare drugs for use in governmental facilities and to save on foreign exchange.[3] In 1942, when the MOPH was formed, it was transferred there and eventually combined with the Division of Medical Depot of the Department of Medical Sciences. Currently, the GPO produces 384 items which, it is estimated, constitute nearly half of the drugs and vaccines distributed to governmental hospitals and health centres.

Since 1950, the activities of the above Departments have been expanded by the assistance of and co-operation with the following international and foreign organisations: the *World Health* Organisation, the United Nations Childern's Fund, the United States Agency for International Development, the Rockefeller Foundation, the China Medical Board of New York and several governments under the Technical Co-operation Scheme of the Colombo Plan. The projects which have benefited by the international and foreign aids are malaria eradication, yaws control, tuberculosis control, maternal and child health including family health, community health development and village sanitation, environmental health, vital health statistics, medical education, trachoma, leprosy control, health education of the public, nursing and mid-wifery education, nutrition promotion and training of personnel.

Field Administration: Local Health Administration

Traditionally, the numerous functions of the MOPH just summarized were carried out under higher centralized authority, but in recent years, stress has been put on the delegation of responsibilities peripherally towards the local level.[4]

Each of the 73 Provinces has an Office of the Provincial

Ministry of Health's Service Institution at Provincial Level

Regional:	9 region	Regional Hospital	(14 hosp.)
Provincial:	73 provinces	Provincial and district hospital	(73 hosp.)
District:	628 Amphone	Medical and health	(323 district centre hosp.)
Tambom:	5608 Tambom	Health Centre	(4204 centres)
Big Village		Mid-wifery centre	(2271 centres
Villages:	56,282	Village Health post	

Field Offices

The Ministry of Health has field offices spread throughout the country. There are 14 Regional Hospitals, 73 Provincial Hospitals, 323 District Hospitals, 4,204 Health Centres, 2,271 Mid-wifery Centres and Village Health posts.

Chief Medical Officer

The PCMO is a public health physician, who is responsible for supervision of both preventive and curative functions of the MOPH throughout his province. Thus, he oversees the Provincial General Hospital of which there is at least one in each province and sometimes two, making a total of 88. These hospitals vary in size from 60 to as much as 800 beds. The PCMO is also responsible for the technical supervision of the work of the District Health Offices in the province. These Offices are headed by a District Health Officer (not a physician), who is typically a sanitarian with additional training in general public health administration.[5]

Within some, but not all of the districts, there are District Hospitals of 10 to 30 beds, staffed by at least one physician along with nurses and other health personnel. Also, within some but not all of the sub-districts or communes (tambons) there are health centres staffed by nursing and other allied health personnel (but not physicians). In some but not all of the villages, especially the larger ones, there are mid-wifery stations, staffed simply by a trained auxiliary midwife. The last two types of health facilities come under the general supervision of the District Health Officer, but the District Hospitals, being staffed with physicians are more particularly the direct technical and administrative concern of the PCMO.[6]

The PCMO is appointed by the central Under-Secretary of State for Public Health, and is technically responsible to him. He may be advised and assisted also, however, on various technical problems by specialists from the several other departments of the central MOPH, for example, on problems of administrative area, the PCMO is administratively responsible to the Governor of his province, who is appointed by the Department of Local Administration of the Ministry of Interior. Provincial Governors are important officials in Thailand, and it is evident that PCMO must exercise great discretion in combining his technical responsibilities to the central MOPH with his administrative responsibilities to the Provincial Governor.

In the same way, the District Health Officer, while technically responsible to the PCMO is administratively responsible to the generalized District Officer. The latter official, like the Provincial Governor is part of the network of authority of the Ministry of Interior. The most recent development in the network of local health services under the MOPH is the "programme of training and activity" of "village health volunteers" (VHV) and "health communicators" (HC) in selected villages throughout the nation. Starting with the movement to limit population growth by encouraging family planning (FP), this programme has broadened to encompass the provision of general primary health care. These village people are part-time health workers who depend for their livelihood on some other occupation. They are not considered part of the bureaucratic structure of the MOPH or any other Government agency.

Thus, it is evident that MOPH, both centrally and at the several peripheral levels, has a very wide range of functions. They embrace both preventive and curative services, and they involve liaison with various officials of provincial and local Government within the nation-wide network of the Ministry of Interior. Even so, as we shall see, there are numerous health activities under the private sector. On the whole, the scope of MOPH authority does not extend to these other activities; when it does the relationship is quite indirect. The Ministry of Public Health must ensure cooperation and co-ordination among allied agencies to achieve good results. It needs to develop an effective information system network to involve all allied agencies.

HOSPITAL ADMINISTRATION

Since many health problems require a level of medical treatment and personal care that extends beyond the range of services normally available in the patient's home or in the physician's office, modern society has developed formal institutions for patient care intended to help meet the more complex health needs of its members. The hospital, the major social institution for the delivery of health care in the modern world, offers considerable advantages to both patient and society. From the standpoint of individual, the sick or injured person has access to centralized medical knowledge and technology so as to render treatment much more thorough and efficient. From the standpoint of society, hospitalization both protects the family from many of the disruptive effects of caring for the ill in the home and operates as a means of guiding the sick and injured into medically supervised institutions where their problems are less disruptive for society as a whole.[7]

Today, a hospital is a place for the definition and treatment of human ills and restoration of health and well-being of those temporarily deprived of these. A large number of professionally and technically skilled people apply their knowledge and skill with the help of complicated equipment and appliances to produce quality care for patient. The excellence of the product—the *raison d'etre* for a hospital, therefore, depends on how well the human and material resources are applied to promote patient care.

Functions

(a) Patient Care

The first and foremost function of a hospital is to give care to the sick and injured and restore the health of diseased persons. Ethically, his care should be given to all without discrimination of social, economic or racial nature. However, the hospitals as national investment in people's health and as centres for scientific practice of medicine, must do many more things than 'produce' medical care. To quote Perry: "The success with which a hospital contributes towards meeting the patients' needs can be measured by the fullness of the life he is able to lead on leaving it."[8]

(b) Training

Education and training of doctors and nurses have traditionally been carried out in hospitals. It is a workshop wherein the student learns by seeing what his superiors and peers do. Radiology, laboratory, radiotherapy, highly advanced surgical techniques demand a variety of skills and knowledge, all of which cannot be mastered by the doctor specialists. These activities have created the need for a large number of skilled technicians who are today the vital support to the specialist whether he is the surgeon, physician, diagnostician or therapeutist.

These people are indispensable for the all-round excellence of all specialist work. To develop these technical skills, a programme should be organized by the hospital under the direction of people who have the required experience, knowledge and attitude to teach others. The purpose of in-service education and training programme is to develop such knowledge and skills in all categories of paramedical personnel as are required to make them fit for the job they hold and keep them attuned to the growing needs of their jobs.

(c) Medical Research

The third important function of hospital is to give support to medical research. A good hospital, where the quality of professional work is excellent, is an ideal ground for medical research. As a matter of fact, excellent professional care of patients largely result from the fruits of research into new problems. An attitude of enquiry and investigation should permeate through the day-to-day care of patients. The hospital can develop facilities for research with comparative ease and speed if the staff and administration are properly motivated. True, elaborate research is expensive. There, nevertheless, remain clinical investigations of applied nature that call for little capital investment. Responsibility for creation of new knowledge is that of any enlightened profession. It is in a hospital that opportunities exist, if not abound, for organized as well as individual initiative for research.

(d) Health Education

The fourth and final object is to support and assist all activities carried out by various public health and voluntary agencies to prevent disease and promote positive health attitudes in the community through health education. Health education, immunization, social and economic rehabilitation are some of the many activities for which the hospital may provide assistance in terms of physical facilities and advisory services to staff. As a matter of fact, in the western countries, this aspect of the hospital as a community health centre is being emphasized more and more. Many ways are being devised to integrate the hospital with the activities of community health agencies.

Administration of such a complex organisation requires blending of technical and administrative competence in the right quantity, at the right time, at the right place, by the right man and in the right way or process. Each hospital is a distinct entity and as such each has to be tailored to the specific aims to be accomplished, the specific tasks to be performed, the volume of services to be rendered and the type of the community to be served. The basic purpose of the hospital is "better patient care" and return the patient back to the community as a productive unit of that community. Hospital administration is an activity to secure better output through optimum utilization of inputs. It is not so easy, as it might seem, to determine the number of hospitals and the number of beds within them, in Thailand. Various reports from different agencies tabulate the hospital resources of the specific agency but an overall tabulation of hospital bed resources, of multiple sponsorships, is not currently available.

In Thailand, there were 491 hospitals and other establishments for in-patient care, with a total of 45,393 beds.[9] Thailand had 60,590 hospital beds or 1.41 beds per 100 population.[10] This may be compared with Malaysia (Thailand's neighbour to the South), which in 1993 had a ratio of 2.63 hospital beds per 100U population. The problem is to determine the classification of these hospital resources by:

(a) type of hospital, i.e. general or for various special purposes, and
(b) sponsoring or the ownership of the facility.

(a) Types of Hospitals

The most detailed categorization of hospitals, by type, is reported in a Ministry of Public Health Publication Institutions containing beds were classified into four types as on the next page.[11]

In later years, the health centres with beds (also known as first-class health centres) were redesignated as "district hospitals", those without beds (formerly called second-class health centres) were simply considered as

Type of Facility	Number	Number of Beds
Hospitals	279	52,005
Health Centres (most with beds)	329	193
Maternal and Child Health Centres	5	575
Midwifery Centres	48	402
Total	661	56,175

"health centres." Accordingly, the facilities that are now designated as district hospitals of the Ministry of Public Health numbered 329 and had 3,168 beds, or an average of slightly less than 10 beds each.

Type of Bed Service	*Institutions*	*Beds*
General Hospitals	248	39,722
District Hospitals	329	3,169
All General Facilities	577	42,891
Specialized Hospitals	31	12,283
Maternal and Child Health Centres	5	575
Midwifery Centres	48	402
All specialized Facilities	84	13,260
All Types of Facilities	661	56,151

Focusing on the hospitals in the above tabulation, those considered "general hospitals", i.e. serving all types of patients, numbered 248, with 39,722 beds. This meant a ratio of general hospital beds of 0.9 per 1000 population. Hospitals for specialized conditions numbered 31, with 12,283 beds. In addition, all the beds in district hospitals (previously first-class health centres) are "general." Correspondingly all the beds in "maternal and child health centres", "midwifery centres" may be considered as "specialized." Thus, breakdown of the above listing of institutions, by type of health service, comes out as follows:

The discrepancy of 24 beds (56,176 minus 56,151) between the two tabulations is explained by the omission from the second tabulation of "second-class health centres", a few of which contained a total of 24 beds. Specialized hospitals are of several sub-types which may be identified as on the next page.

Thus, in summary, of all facilities with in-patient beds in Thailand, 84 with 13,260 beds or about 13 per cent of the facilities and about 24 per cent of the beds are in specialized facilities. The majority of these beds are in facilities related to mental disorder—17 institutions with 8,503 beds. Another 2320 beds are for leprosy patients from though most people with this disease have relatively mild cases that are hospitalized. The remaining

Type of Specified Hospitals	Number	Beds
Mental Disease	14	7,483
Mental Deficiency	2	520
Narcotic Addiction	1	500
Leprosy	4	2,320
Tuberculosis and Chest Diseases	2	584
Tropical Diseases	1	100
Infectious Diseases	1	230
Eye Diseases	4	46
Maternity	1	50
Pediatrics	1	450
All Specialized Hospitals	31	12,283

beds are in facilities for various diseases of demographic groups, mainly mothers and children.

From the viewpoint of the number of different patients served, the general hospital with 76 per cent of the beds are most important. The great majority of these are under the Ministry of Public Health at the provincial and district levels. In contrast to the specialized hospitals, the average length of stay of patients is relatively short. In 1975, it was only 5.9 days in all provincial hospitals (that is, at the provincial level, not district hospitals) and 10.3 days in the Bangkok City hospitals (but not counting the large medical school teaching facilities.[12] Thus, there is relatively rapid turnover in the use of general hospital beds. In most of the specialized hospitals, the average patient stays for several months or years.

(b) Hospital Sponsorship

Highly relevant to hospital planning, as well as to the whole distribution of health services, is the sponsorship of hospitals. Institutions under governmental control, particularly the Ministry of Public Health, are more readily subject to planning in relation to general population needs. Sponsorship is important mainly with regard to general hospitals. Of specialized hospital beds, only a handful—hardly 5 per cent are not governmental in sponsorship.[13]

Some of these figures requires explanation. The Ministry of Public Health data do not count beds in district hospitals which were identified as "first-class health centres" if these 3,193 beds are added the MOPH total becomes 26,456 beds. The other Ministries include the large teaching hospitals in Bangkok (Sirirat Ramathibodi, and Chulalongkorn Hospitals) under the State University Office as well as hospitals under the Ministries of Defence, Communications, Interior and other branches of Government. The 13 hospitals of state enterprise include those of the railway system, the tobacco monopoly and other organisations.

Sponsorship	*General Hospitals*	*Number of Beds*
Ministry of Public Health	87	23,262
Other Ministries	63	11,463
State Enterprises	13	574
Municipalities	6	1,243
Private	79	3,180
All General Hospitals	248	39,722

It should not be inferred that care in Government hospitals is without cost to the patient. For drugs, laboratory and X-ray examinations, and various supplies, the vast majority of patients using public hospitals must pay. The very poor are theoretically exempted, but in practice few qualify for this completely free hospital care in public general hospitals.

Health Centres

Before 1975, these were classified as follows:

Class I: Medical and Health Centres
Class II: Health Centres
Class III: Midwifery Centres

Class I facilities typically had a few beds for accidents, maternity, or other conditions pending referral to a hospital; at least one doctor was on the staff. Class II units had no beds and were staffed entirely by auxiliary health personnel. Class III units were staffed solely by midwives (not nurse midwives) and sometimes also with an assistant sanitarian.

Since about 1975, there has been a gradual upgrading in the status of these types of units, and a fourth echelon of primary health, care has been added. Class I "medical and health centres" are now designated as district hospitals with 10 to 30 beds, it has been easier to have them staffed with a doctor, since the mandatory 2-year period of rural services has been required of all new medical graduates.

The Class II health centres, now simply designated as health centres, have increased in number and in staffing. Many of them are now staffed with middle-level, personnel-nurse practitioners or wechakorn and their allotment of drugs and supplies has been increased.

The Class III units or midwifery centres have also been increased in number, and the scope of functions of the midwives has been broadened to encompass general family health (including family planning) and some basic primary health care for first aid to patients with minor illness or injury. The time of rural midwives is now devoted more than half to services other than attendance at child births and maternity care.

Finally, in a number of demonstration projects, a fourth echelon of "village health post" has been established where very briefly trained health volunteers—backed up by health communicators—offer basic primary care closer to village dwellers than any of three previous levels of health centres. This level of peripheral primary care facility has not required new construction, since the services are rendered directly in the home of the volunteer or, if he is a shopkeeper, in the store. Whether this type of facility will be spread throughout the country depends on evaluation of its effects in the selected demonstration area, especially that in Lampang Province. Unfortunately, there is a serious problem of underutilization of all four levels of health centres in relation to the health needs of the population theoretically served.

Deficiencies in Coverage

Health planning in Thailand has for several years contemplated coverage of the population with the several types of hospitals and health centres described above, according to certain designated ratios. These have, as a minimum, simply corresponded to the structure of the political subdivisions of the nation: provinces, districts, communes and villages. Although these constitute very rough guidelines, since each of these geo-political areas have different total populations, it is helpful to examine the coverage of the nation at present along these lines. The established facilities were as below:[14]

Types of Facility	*Facilities Established*	*Percentage coverage*
Provincial Hospitals	89	100 plus
District Hospitals	317	56.6
Health Centres	4,047	73.0
Midwifery Stations	1900	3.9

As indicated above, the provinces are relatively abundantly served by provincial hospitals in the capital cities, and in several provinces, there are two such hospitals. Many of these are old structures, which require renovation, but it is clear that the needs are more urgent at the more peripheral areas, close to Thailand's large rural population.

The coverage of 55.6 per cent indicated for districts, with district hospitals, is somewhat of an exaggeration, if one considers the adequacy of staffing. Of the 317 district hospitals, 62 are not yet stationed to the minimal standard. If the coverage is adjusted to take account of staffing, district hospitals would number 255 and the coverage would decline to 48.2 per cent. The great majority of these district hospitals (165 of them) have 12 beds, and nearly all the remainders have 30 beds.

Progress has been particularly rapid at the commune (tambon) level. The coverage at this level with health centres was reported as 57 per cent and it has now risen to 73 per cent. On the other hand, the coverage level of only 3.7 per cent for midwifery stations would seem to be based on an unreasonable criterion. Since the average village has only 500 to 600 population, one should not expect a midwifery station in every village; a cluster of two or three villages aggregating to about 2,000 population would actually be more consistent with planning objectives. On this basis, the coverage now achieved would be between 8 to 12 per cent.

With respect to the fourth level of "village health posts" for primary care, staffed by health volunteers, the objective is indeed to cover every village in the nation. Unfortunately, different sources in the Government report different number of facilities actually in place and in operation. The data is given above were obtained, as indicated, at the Thai Ministry of Public Health but they differ from figures reported in publications from other sources.[15]

Administrative Set-up

All hospitals—both general and specialized—under government sponsorship are administered or supervised by a physician who is assisted by various managerial and nursing personnel. The numbers and backgrounds of those associated vary, of course, with the hospital size (number of beds). The Hospital Director or "Chief Executive Officer" of the hospital is appointed by the Central Government authority responsible for the hospital. Thus, in Ministry of Public Health hospitals, both at provincial and district levels, this would be the Minister, ordinarily on recommendation of the Director of the Department of Medical Services. In hospitals under other Government agencies, such as the State University Bureau (which controls the large teaching hospitals in Bangkok) or those serving various state enterprises, the Hospital Director is appointed by the top official of that agency.

Most of the other supervisory personnel in each hospital are also appointed by the central authority, on the recommendation of the Hospital Director. Appointment cannot be finalized, however, until the Civil Service Commission has determined that the individual meets the requirement officially listed for the position. In fact, for any technical position in a hospital, such as a laboratory or X-ray technician, such review by the Civil Service Commission is required. In one case, in which one X-ray technician trained by a radiologist and considered very well qualified could not be appointed because she had not taken certain formal courses required in the rules of the Civil Service Commission.[16]

The entire staff of the public hospital is responsible ultimately to the Hospital Director, although this may be through an intermediary, such as the "Chief Nurse" or the "Secretary" (or business manager). The physicians on the hospital staff are always responsible directly to the Medical Director.

Staffing Patterns

In contrast to hospitals in the United States—although in common with hospitals in most developing countries—the physicians on all public hospital staffs are appointed to salaried position designated on an "organisational chart." Thus, the doctors are members of a "closed staff", and no physician who is not a member of this staff may admit a patient to a hospital bed, except, of course, in obvious emergencies. Thus, a patient may be referred to the hospital by a health centre doctor or a doctor in private practice, but after admission, the case is entirely the responsibility of a hospital doctor. After discharge, a report is supposed to be sent to any outside physician serving this patient, but such reports are evidently not always sent.

Probably the commonest practice of admission of a hospital patient is through "self-referral"—that is, the patient simply coming directly to the hospital out-patient department (OPD) on his own initiative. There, an OPD physician decides on whether admission to a bed is necessary. The case then becomes the responsibility of a hospital doctor, if it is a large hospital—such as at the provincial level or in Bangkok this doctor will be in one or another clinical departments (such as surgery, medicine, obstetrics, pediatrics or some other. For a private patient, that is, someone occupying a private or semi-private hospital room, the arrangements are different. Such a patient is admitted on the request of the hospital staff physician who has served this patient in his private practice. This physician, then takes care of the patient throughout his hospital stay. It should be explained that officially a government doctor may not charge for services rendered in a public hospital, even for patients in private rooms.

The usual custom, however, is for the physician to charge a certain fee for the services rendered in the private office or "clinic", when a patient is scheduled to be treated in the hospital with surgical or other procedures, the fee charged is simply calculated to cover the services rendered in the hospital as well. It need hardly be mentioned that these practices have developed in Thailand, as in certain other developing countries, because the official medical salaries for hospital work are so low (These salaries are standardized by the Civil Service Commission for all public hospitals, including those of state enterprises or the municipal hospitals of the Ministry of Interior, as well as in MOPH facilities). Earnings per hour in private practice are five to ten times higher.

In all MOPH hospitals, there are certain official standards for staffing, varying with the size and role of the institution. In the average Provincial General Hospital, for example, the standards call for one doctor to every 15 beds. For larger "regional hospitals" expected to serve several provinces for highly specialized services, the doctor to beds ratio is theoretically 1 : 10. In practice, however, these standards are not yet being implemented; currently, the ratio of doctors in Provincial Hospitals generally is about 1:20 beds.[17]

Likewise, for nursing personnel, there are official standards, although they allow for flexibility in the proportions of professional nurses (with RN credentials) and auxiliary nurses. In Provincial Hospitals the standard calls for a ratio of five nursing personnel (of various level) to nine beds. This standard is currently attained, however, in only a small fraction of these hospitals.[18]

In District Hospitals, where the patients have less serious conditions, but at which it is expected that out-patient and preventive service will require a good deal of staff time, the personnel standards differ. For the typical District Hospital of 10 beds, there is required one doctor who takes clinical responsibility for all in-patients and out-patients, as well as being the Hospital Director. Other personnel in a 10 bedded District Hospital, according to official standards, should include:

Nurses: 8, of whom one has RN qualification.
Administrators: 3, of whom one is Secretary, plus 2 clerks.
Technician: 1 for laboratory tests.
Sanitation Control: 3, who also do communicable disease control. Health Promotion: 4, including a health educator, public health nurse and others.
General Maintenance: 8, including a driver, a mechanic for repairs, etc.

For large 30-bedded District Hospitals, in addition to proportionately more doctors (3 or 4) and the above types of personnel, there should also be a pharmacist and a dentist. As in Provincial Hospitals, however, these various standards are seldom achieved at present. According to a high MOPH official, only about 10% District Hospitals currently meet these standards.[19]

In District Hospitals of 10 beds, these are typically set-up in two wards (for men and for women); there are not ordinarily any private beds. Provincial Hospitals have their public beds in wards of about 6-8 beds each, with between 5 and 15 per cent of the total beds reserved for private patients. The occupancy levels at these two types of hospitals are very different. District Hospitals typically are reported to have occupancies of under 59% although it would be more accurate to say under 25%. The explanation would not seem to be mysterious; on the relatively rare occasions when rural people feel sick enough to seek admission to a hospital (considered a fearful experience) they want to be treated in a hospital with various medical specialists and advanced equipment. Thus, they usually by-pass the District Hospital and go directly to the Provincial Hospital, (it may turn out that the case is simple and could have been handled at the District Hospital, but it is simpler to give care than to send the patient back).

Assessment

(i) Provincial Hospitals, therefore, have very high occupancy levels as a rule—from 75 to over 100 per cent. Sometimes two patients must be put in one bed and extra beds crowded together in the wards or even the corridors, are common. It is also not uncommon to see the public wards terribly overcrowded, while the private rooms are half-empty. In view of this situation, the MOPH has attempted to build up the District Hospitals—especially since young doctors are now available to staff them under the mandatory public service law to reduce the pressures on Provincial Hospital. So far, the desired effect has not been participated perhaps if referral from a District Hospital or Health Centre becomes obligatory for acceptance in a Provincial Hospital (except of course in obvious emergencies), the occupancy problem would be corrected.

(ii) The training of Hospital Secretaries for their administrative Responsibilities on budgeting, personnel, kitchen and laundry maintenance, house-keeping, etc. is surprisingly limited. It is done through a one or two-week course given by the MOPH in Bangkok. The Mahidol University Faculty of Public Health offers a course in "hospital administration" but this is limited to physicians or other professionals with a doctorate degree. Some reflection of this weakness in training may be the deficiencies in ordinary sanitary maintenance that characterize many Provincial Hospitals, by this may also be due largely to the relatively tight budgets on which he must depend, with inadequate nursing and house-keeping personnel.

(iii) Another comment about public hospitals in Thailand is called for the policy of making charges for drugs and diagnostic procedures to all but the very poorest patients. In practice, even though many patients have very low incomes nearly everyone pays something. Further indirect evidence of the deterrent effect of these costs is the very low rate of hospital utilization in Thailand as a whole. Based on 1973 data although published in 1974, the Thai population uses the general hospitals of the MOPH at the very low rate of 64 patient days per 1000 persons per year.[20] This may be compared with a rate of some 1800 days per 1000 in a developed country like Canada, but even to 500 days per 1000 in a developed country like Canada, but even to 500 days per 1000 in Government hospitals of neighbouring Malaysia.

(iv) A final aspect of the MOPH hospitals is their accessibility of the population. A study of this was made, simply by relation Provincial Hospitals to the geographic centres of numerous political districts (Amphoe) whose population they served. The nation was analyzed in terms of its 5 official districts, plus 73 additional areas sometime considered "small district", making a total of 643 area, these 358 were found to have "good" for reasonable access to a Provincial Hospital, meaning that the district contained a Provincial Hospital or was adjacent to a dist its population were within 50 kilometeres of it. In a second category were 111 districts not contiguous with a district, containing a provincial Hospital, but with a population mainly (but not entirely) under 50 kilometers distance from it; these were termed "intermediate." Finally, these were 174 districts with "poor access" or "isolated" from a Provincial Hospital being located where most of the population were over 50 kilometers away from such a hospital considering the many poor roads and inadequate public transportation, one can appreciate the difficulties faced by residents of these 174 districts in reaching Provincial Hospital.

Provincial Hospitals

Provincial hospitals, located in the capital town of every province in the country, by far account for the largest number of general hospital beds overall, as well as for hospitals within the control of the Ministry of Public Health. Ministry sources indicated there were 89 hospitals "labelled provincial hospitals" for the country's 72 provinces. Although a province normally only has one provincial hospital, indicated in the capital town, the excess number of provincial hospitals is a result of more than one general hospital being located in each of several larger provinces with dispersed populations. The average size of a provincial hospital remains about the same as in 1974, or slightly more than 250 beds per hospital. However, they range from as small as under 100 beds, to several hospitals now being expanded and upgraded as regional referral facilities with 600 to 700 beds, the size of the hospital varies roughly with the size of the provincial population it serves. The number of physicians varies with the size of the hospital, and MOPH standards suggest one doctor for every 15 beds in a provincial hospital, and one doctor for every 10 beds in the regional facilities. However, some of the smaller provincial hospitals in more isolated provinces have only four or five doctors in residence (range in 1978,3-35 doctors/hospitals with an average of 10.5 doctors per hospital and the overall ratio throughout the country is about one physician for 20 beds.[21]

A Case Study of Lampang Provincial Hospital

In 1942, a 25-bed hospital was built under the sponsorship of the Lampang Municipality on a 20 acre plot. In 1950, the Department of Medical Services in the Ministry of Public Health took over responsibility for the hospital, purchasing adjacent land and adding new buildings and departments. The in-patient departments currently include: surgery, medicine, pediatrics and obstetrics-gynecology. The out-patient departments are obstetrics, gynecology and family planning, pediatrics (including well-baby immunization) clinical, ear, eye, nose and throat minor (EENT); minor surgery (including orthopedics), and medicine. As in most provincial hospitals, some community health activities, such as family planning, well baby and immunization) clinics, have been integrated into the out- patient departments.

Issues and Problems

(i) It is clear that although the budgets of both have increased each year, the operational resources available to the Provincial Health Office are small in comparison to those available for the Provincial Hospital. If capital funds were also added to these budget totals, the difference between the hospital and the Provincial Health Officer would be even greater. The difference between the two in resources available is emphatic when one considers that: the Provincial Health Office is responsible for seven district hospitals, about 70 district health centres, 35 midwifery centres, a variety of special purpose programme, and the primary health care volunteer network. The provincial hospital is a single facility.

(ii) As in all provinces of Thailand, the Director of the Provincial Hospital is nominally under the authority of the Provincial Health Officer. However, the Provincial Health Officer has little role in co-ordinating hospital activities and exercises no control over the Provincial Hospital's budget or administration, which flow through a separate line from the Ministry of Public Health. There has traditionally been no routine system of reporting hospital activities to the Provincial Health Office. These are a few factors which suggest a relative autonomy of operation of the Provincial Hospital within the provincial health care system.

(iii) In the near future, the Provincial Hospital's size may grow to 750 beds as it assumes regional hospital status. In recent years, as the hospital slowly increased bed capacity under its phased expansion plan, the in-patient load has not significantly increased. This is due, in general, to a much more slowly increasing hospital staff. As the new hospital units open in the near future, the problem of staffing will become extremely acute. It will most likely be some time before sufficient staff can be made available to, appropriately match the increased bed capacity. This suggests that there will be great pressure on current hospital staff to assume responsibility for the new capacity, and the increase in size and status of the hospital will undoubtedly open up new opportunities for advancement in the clinical departments. A major concern is that the already considerable pressure on the Community Health Department staff will become more pronounced as the department expands its role and that many of the very competent staff will be attracted to the new clinical positions available with more career potential.

(iv) Provincial Hospital and Provincial Health Office Administration still remain basically separated and uncoordinated. Informally, a number of staff within the provincial health headquarters were shifted to the Community Health Department in the hospital. However, administrative problems are encountered, the provincial health staff, who were never really under the authority of the Community one Health Department Chief, shifted back to the Provincial Health Office.

(v) The Provincial Health Office is directly responsible for district hospitals, but there is no official link between the Provincial Hospital and the district hospital's technical support and resources could possibly be provided to district hospitals by the Community Health Department, but there is no official channel to institutionalize this. A further complication is that the district hospital itself is only responsible for the geographic area of the sub-district in which it is located, and is not responsible for health care in the full district. Health centres within the district and their staff fall under the responsibility of the non-physician District Health Officer. If a strong technical support and supervision network is to be established, a more appropriate arrangement might be the Community Health Department providing technical and administrative support to the district hospital, and the district hospital in turn providing some kind of support for wechakorn and other personnel in the sub-district health centres with overall co-ordination at the Provincial Health Office. This might also provide the means for rotating junior hospital staff into district hospitals or districts which do not have a physician at present, which would provide technical input to the district, as well as give experience and understanding to the hospital physicians in the needs of the rural health care.

Expanding Role of the Hospital

With the help of foreign aid and consultation, the hospital role was extended to the following:

(1) Temporary extension of the hospital out-patient department to district health centres.

(2) Establishing a Community Health Department in the hospital which eventually would have responsibility for direct support of rural health services.

Extended Out-patient Services

In the first phase hospital out-patient department services were extended to the district health centre in Hang Chat, the first district to which integrated services were introduced. Since the district health centre had no physician in residence, an immediate priority was to add one to the staff. The simplest approach to filling the position, and to initiating involvement of the hospital in rural health care, was to rotate provincial hospital physicians through the centre in Hang Chat at two-month intervals. The rotation programme continued for almost two years, providing services during the clinic hours five days a week, until the new district hospital was completed and staffed by a permanently-assigned physician. During the period that provincial hospital physicians served in the Hang Chat health centre, the utilization of services there increased sharply in the years before physicians were rotated through Hang Chat, the average number of patients seen per month had been about 125. However, shortly after the physician rotations began, the monthly average more than doubled. Since the hospital physicians were only in transient assignments, their role was generally limited to providing medical care services and they did not have sufficient time or opportunity to lead the district health team. With the completion of the district hospital in Hang Chat, the permanently assigned physician assumed this responsibility.

Development of the Community Health Department

A community health department was proposes as a mechanism to effectively link the Provincial Hospital to the Provincial Health Office and rural health services. The hospitalized planner undertook the initial organisation of the department, and became the department chief. An old building separate from the Provincial Hospital main buildings, was assigned to the Community Health Department.

The Community Health Department established in the Lampang Provincial Hospital was the first of its type in Thailand, although there were already a number of community health or community medicine departments in teaching hospitals associated with the medical schools. However, the function of community health departments in medical schools has been primarily to train medical students and other health professionals. Each medical school faculty has generally chosen one rural district, served by a district hospital and outlying health centres, through which small groups of medical students have rotated for periods of upto six weeks. The field work in the rural district is occupied with class room lectures and is expected to prepare the newly trained physician for future work in rural areas.

Developing a community health department in a non-teaching provincial hospital was a complex talk. The objectives of such a department are somewhat different from those of a medical school department. The medical school normally selects small areas to be used as a field training site for students. The objective in Lampang, on the other hand, was to make the Community Health Department the centre for stimulating and co-ordinating health services in all rural districts, rather than in one selected area. Training is also an integral part of the department's role in linking the hospital with rural health centres. The Ministry of Public Health has recognized the need for community health departments in general hospitals and has planned to establish such departments in other provincial hospitals in Thailand. The Department of Community Health was initially headed by the Project's hospital planner, assisted by a public health nurse/ health educator, a social worker, an epidemiologist/statistician and secretary.

With a seriously limited number of available staff positions and resources at its disposal most of the early activities of the department were focused inside the hospital. These were:

(1) Organizing educational activities for the prenatal, well-baby postnatal and family planning clinics;
(2) Implementing educational activities and discharge counseling programmes in the various wards;
(3) Producing a variety of educational brochures and leaflets for distribution in the various out-patient clinics;
(4) Improving the public address system for broadcasting health messages periodically during the day;
(5) Improving environmental sanitation on the hospital premises; and
(6) Co-ordinating collective of hospital statistics and epidemiological reports normally sent to the Provincial Health Office.

While concentrating on activities inside the hospital during the initial period, the department's chief looked for opportunities to link the department with peripheral rural health services. In mid-1977, one such opportunity presented itself; the organisation of a mobile vasectomy clinic. Under this programme which is a part of the National Family Planning; Project, teams were set-up within Provincial Health Offices in a number of provinces to provide vasectomies to village in rural locations. This was an ideal activity for the Community Health Department to expand rural services, as the chief of the department was a skilled surgeon specializing in urology. With assistance from the vasectomy training team of Ramathiborli Medical School, the first mobile clinic was organized in Hang Chat District in October 1977. The response was much greater than expected-1SO rural villagers had a vasectotny in the first two days of the clinic, confirming the acceptability of vasectomy in the rural areas. After the first clinic, the mobile team travelled to rural locations twice a month. A motivation team worked with local village leaders and health volunteers prior to the mobile team's visit.

The Family Health Division of the Ministry of Public Health provided a mini-bus for the mobile team as well as costs of supplies and per diam for participating staff. The mobile vasectomy team achieved important results during its first year of operation. Nearly one thousand vasectomies were performed compared with less than a hundred performed in the hospital in previous years.

The mobile clinic has filled a major gap in the generally successful National Family Planning Project. It seems apparent that many rural people are interested in having a vasectomy. But the Provincial Hospital where vasectomies have been most readily available, is not easily accessible to rural population. Bringing the service closer to their homes (the mobile clinics have been operated from rural health centres) has made it more convenient, and the high quality of service provided has reinforced acceptance among rural villagers. Chart 8.1 summarizes the current overall functions of the Community Health Department and plans for future additions. Chart 8.2 outlines the specific responsibilities of each unit within the Department.

CHART 8.1

Current and Future Functions of the Community Health Department, Lampang Provincial Hospital, 1979

Community Health Department		
Hospital-based Services	• Community-based services	• Support for Perripheral Services
Immunizations	• Jail Health	• Medical referrals
Nutritions	• School Health	• Mobile clinics
• Health Education	• Community Information/ Education	• Special Services
• Communicable disease control and surveillance	• Mobile health services	• Technical Supervision
• Out-patient medical care	• Co-ordination of health activities in the Lampang municipality	• Technical supervision
• Out-patient medical care	• Co-ordination of health activities in the Lampang municipality	
• Environmental sanitation		
• Social Welfare		
• Drug addict care (out-patients)		
• Medical Care by radio or isolated areas		
• Malnourished children's ward		
• Ward for contagious-diseases		
• Drug addiction ward		
• Geniatric services		

Source: MOPH, Govt. of Thailand.

Assessment of the Working of the Hospital

The assessment of the Hospital is based upon both primary and secondary data. Patient opinion survey was designed and 100 patients were interviewed, on random basis, for two weeks. Three questionnaires were designed to solicit the opinions of the employees in the hospital to ascertain their views on hospital functioning. The sample for questionnaires

CHART 8.2

Responsibilities of the Community Health Department, Lampang Provincial Hospital, 1979

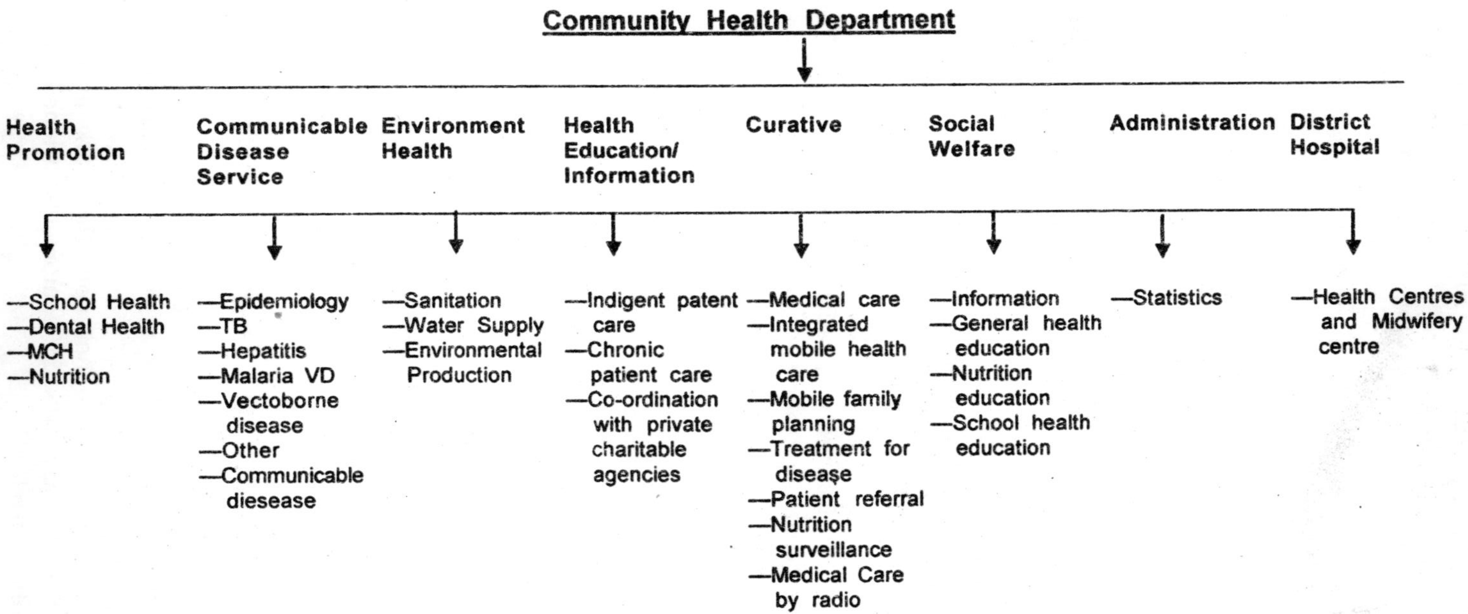

1 and 2 included all the physicians (32); Dentists (2); Pharmacists (3); while Nurses (25); Nurse Aides (25) and Other Staff (SO) were selected on random basis. Besides, the record of the hospital was studied to analyze the functioning of the hospital.

The answers to the patients' opinion surveys have been analyzed in percentages and are given in Table 3. The analysis of the table indicates that the patients are satisfied by and large towards the services provided by the hospital as well as with the behaviour of the personnel working in the hospital. However, the following difficulties were mentioned by the patients and their relatives. We present here these and their probable solutions.

A. Problems of Outdoor Patients

(1) Though it is a fact that in the present decade of reforms communication with the District and Sub-divisional towns hits improved tremendously still there are remote and inaccessible areas from where patients find it difficult to come in time to get medical facilities at the outdoor. As such they have to wait for the next day for getting Medical facility unless the case is a serious one. This communication difficulty poses problems both for the patients and the staff of the hospitals.

(2) The facilities for investigation at the outdoor is very meager, as such the cases cannot be investigated properly.

(3) Even though the facilities exist, as the staff strength is very meagre, the cases cannot be investigated and treated with greater speed and care.

(4) The supply of medicines falls short of the requirements because the budget provision for each hospital is fixed. Unless and until more budget provision for supply of medicines to different hospitals is made to cope with the rise of population and rush at the outdoor, most of the patients will have to go without medicines. Sometimes, the most essential and cheap items of medicines are not supplied while costly and rarely used medicines are given.

B. Problems of Indoor Patients

(1) There is shortage of staff. As such the admitted cases cannot be looked after properly.

(2) Bed strength is meagre in comparison to the demands of admission cases—resulting in refusal of admission of genuine cases.

(3) Operation theaters are not upto the mark in most of the hospitals as they lack in equipments, trained O. T. staff, electrification, etc.

General Problems

(1) Huge Cost of Transportation

It was found that villagers used up quite a lot of money in bringing themselves to be examined by the doctor, which was due to the difficulty in transportation and the expenses by the relatives who come along with the patients. The expense of one visit, in average, for a villager at about 11 kilometers away from the district hospital is:

	Cost of transportation	*Cost of medicine*	*Cost and expense of the relatives*	*Total*
An out-patient	40	30	250	320
An in-patient	40	50/day	400	490/day

Note: The currency is in the Bahts.

Many villagers have faced troubles in transporting themselves to the district hospital and provincial hospital, especially during the night time. For the poor, the problems are much more serious as they have to manage their scarce money for food rather than medicines. It is suggested that the Government may help to set-up a village health fund from the villagers for supporting the volunteer in giving all services in primary health care to their members in the village. The fund needs to be controlled by a group of self-selected villagers called "Village Health Bank Committee."

(2) Lack of Functional Literacy

In the study, we also found that most of the poor patients did not want to see the doctor when they got ill, they would let the disease become complicated until they thought that they would die if no doctor was consulted. Usually it was too late for the patient to receive the proper treatment, and it would mean much larger amount of money in treating such a patient.

It is suggested that there is a need to co-ordinate health functions with other socio-economic factors. The first step in this context is to set-up a fund in the village and a programme for training of the health volunteer to make use of that fund in elevating the health status of the villagers.

(3) Absence of the Involvement of the Community

Most of the people contacted were of the view that the Health Administration never takes the people into confidence. To achieve its aim, a health team must be able to promote community participation, i.e. to help people to rely as much as possible on their own efforts and resources for their health needs. A health team must:

- understand and communicate with the community;
- encourage community participation in identifying problems and seeking solutions; and
- work in the community.

To establish good relations with the community a health worker or health team follows these steps:

(a) listen, learn and understand;
(b) talk, discuss and decide; and
(c) encourage, organize and participate.

(4) Neglect of Rural Areas

Most of the people contacted were of the view that rural people are discriminated and neglected as compared to the urban population. The Health Department must provide more services to the rural people as they cannot afford to be examined by private physicians. To quote Neutra:

> "We can foresee a time when our technical civilization, will keep its promise and serve not only the strictly urban variety of mankind. ...People who populate vast stretches of the earth, will then no longer feel themselves to be second rate citizens."[22]

(5) More Emphasis on Preventive than Curative Measure

It was observed that most of the members of health team take more interest in curative than preventive measures. The hospital may attend to curative services but its ultimate aim should be preventive and promotive. To quote Mackintosh:

> "The appropriate field of study of a hospital is not sickness in the narrow senses but life in the broad sense. Sickness is an incident grave, troublesome or restful — the life of a person, but to the hospital and its staff sickness is a challenge, a focus of enquiry from which prevention should radiate as well as the cure of the Individual."[23]

(6) Lack of Willingness of the Health Experts to Serve in the Villages

Perhaps most formidable obstacle to the setting up of a comprehensive system of medical care in the rural communities of under-developed countries is the small number of medical practitioners who will agree to settle in such areas. We have to examine this problem through effective manpower planning. As long as Government cannot offer salaries comparable with the fees paid in the private sector it would be unrealistic and unreasonable to require physicians to accept full-time appointments in public hospitals. Moreover, members of the medical profession in the developing countries prefer to remain in the large towns since the majority of the people can afford to pay higher medical fees.

A questionnaire was issued to employees to understand the process of decision-making. The responses are given in Tables 8.1 and 8.2, The analysis of the tables indicates that there is centralization and no Delegation is given to the employees to take decisions. Besides, there is no participation in decision-making. Speedy and realistic decision-making is one of the essentials of efficient administration. In a big and complex organisation, the number of decisions to be taken from time to time is so large and the points at which the decisions are to be implemented are so many that it becomes necessary to distribute decision-making powers among a number of personnel/organs, rather than concentrate in one person/organ. This is expected to prevent the emergence of bottlenecks which bedevil highly centralized power structure.

TABLE 8.1

Patient Opinion Survey in Percentages based upon Questionnaire No. I

Sl. No.	*Service Facility*	*Very good*	*Good*	*Satisfactory*	*Bad*	*Hopeless*	*No Reply*
1.	**Service**						
1.1	Medical Treatment	5	50	25	5	5	10
1.2	Dispensary	5	22	53	10	5	5
1.3	Laboratory	10	40	25	15	10	.
1.4	X-Ray	12	23	54	4	..	7
1.5	Physiotherapy	10	20	56	7	4	3
2.	**Behaviour**						
2.1	Receptionists	15	20	32	6	5	22
2.2	Senior Consultants	11	22	44	12	8	3
2.3	Junior Consultants	13	19	51	13	..	4
2.4	House Surgeons	16	21	49	9	3	2
2.5	Registrars	17	24	52	5	2	..
2.6	MRD Staff	7	28	55	8	1	1
2.7	Matrons	9	51	28	7	3	2
2.8	Ward Sisters	6	48	39	6	..	1
2.9	Duty Sisters	12	41	29	11	4	3
2.10	Male Nursing Staff	10	38	47	2	1	2
2.11	Class IV Employee	11	23	56	2	1	7
3.	**Availability of**						
3.1	Medicines	12	55	26	4	3	..
3.2	Injections	8	31	51	3	5	2
3.3	Dressing	11	33	49	5	2	..
3.4	Linen	9	30	41	9	5	6

4. Cleanliness						
4.1 Officers	20	28	43	4	3	2
4.2 Verandahs	7	32	41	11	6	3
4.3 Wards	6	23	48	18	2	3
4.4 Lawns	10	31	40	10	6	3
4.5 Stores	8	32	41	5	6	8
4.6 Bathrooms	9	31	39	11	5	5
4.7 Latrines	11	20	31	20	10	8
4.8 Urinals	10	31	49	5	2	3
4.9 Linens	11	22	51	5	6	5
5. Food						
5.1 Cooking Standards	9	31	50	6	2	2
5.2 Variety	10	24	51	7	4	4
5.3 Quantity	11	25	49	9	.	6
5.4 Services	12	23	48	9	8	2
6. Amenities						
6.1 Light	10	20	55	10	5	..
6.2 Fans	15	22	47	10	6	...
6.3 Drinking Water	8	21	45	15	11	2
6.4 Canteen	9	25	46	12	5	3
6.5 Postal	11	26	47	8	7	1
6.6 Telephones	8	24	45	15	8	.

Besides the respondents were of the view that participation should be encouraged. Participation is an individual's mental and emotional involvement in a group situation that encourages him to contribute to group goals and to share responsibility for them.[24] An employee's participation would build his morale and ultimately his efficiency. An ILO document mentions that the individual worker "is not just a cog in the very big wheel, but that his personal effort is essential for the achievement of the overall production plan."[25]

The research theory in social organisational psychology has also suggested that participation in group decision-making enhances satisfaction among members and removes tensions. Michael R. Cooper and Michael T. Wood have shown that satisfaction is affected by the participation. Satisfaction was greater when participation was complete than where it was partial.[26]

There is a need to practice 'Management Objectives' to ensure fruitful participation. Management by Objectives shifts the focus to goals, to the purpose of the activity rather than the activity itself. It is a process whereby the superior and subordinate personnel of an organisation jointly identify its common goals and ensure performance. The Manager must encourage the development of such concepts among employees. The response in

TABLE 8.2

Hospital Communication and Decision-making Process: Employee's Response

Sr. Code	4	3	2	1
CD 1	-	-	60	40
CD 2	-	-	80	20
CD 3	-	-	10	90
CD 4	10	30	40	20
CD 5	-	-	40	60
CD 6	-	-	40	60
CD 7	-	-	50	50
CD 8	-	-	20	80
CD 9	-	-	10	90
CD 10	-	-	15	85
CD 11	10	20	40	30
CD 12	-	-	10	90
CD 13	-	-	10	90
CD 14	-	-	40	60
CD 15	-	-	10	90
CD 16	-	20	10	70
CD 17	70	10	10	10
CD 18	-	-	40	40
CD 19	-	20	40	40
CD 20	-	20	40	40

Table 8.3 has been presented to depict the management working environment in the hospital. The respondents were the same as selected in earlier questionnaire. Majority of them rate all activities below average. We must encourage employees' satisfaction to ensure fruitful results. A climate of creativity must be developed and maintained by management. Maier and Hayes say that "the optimal climate for creativity is whatever human conditions' optimal for individual freedom and self-expression in social setting.[27] Most of the respondents were critical of the top persons in the hospital. The success or failure of an organisation depends, to a great extent, upon the administrative capability and motivation of its top leadership.

Administrative capability is "the capacity to obtain intended results through organisation.[28] Katz says, "Administrative capability for development involves the ability to mobilize, allocate and combine the actions that are technically needed to achieve development objectives.[29] Leaders must be the persons with vision, initiative and desire to achieve the operational goals with dedication and perseverance. The greatest efficiency and productivity will flow from the efforts of those who find satisfaction in their work and conditions of service, who sense an awareness of usefulness

TABLE 8.3

Percentage Response Based on Questionnaire

Needs	*Priority Ranking*					
	1	*2*	*3*	*4*	*5*	*6*
Security of Job	12	18	30	35	4	1
Salary	50	20	10	5	2	3
Promotion	42	31	14	8	3	2
Appreciation Recognition of work power and respect	32	26	16	12	8	6
Development of personal worth	1	4	10	15	30	40

of their function, who feel encouraged to move ahead and to meet new challenges, who perceive their working environment as one in which high standards of performance are maintained and rewarded and not one in which indolence and incompetence can be ignored or even protected and rewarded.

In order to determine personality characteristics of a selected sample of hospital employees, a questionnaire as shown administered to 50 respondents.* [* Physicians (16), Dentists (2), Pharmacists (3), Nurses (10), Nurse Aides (5), Other staff (14)] The respondents were asked to rank following six needs in order of priority:

(a) Security of Job,
(b) Salary,
(c) Promotion,
(d) Application and recognition of work,
(e) Power and respect, and
(f) Development of personal worth.

The selection of respondents was based on stratified random sampling where employees belonging to various wards/departments and of different official statuses were chosen. The response in terms of percentages is given in Table 8.3.

Analysis of data given in Table 8.3 reveals that maximum number of employees give higher weightage to salary and promotion and their next consideration is security of job/recognition of work. Thus, the management must give due consideration to this aspect. It is true that the importance of pay or compensation is very great for every employee. The standard of living and the social prestige of an employee depends to a great extent on the pay he draws. Manson Haire remarks, "Pay in one form or another is mainly one of the mainsprings of motivation in our society."[30] Thus, an adequate and sound salary, structure, together with other working conditions, is the *sine qua non* for the organisational effectiveness. However, we must be clear that no compensation plan can satisfy all the employees. The true efficiency in an organisation can be promoted only through dedication and loyalty of its staff members. We must inculcate pride in the job among the staff members of an organisation, i.e. doing job with their best ability to achieve excellence in their own fields. Only such individuals who aspire to fulfil their self-actualization needs can bring about creativity, innovation and development in the structure and functioning of the organisation. The administration must provide congenial and creative environment for them as they are the builders of the organisation. To quote Nehru, "No administrator, I suppose, or anyone else for the matter of that, can really do first class work without a sense of function, without some measures of a crusading spirit. I am doing this, I have to achieve this, as a part of great movement in a big cause. That gives a sense of function not the sense of individual, narrow approach of doing a job in an office for a salary or a wage, something connected with your life's outlook or anything, perhaps being interested as people inevitably are, on one's personal preferment in that particular work."[31] Based upon discussion and facts, we maintain here some other areas and their solution.

Escalating Costs

The budgets of hospitals are increasing beyond proportions over the years which is beyond the capacity of poor countries like Thailand. The whole of the health budget is spent in maintaining few hospitals neglecting the vast population needing health and medical care. According to H.A. Goddard:

> "In the management of administration of any enterprise, the quality, quantity, timing and cost of the work necessary to reach the objectives of the enterprise are inter-related factors which must be given constant attention. In the resources for health work in trained persons and in finances were unlimited, the need for constant attention to these factors would not be so great. But the limitation in the number of trained personnel and the lack of adequate financial resources are major obstacles to greatly improved health in the world today. We must, therefore, husband our resources carefully to accomplish as much as possible with what we have available."[32]

Absence of Cost-consciousness among Hospital Staff

A serious problem in health care administration is the absence of cost-consciousness among the staff of public health administrations. All over the world, health, service staff—even of the highest professional cadre—are taught little about the economics of health services and know little about the costs of the equipment and supplies they use. Doctors tend to employ what is new without regard to cost. It is a fashion to prescribe costly drugs. They are also subjected to considerable sales pressure from manufacturing firms. A cheaper drug or cheaper equipment may give just as good a result for the vast majority of patients. Cost-consciousness is not just a matter for central administrators or planners but should be inculcated in all those working in health care. More people can be provided with services if no services cost more than that is a must to provide the necessary level of care. The price paid for high-cost technology for a few is no technology at all for the many. Another aspect of this problem is the use of hospital non-judiciously.

Absence of Co-ordination

At present, all hospitals whether at the state, district or local levels, are working in isolation and their services are not provided in a co-ordinated manner. Most of the patients visit all these hospitals and are examined afresh by all of them resulting in wastage of efforts and resources. The medical staff prescribe medicines to patients without having a proper awareness of his previous treatment.

How can we get out of this chaos to design a system of patient care? The answer is introduction of Regionalization. Regionalization connotes the development of graded patient care within a defined geographical or functional area from lower to higher levels adapting the health services to the characteristics and needs of the area and thus ensuring the optimum utilization of resources. The essential characteristics of regionalization are:[33]

(a) Two-way flow of patients.
(b) Two-way flow of records.
(c) Two-way flow of services.
(d) Two-way flow of personnel.
(e) Mobile units.
(f) Centralized administration and decentralized execution.
(g) Co-ordinating Education Programme for the Region.
(h) Communication and Transport between components.
(i) Co-ordination with other community health services.

Thus, regionalization would ensure the best utilization of time of the specialists and provision of comprehensive health care to the patients nearer their homes with all the benefits of specialities. The regional area should neither be too large nor too small but should be such as to ensure adequate span of attention. It would also automatically develop referral system scientifically. The referral system presents the following five aspects:[34]

(a) It has to be built into the organisational structure of the medical services of a country. The rule should be that only when one unit cannot provide what a patient needs should the patient be referred for the next higher unit in the chain.
(b) The referral system has to be organized both internally and externally. 'Internally' means that patients in the hospital have

to be referred from the in-patients to the out-patients department just as soon as their health situation permits. The 'externally' referred system exists among the several institutions on different levels of the hierarchy.

(c) The referral system, must be established for the purpose of diagnosis and treatments and used for both in-patients and out-patients.

(d) It is a two-way system. Patients should be referred to higher level institutions for diagnosis and treatment when necessary, but they should also be referred to the referring institution as soon as possible.

(e) The referral system concerns not only patients and diagnostic facilities but also the personnel of the medical services. This is also a two-way system, so that human to knowledge and skills are utilized fully and are continually developed through consultations and the interchange of ideas and experience.

The specialists from the regional hospital must come to the District hospital and the specialist from the District hospital to the health centre on a regular basis as consultants to hold specialist clinics and give guidance; the medical and para-medical personnel should go to the higher level institution regularly for in-service training.

Lack of Administrative Capability

Hospital administration is a science as well as an art. The hospital administration has become complex and requires administrative capability to solve its managerial problems to provide the optimum care to the patients. It is, therefore, necessary that the peons charged with the efficient running of the hospitals are trained in the managerial techniques and tools which may be applied by them for getting the best out of the resources available.

Lack of Effective Public Relations

Hospitals should try to establish cordial, equitable and, therefore, mutually profitable relations between the hospitals and their beneficiaries. The patients mostly complain of discourteous behaviour of hospital staff especially at the lower level. This irritates the patients and their relatives. The test of the efficiency of a hospital is the satisfaction of the beneficiaries. The sympathetic and courteous behaviour of hospital staff would have a soothing and lasting effect on patients and their relatives. It is suggested that all hospital personnel must inspire confidence and put the nervous patients and relatives at ease.

"The hospital today is more than the combination of medical and therapeutic treatment by specialists, greater and refined medical and surgical knowledge and ever better and more effective facilities and equipment. It includes these factors as the core of its efficient operation but an additional dimension—one which is too often ignored or at least minimized—is the human and social element in the structure of the organisation."[35]

Lack of Dedicated Staff and Government Organisational Structure

The ideal of service must be encouraged among the personnel responsible for health care. It is the responsibility of the hospital authorities to set the pattern for the philosophy of patient care. It was rightly mentioned by Gardner:

> "No society can reach heights of greatness unless in all fields critical to its growth and creativity there is an ample supply of dedicated men and women."[36]

The patients also complained of the lack of co-ordination between supportive services and the medical services. Most of the patients complained of the non-availability either of their X-ray report or other laboratory reports. They go on wasting their time in tracing their reports. Besides, many patients complained that preferential treatment is given to friends and relatives of the hospital staff. Many patients complained of the non-availability of medicines. Besides, patients are referred to other departments which results in great delays for the treatment to be given to them because of unsatisfactory co-ordination among the various departments of the hospital. It is suggested that:

(1) To encourage polite and courteous behaviour of the staff towards the patients, orientation and in-service training opportunities should be provided to the staff.
(2) Out-patients should be properly guided by the doctors issuing prescriptions regarding the procedure to be followed to get their blood, urine, stool, etc. samples tested.
(3) Laboratories may be modernized and out-dated equipment replaced as early as possible to improve the accuracy of the test results because these tests form the basis of the medical treatment which the patients are to be imparted.

Further, it is suggested on the basis of the observations by the authority that the patients may be issued the slips on arrival on which may be indicated the probable time of his examination by the doctor. The following steps could also be taken to improve matters:

(a) Effective co-ordination should be established between the medical services and the supportive services to ensure promptness and clarity.
(b) Effective co-ordination and co-operation must be ensured among the various departments of the hospital to help the patients in

diagnosing their ailments. It is suggested that a medical board may meet once a week where all the specialities may be represented and the patients needing the attention of more than one speciality may be asked to attend the board.

(c) A receptionist well-versed with the functioning of hospital system may be appointed to guide the patients to approach the hospital properly.

(d) There is a need of play cards and signboards to guide the patients and their relatives.

(e) Provision of cheap and quality goods to be used by the patients or their relatives.

(f) Arrangement of stay of the relatives in rest houses specially constructed for the purpose.

(g) Hospital beds may be given to patients according to the severity of the diseases rather than other trifle considerations like obliging the VIPs.

In brief, the functioning of the hospital should be organized and re-organized to serve the patients most efficiently. All the personnel engaged in patient care must keep the following definitions of the patient in their minds:

1. The patient is the most important person in the hospital.
2. The patient is not dependent upon us—we are dependent on him.
3. The patient is not an interruption of our work—he is the purpose of it.
4. The patient is not an outsider to our business—he is our business.
5. The patient is a person and not a statistic. He has feelings, emotions, biases and wants.
6. It is our business to satisfy him.

We must attend to all these problems to ensure efficiency of the hospitals. These problems also emanate from a number of constraints on hospital authorities, e.g., shortage of staff at all levels, absence of proper accommodation to provide space to the ever increasing number of patients, shortage of funds, shortage of medicine, shortage of equipment, political and administrative interference, etc. which need to be attended to by the Government to provide satisfactory hospital services. Besides, the patients and their relatives must co-operate with the hospital authorities to make the best use of the available resources. Thus, we shall to have a three-pronged attack—increasing internal efficiency, mobilizing Government support and enlisting people's co-operation to ensure the reputation, prestige, credibility and viability.

Notes and References

1. Members are elected by People.
2. Ministry of Public Health in Thailand, Bangkok, 1973. This is a piece of doctoral Research by Krienkrai Klimoboul, first Secretary, Thais Embassy, under the guidance of the Author who visited Thailand alongwith the study.
3. Chareon Chittasombat, Presentation of the Government Pharmaceutical Organisation, Bangkok, Conference on Health Economics, May 1974.
4. Chalad Tirapat, Medical Referral System in CBD Project, Bangkok, Mahidoi University, Public Health Faculty, April, 1977.
5. Uthai Sudsukh, Director of the Rural Health Division, Officer of the Under-Secretary of State MOPH, Personal Interview, Bangkok, November 1978.
6. Debhanom Maungman, New Approach to Rural Health Care in Thailand and its possible application to other Development Countries, New Delhi, WHO, South-East Regional Schools of Public Health, 1-3, Nov. 1978.
7. WHO: Technical Report Series, 1968, 396, p. 6.
8. Elen, I. Perry: Ward Management and Teaching, Bailliere, Tindall, London, 1978, p. 2.
9. World Health Organisation, "Thailand", in Fifth Report on the World Health Situation, 1969-74, Geneva, 1975, p. 151.
10. World Health Organisation, Regional Office for South-East Asia, Basic Statistical Information Relating to Health, in WHO South-East Asia Region, New Delhi, July 1978, p. 5.
11. Ministry of Public Health, Division of Public Health Statistics, Public Health Statistics, 1973-74, Bangkok, 1975, pp. 263-67.
12. "Ministry of Public Health", Department of Medical Services, Statistical, Statistical Report, 1975, Bangkok, 1978, p. 25.
13. Official Records of the Ministry of Public Health, Thailand.
14. Narong Sabudi, Director of Divisions of Provincial Hospitals, Ministry of Public Health, Personal Interview, Nov., 1978.
15. World Bank, Thailand, Appraisal of a Popoulation Project, Report No. 1663—TH, 18 January, 1978, p. 7.
16. Prawase Wasi, Professor at Siriraj Hospital Medical Faculty, Personal Communication, November 1978.
17. Narong Sabudi, Director of the Division of Provincial Hospitals, Ministry of Public Health, Communication, November 1978.
18. *Ibid.*
19. Samboon Vachrotai, Director of the Department of Health, Ministry of Public Health, Personal Communication, November 1978.
20. South East Asian Medical Information Centre, Seamic Health Statistics, 1978, Tokyo. The rate in the text has been derived from this source.
21. Prawasee Wasi, 9.21.
22. R. Neutra (1948), Architecture of Social Concern in Regions and Mild Climate, Sao Paulo.
23. S.M. Machintosh (1951): What is a Hospital for? WHO unpublished document, WHO/PHA/4.
24. Keith Davis, "The Case for Participative Management", *Business Horizons*, Vol. 6, No. 3, 1963, p. 141.
25. ILO: International Labour Confernece, 33rd Session, Provisional Records, p. 34.
26. Cooper R. Michael, and Wood, T. Michael, "Member Participation and Commitment in group decision-making on influence satisfaction and decision.
27. Norman R.F. Maier, and John, J. Hayes: Creative Management, New York, John Wiley and Sons Inc., 1962, p. 36.

28. Saul M. Katz, "A Methodological Note on Appraising Administrative Capability for Development", in Appraising Administrative Capability for Development, (UN Publication Sales No. E.60 11, H.2) p. 8.
29. *Ibid.*, pp. 99-100, 24, Manson Haire, *et. al.*
30. IIPA, Jawaharlal Nehru and Public Administration, New Delhi, 1975, p. 88.
31. H.A. Gaddard, Principles of Administration applied to Nursing Service, World Health Organisation, Geneva, 1958, p. 34.
32. Timmappaya, Regionalization of Health Care.
33. WHO, SEARO: SEA/RC 23/1, pp. 39-40.
34. Mary D. Shanks and Dorothy A. Kennedy, The Theory and Practice of Nursing Service Administration, McGraw Hill, London, 1965, p. 95.
35. John W. Gardner, Excellence, New York, 1961, Harner and Brothers, p. 154.
36. Edythe Alexander *et al.*, Nursing Service Administration (ed.), New York, C.V. Mosby Co., 1962, p. 63.

9

CHAPTER

Functions and Role of Chief Executive in Secondary and Tertiary Hospitals

In the health system, the top level positions are occupied by Director-General of health services at the Union Level, Director of health services at the state level and district health officers at district level. These top-level health functionaries are called technical chief executives in their respective jurisdiction. Since most of them occupy these higher offices on the basis of seniority, they may not possess insight, vision, depth, and creative intelligence to tackle the health issues. It is very important that Government must select persons with right qualities of head and heart to occupy these positions to inject dynamism in health services. An organisation is like a ladder. At the top of the ladder is the chief executive.

In the sacred book, Bhagvad Geeta, Chapter III, Sloka 21, it has been rightly said that whatever a great man (chief executive) does, that very thing other men also do; whatever standard he sets, the generality of men follow the same.

The success of the organisation depends, to a great extent, upon the personality, interest, ethos, perception and attitude of its chief executive. Therefore, there is a need for great care and forethought before appointing the chief executive of an organisation.

Medical Qualities for Superintendent/Director

A Medical Superintendent/Director is the head of a hospital depending upon the size and complexity of a hospital. Secondary Health Care hospitals are manned by medical Superintendents while tertiary health care has a higher-level post called Director. These posts require both technical as well as administrative knowledge to run the hospital efficiently. Since medical superintendents/Directors are from medical background, they lack administrative skill resulting into poor performance.

The success or failure of the organisation depends to a substantial extent upon the capacity, capability, motivation and perception of the chief executive and his top team. The chief executive has to facilitate the accomplishment of desired objectives with the least friction and the most satisfaction to those for whom the task is done and those engaged in the enterprise. According to Edwin E. Chiselli (American Pshychologist, Vol. 18, No. 10), talented chief executives are well endowed intellectually, gifted with the capacity to direct the efforts of others, self-stimulated to action, confident in their abilities and striving for a position where they can most fully utilize them. Top executives are to provide leadership to the organisation. According to Haimann, "Leadership is the process by which an executive or a manager imaginatively directs, guides and influences the work of others in choosing and attaining specified goals by mediating between the individual and the organisation in such a manner that both will obtain the maximum statisfaction."[1]

To quote Keith Davis, "Leadership is the ability to persuade others to seek defined objectives enthusiastically. It is the human factor which binds a group together and motivates it towards its goals."[2] It is said that a critical part of health and medical reform to promote health executive development and the role that executives play in productivity. Effective management must start from the top and work downward. Standards and reasonable health and medical objectives should be developed from a high degree of involvement and inter-relationship at each level so that no instruction is given or goal set which is not shared and reasonable. In the final analysis, the work performed by an employee at the lowest level cannot be more effective than the work performed by the person setting the goals.[3]

Without the right health and medical chief executives, administration will not merely retard the development process but may even retard the health and medical development effort. The quality of the men placed in top positions is more important than laying down of rules and methods of operation.

The hospital administrator is the key executive of the hospital. Success or failure of the hospital depends to a great extent upon the competence, capability, perception, ethos and dedication of hospital administrators. The most important qualification is technical knowledge and administrative knowledge. Either he should be a postgraduate in hospital administration or has attended courses in hospital administration.

Let us discuss the essential qualities required for medical Superintendent/Director in the field of Administration. So, that they can be effective health and medical leaders.

The secret of right action in reality is not a secret. It does not lie in any formula that we repeat. There is no magic by means of which we can follow the path of idleness and yet make our life productive. No! The secret lies in our own motives, in our power of application. It is not the strong physical vehicle which makes the productive human being; it is skillfulness in action, knowing how to adjust ourselves quickly, how to perform a task with the least expenditure of energy. This is what gives immediate success.[4]

Robert M. Hutchines states, "Thus, all organisations can function and achieve excellence provided all its members strive to pursue the goals of the organisation earnestly, sincerely, whole-heartedly and with dedication."[5]

Our thought is the seed, which determines the fruit of our action. If the seed is good, then the flowers and fruit, which come from the seed, must be good and must prove beneficial to ourselves and others. But if we plant in our hearts a poisonous seed, it will harm not only ourselves but all who come in contact with us. Human life is a great responsibility. Only a thoughtless man will say: I cannot help what happens, I am not responsible. We are constantly influencing ourselves and our fellow-beings by what we think, because our thought shapes our inner nature and we radiate consciously or unconsciously what we are. Let us be wakeful then. Let us be thoughtful in whatever we do. Let us be faithful to our true self; for all blessings must come to us, if we prove ourselves true to our higher nature. (see Chart 9.1)

Work Culture

Health and Medical Leaders must create work culture and not psycho-fancy. Work culture is at the lowest ebbs these days. Bata K. Dey in his Article, 'Work Culture in India—Achievements and Failure' rightly says that culture is not something, which can be imported or transplanted; it must grow from within; it grows, and it does, in fertile soil and congenial climate. Gap in capital equipment or technology can be filled by import. You can even buy management, but not dedication, commitment, culture. How to create that is a million dollar question. An inexpensive answer to such a costly question is that, work culture tends to be congruous with, and is an extension of, the societal, indeed national culture. And the latter, at the moment, is the elusive commodity, despite this country's ancient civilization and old culture. The search is on. And we shall succeed.[6]

Murtaza Mithani, Chairman and Managing Director of Wintech Group in his article, "The High Road", in *The Tribute*, dated June 28, 2000 expects his employees to be committed to their work." As the head of an organisation, I, expect my employees to be innovative, competitive and flexible. They should possess total commitment, be actively involved in every day work, and have no hastiness while interacting. He wants his team to be able to work in synergy with various departments. Failures and challenges should be treated as a stepping-stone to success. Think big, create your own space and help yourself." The health and medical leaders must create a work culture and among health and medical personnel to provide decent health care delivery.

Need of Commitment and Empathy

Quality needs teamwork and mutual understanding. Personnel in health and medical care must work in a team to achieve quality. S.J.

CHART 9.1

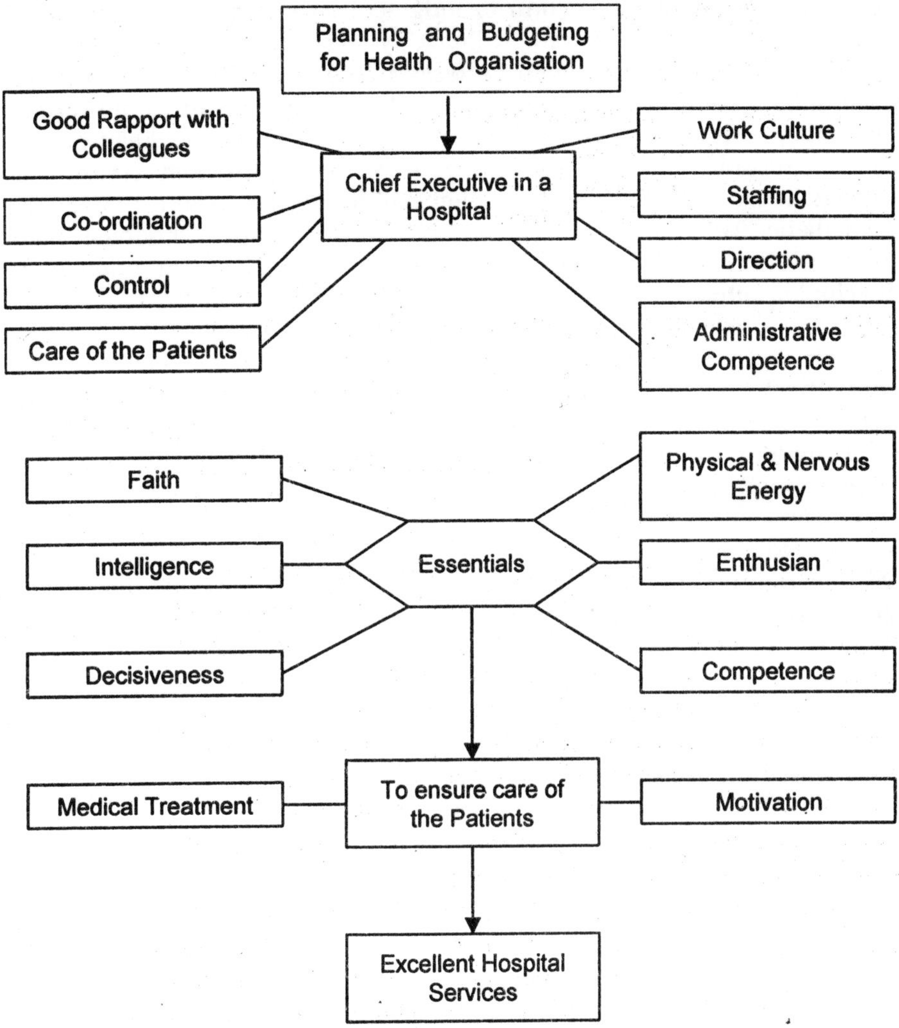

Maricodoss mentions two ingredients of teamwork commitment and empathy. These can be developed by sound health and medical leadership. To quote him:

Commitment is a deep and profound value of emotional intelligence. It means aligning oneself with the goals of a group or organisation. It is applying oneself completely for a cause. People possessing this competence readily make sacrifice to meet larger organisational goals. Hence more than the individual interests, the group's mission or interest takes priority. It is very deep to the extent of sacrificing oneself. It also involves taking sides or taking stance.

Emotionally balanced people are generally empathetic and not sympathetic. Sympathy perpetuates oppression and makes people dependent. Sympathy is a form of judgment. We should therefore avoid being sympathetic towards others. Empathy means understanding the issue or concern that lie behind another's feeling. It is an ability to look at things from other's point of view or to read another's emotions or to put oneself into other's shoes and think from their angle. Avoiding pretension, it enables sensing and responding to a person's unspoken concern or feelings. It can be called the foundation skill for all the social competencies. Empathetic listening is a tremendous deposit in the Emotional Bank Account. Empathy includes understanding others, service orientation, developing others, leveraging diversity and political awareness.[7]

Azim Premji in his article "Leader for the Knowledge Era" rightly suggests that leaders must build star performers and teams. They must not only attract the best of minds to join the organisation but create a strong sense of ownership in them. Ownership is not just offering stock options. It has more to do with an emotional engagement and integration with the organisation.[8]

The most important quality on which actual role of medical and health leadership would depend is the integrity. In this context, Peter Drucker rightly observes that a person who does not have the integrity of character is unfit to be a manager and a gentleman. According to Ordway Tead, the Chief Executive, besides integrity, must possess the following qualities:

(i) Physical and nervous energy;
(ii) Enthusiasm;
(iii) Sense of purpose and direction;
(iv) Technical mastery;
(v) Friendliness and affection;
(vi) Decisiveness;
(vii) Intelligence, and
(viii) Faith.

Chester Barnard mentions the following qualities:[9]

(i) Vitality and endurance;
(ii) Decisiveness;
(iii) Persuasiveness;
(iv) Stability in behaviour;
(v) Intellectual ability, and
(vi) Knowledge.

In spite of the awareness of the importance of the chief executive in an organisation, the selection process of CEOs in public health sector leaves much to be desired and most of the CEOs are appointed purely on seniority or on political affiliations.

We must induct chief executives in health system from any source and as Paul H. Appleby has said, "The persons capable of serving well at high levels are rare birds, they must be sought wherever they may be found and developed by various methods." The need is to change the frame of mind of these chief executives, to make them more adventurous in style, more determined to change the way things are done, perhaps, braver.

There is a need to link the promotion of those personnel to position of the chief executives of health and medical organisations who are result-oriented. A chief executive who cannot take the right decision at the right time cannot aspire to be a successful executive. Therefore, seek those individuals in the organisations who have proved their worth in achieving productivity. To quote A.P. Saxena; Productivity will only be feasible if administration can provide a corpus of administrators, who are knowledgeable and skilful and have a sense of dedication to the goals of health and medical organisations. Such health and medical administrators will have to fulfil several roles. These will include:

(a) As experts who are capable of identifying problems and providing solutions, who will recognize priorities of productivity tasks and apply their expertise to these tasks;
(b) As change agents who know the conditions and directions of change, understand their roles and can direct efforts toward change, keeping the key focus on productivity; and
(c) As leaders who organize and mobilize people and resources, both physical and financial to fulfil the productivity tasks.[10]

There must be a regular appraisal system to screen the functioning of the chief executives. The appointing authorities must be prompt in taking quick decisions regarding the services of the chief executive on the basis of performance appraisal.

C. Rajagopalachari in his lecture delivered under 'Sardar Vallabhbhai Patel Lectures Series' on 14th August 1955 said that character is by no means enough. But without it, let it be remembered, nothing else will be of any avail. It is like daylight, which we are apt to forget on account of its very importance. Therefore, there is a need to ensure that men of right character occupy high positions.

Let me quote a few words a thousand years old, they are as true toady. "The efficiency of the army consists partly in the order and partly in the general, but chiefly in the latter, because he does not depend upon the order, but the order depends upon him." Therefore, there is a great need to select and develop the right chief executives to produce social change and modernization in health system.

If the ideal of health administration is to provide better medical care to the people then we shall have to see that in a given situation we make the best possible use of our resources in terms of personnel and finances to achieve optimum results. For instance, in a developing country life India, the health administrator should normally be concerned with the following:

(a) that the patients are treated as close to their homes as possible in the smallest, cheapest and simply equipped unit such as a sub-centre which is capable of looking after them adequately;
(b) that the medical services should be organized and administrated in such a way that the quality of medical care improves gradually;
(c) that medical care services should be organized from the bottom-up and not from the top-down;
(d) that the services planned should meet the needs of the people;
(e) that the members of the health and medical personnel function as a well-knit team; and
(f) that new categories of health personnel such as multi-purpose health workers and community health workers should be given suitable training and support to provide simple medical care and preventive services to large sections of the community.

Generating Ethical and Moral Values

Chief Executives need to develop ethical and moral standards. Public services must also develop the normative linkages, i.e. they must develop professional standards which should help them in their best performances. Standards are contagious. They spread throughout an organisation, a group, or a society. If an organisation or group cherishes high standards, the behaviour of the individual who enters it is inevitably influenced. They should not develop an excessive sense of self-importance or arrogance. As has been said in the Gita, "We should purse the path of excellence without fear or favour and work ceaselessly to achieve the objectives." Good organisation building has to create around it a bracing atmosphere, a prideful tradition of integrity, excellence and fellowship. Human beings breathe an ethos around them almost unconsciously, these traditions make for that ethos."[11]

Functions of the Chief Executive of Health and Medical Organisations

The functions of the chief executive are increasing at a very fast rate in keeping with the complexity of the health and medical organisation, like the evolution of man from a one-cell animal to a complex and specialized human being. With the growth in complexities, many tools, techniques and instruments have been developed, which can help the chief executive in attending to his modern and complex functions in an efficient manner.

Health system is becoming complex as new problems like non-communicable diseases, disease of modern lifestyle, etc. are raising their head. So the health executives must be well equipped to tackle these problems before these become explosive. Let us enumerate some of the important functions of the health and medical executives.

I. Allocating Work among Line, Staff and Auxiliary Agencies

The chief executive carries out his work through line, staff and auxiliary agencies, as he cannot discharge his functions individually with speed and efficiency.

Line Agency

Line organisation is the oldest and the simplest form of structure. The 'term' line has been borrowed from the military organisation. Line agency is concerned with the carrying out of the primary objects of the organisation and,. thus, deals directly with the persons concerned. The citizens come directly in contract with line agencies. The following are the characteristics of a line agency:

(a) Authority flows from top level to the lower levels through delegation and decentralization to ensure the carrying out of activities at each level commensurate with responsibility.
(b) It consists of direct vertical relationships through various levels of the hierarchy of the organisation.
(c) A superior exercises inherent authority to guide the operations of the persons at lower levels.
(d) All the persons engaged in line operations are directly involved in the fulfilment of the objectives of the organisation.
(e) Lower levels report regularly to the upper hierarchy to keep the top persons duly informed.[12]

In health and medical organisations, the Chief Executive operates through medical and health personnel, as they constitute the key persons in providing medical and health care delivery system.

Staff Agency

The 'staff' idea also took birth in the army where it was observed that, with the growth of the army, the commander could not function only on the support of line agency. The 'line' was supplemented by the 'staff'. The staff refers to the officers who provide advice to line as to how to achieve results. The 'staff' became the think tank of the line agency. The larger the organisation, the more is the need for the staff. Henri Fayol rightly stressed the need of staff, "Whatever their ability and their capacity for work, the heads of great enterprises cannot fulfil alone all their obligations. They are, thus, forced to have recourse to a group of men who have the strength, competence and time, which the head may lack. This group of men constitutes the staff of the management. It is a help, or reinforcement; a sort of extension of the manager's personality to assist him in carrying out his duties. The staff appears as a separate body only in large undertakings and its importance increases with the importance of the undertakings."[13]

Pfiffner and Presthus, mention the following as staff functions:

1. Advising, teaching, consultation.
2. Coordination, not merely through plans but also through human contacts, trouble-shooting and winning over opposition at all levels of organisation.
3. Fact-finding and research.
4. Planning.
5. Contact with other organisations and individuals to know what is going on.
6. Assisting the line without infringing its authority.
7. Sometimes exercising delegated authority from the line commander.[14]

The information technology has made the staff agency indispensable as these agencies through the analysis of information help the line agency in policy-making, planning, decision-making, co-coordinating, control, etc.[15] For example, the Planning Commission in India helps the Union and State Governments in optimizing their resources through planning. Similarly, University Grants Commission helps the Union and State Governments in controlling standards of the university education. Science and technology is providing great opportunities to Governments to provide good services to the people and raise their standard of living. Staff agency can help the line agency in making use of science and technology. L.D. White mentions the following advantages, which can accrue to top line personnel through staff help:

(1) To ensure that the chief executive is adequately and currently informed;
(2) To assist him in foreseeing problems and planning future programmes;
(3) To ensure that matters for his decision reach his desk promptly, in condition to be settled intelligently and without delay, and to protect him against hasty or ill-considered judgments;
(4) To protect his time;
(5) To exclude every matter that can be settled elsewhere in the system; and
(6) To ensure means of ensuring compliances by the subordinate with establishment policy and execution direction.[16]

In tertiary hospitals, medical superintendent, Deputy Director Finance, Deans, etc. help the health and medical Chief Executive.

Auxiliary agencies also help the line agency in the performance of its duties. These are institutionalized services to the line agency. Besides, the auxiliary agency provides expert services in its area of operations economically. Some of the experts make no distinction between staff and auxiliary agencies. Others make the following distinctions:

(i) Auxiliary agencies are operating services while staff agencies are engaged in thinking, planning, research, etc.
(ii) Auxiliary agencies are not directly involved with the major policies of the organisation while the staff is engaged in policy formulation and other advice regarding functioning of the organisation.[17]

Such services make the cost of the product cheaper because of large scale operation and expertise developed. Such organisations in a hospital or health organisations are drug stores, sterilization units, dietary arrangements, etc.

2. *Ensuring Authority and Responsibility Through Active Involvement of all Health and Medical Functionaries*

Authority is the right or power of a person to command other people to do things and to get work done from them. Responsibility means a charge for which one is responsible or accountable. Since it would not do just to hold a person responsible for performing a task without first giving him/her the authority necessary to get the job done, responsibility should always be coupled with commensurate authority. This parity is not mathematical but rather co-extensive both related to the same assignments. According to Ernest Dale, "Authority should be equal to responsibility. That is, if a man is responsible for results of a given operation, he should be given enough authority to take the action necessary to ensure success."[18]

The trend today is to make use of authority in collaboration with colleagues-developing team work. Teamwork is a plan of health care to provide optimum care. Every health functionary should be a team member. The team leader must ensure effective communication to ensure effective participation.

Thus, the fuller staff participation is important both as a means of tapping the practical and intellectual resources of all the health personnel for the benefit of the health organisation and as a way of making work in the organisation more meaningful for everyone.

Such participation though theoretically available in one from or the other is practically non-existent. Most of the health functionaries interviewed revealed that the leaders allow superficial participation, indicating the presence of distrust in the minds of the health personnel.

The following advantages would result from the participative management:

- Participation yields personal commitment and involvement toward organisational goals;
- Participation produces the free flow of communications for an informal work force and atmosphere;

- Control systems are primarily of self-monitoring and guidance and not needed for external control;
- Through participation a leader is likely to obtain stronger motivation towards an objective. Even those who disagree will feel compelled to show loyalty by the sheer weight of the group opinion; and
- A high degree of confidence is shown in subordinates which facilitates interpersonal processes.

These qualities—interest, intelligence, and energy—are fundamental to strength of personality. But they must also be in balance. Unless the individual's traits are so combined that they enable one to win and hold the devotion of other colleagues, one will have little chance of meeting the demands made on him or her. The personnel must be able to feel that they know their leader and can trust because he is the leader of their team. More specially, an executive must have that quality about his or her personality, which enables him or her, without sacrificing integrity of purpose, to lubricate human relationships.

3. Effective use of Delegation and Decentralization to Promote Efficiency of Health Systems

The decentralization and delegation can lighten the burden of the health executives and enable them to devote attention to important aspects of planning, policy-making and coordination. They should clearly make use of delegation and decentralization through staff to achieve the objective of best patient care. According to Fayol, "Everything that goes to increase the importance of subordinate's role is decentralization. Everything which goes to reduce it is centralization."[19]

Besides, proper delegation of authority promotes effective control over operations, due to a clear definition of responsibility and action at each level. When decisions are no longer to be referred up the line, the delay in execution is minimized.[20]

The importance of delegation was also stressed by Goddard: "Delegation of responsibility and authority is an important aspect of successful administration, to place the responsibility for decision at the lowest possible organisational level in order to attain decision as speedily as possible. No administrator can do in detail all the work he is administering, for by definition an administrator manages the work of others. Therefore, the principle of delegation of responsibility should be followed to the utmost extent consistent with efficiency and coordination of policy. The responsibility and authority of individuals should be clearly defined in writing, and the authority placed in each position must correspond to the responsibility which the position carries."[21]

4. Administrative Functions and Responsibilities

Administrative functions constitute the major activities of the chief executive. This involves the management of men, money and material. His administrative functions are summed up by Gullick in the word 'POSDCORB'. These elementary functions have become highly complex and developed. The chief executives must understand this complexity with the help of advanced. Techniques and use them to discharge administrative functions. In health and medical organisations, the Chief Executive lack in performing these functions. There is a need of intensive training to make them efficient. Let us mention these briefly as given by Gullick:

(a) Planning, that is, working out in outline the things that need to be done and the methods for doing them to accomplish the purpose set for the enterprises.
(b) Organizing, that is, the establishment of the formal structure of authority through which work sub-divisions are arranged, defined and coordinated for the defined objective.
(c) Staffing, that is, the whole personnel function of bringing in and training the staff and maintaining favourable conditions of work.
(d) Directing, that is, the continuous task of making decisions and embodying them in specific and general orders and instructions, and serving as the leader of the enterprise.
(e) Coordinating, that is, the all-important duty of interrelating the various parts of the work.
(f) Reporting, that is, keeping those to whom the executive is responsible informed as to what is going, on which, thus, includes keeping himself and his subordinates informed through records, research and inspection.
(g) Budgeting with all that goes with budgeting in the form of planning, accounting and control.[22]

5. Administrative Improvements and Reforms to keep the Health System Efficient

The Chief Executive needs to keep his organisation well designed through improvements and reforms to ensure maximum output.

The chief executive may check the organisation intermittently in the context of the essentials of a good organisation.

Proper appreciation and application of principles of organisation can help in the evolution of a framework required for this purpose, and in ensuring that the organisational structure continue to meet the changing overall needs of the enterprise.

6. Control over Internal Management

Internal functioning of health and medical work is deteriorating day-by-day even in institutions of International importance like AIIMS, PGI, Destnet Hospital, etc.

One of the very important tasks of the chief executive is to supervise, direct and control the performance of the organisation within the scope of law, policy and regulations already established to ensure decent delivery of health services. He can achieve effective supervision through a number of methods, viz., setting of service standards, budgetary control, reporting system, inspections, etc. In order to be effective as a supervisor, he must possess three qualities, i.e. job competence, the ability to guide the subordinates and the personal traits like ability to cooperate and motivate others.

7. Public Relations

People talk of high inefficiency in health and medical institutions. There is no body to listen this inspite of the operation of Right to Information Act, 2005.

The Chief Executive is to ensure participation of people in the formulation and implementation of plans and programmes. Imaginative measures are needed on the part of the chief executive to promote and sustain the interests of the citizens in the administration, to give them a sense of participation in the decisions that immediately affect them and to enable them to contribute to better administration.

8. Implementation of Health and Medical Programmes

Words, written or spoken, are of no use unless they are put into action. The emphasis should be more on performance rather than paper planning. Khalil Gibran has rightly said, that "believing is a fine thing, but placing those beliefs into execution is a test of strength. Many are those who talk like the roar of sea, but their lives are shallow and stagnant, like the rotting marshes. Many are those who lift their heads above the mountain top, but their spirit remains dormant to the obscurity of the caverns."[23]

Swami Vivekananda has also mentioned that we must act decisively to regenerate the potentialities of our country. "Let us all work hard, my brethren; this is no time for sleep. On our work depends the coming of the India of the future. She is there ready waiting. She is only sleeping. Arise and awake, and see her seated here, on her eternal throne, rejuvenated more glorious than she ever was, this Motherland of ours." The Union and State Governments are announcing health and medical schemes for the poor frequently but what is the result? Their half-hearted implementations lead the criticism of Government and loss of already short finances.

9. Creating Commitment to the Ideals of the Health and Medical Organisation

No organisation can develop until and unless the top persons working in the organisation are committed to achieve its ideals. An attitude of dedication to the goals of an organisation should be an indispensable trait of the top leaders. This is their primary requisite to operate and function effectively and efficiently to build self-confidence in themselves and, in turn, in the public.

Administrative functions constitute the major activities of the chief executive. This involves the management of men, money and material for which most of health and medical executives are not well grounded. They instead of giving directions are rather dependent upon their junior staff. This needs to be improved.[24]

10. Generating Ethical and Moral Values in Health and Medical Organisations

Chief executives especially in the foiled of health and medical organisations need to develop ethical and moral standards. Health and medical services must also develop the normative linkages, i.e. they must develop professional standards, which should help them in their best performances. Standards are contagious. They spread throughout an organisation, a group, or a society. If an organisation or group cherishes high standards, the behaviour of the individuals who enters it is inevitably influenced. They should not develop an excessive sense of self-importance or arrogance. As has been said in the Gita, "we should pursue the path of excellence without fear or favour and work ceaselessly to achieve the objective." Good organisation building has to create around it a bracing atmosphere, a prideful tradition of integrity, excellence and fellowship. Human beings breathe an ethos around them almost unconsciously, and these traditions make for the ethos." The health and medical leaders must promote it.

Let me quote Josiah Gilbert Holland, who, through this couplet, mentions the required moral ingredients of the top men, especially health and medical personnel.

God, Give us Men!

God, give us men! A time like this demands; Strong minds, great hearts, true faith and ready hands; Men whom the lust of office does not kill;

Men whom the spoils of office cannot buy;
Men who possess opinions and a will;
Men who have honour; men who will not lie.

A chief executive like Director of a AIIMS is not supposed to carry out by himself all the functions entrusted to his care. The actual day-to-day administration is carried out by the permanent heads of the departments like Cardiology, Urology, Orthopaedies, etc. His actual role is that of "a trouble shooter, a supervisor and promoter of the future programme." The chief executive is a leader to motivate and coordinate the work of others. He has staff and line organisation working under him. His great virtue lies not in himself administrating the work but in making others administer. As Prof. Dimock says, "First, he must keep the enterprise on an even keel. Second, he must delegate everything he can. Third, if the programme is going on satisfactorily, he then has the time and nervous energy with which to chart that lies ahead."

The Chief Executive must infuse such a sense of responsibility among his colleagues so that they work whole heartedly to ensure high quality of life through the provision of preventive, promotive, curative and rehabilitative health services. In this way reputation and prestige of health system would shine.

11. Direct access to the people

A health and medical leader has to be accessible to the people he leads. He cannot afford to run his organisation from behind the closed doors of his office. He has to be on the shop floor, working with the rest of his team and leading from the front.

Robert H. Rosen has stressed that a new way of leading is emerging-one, that is lowly, quietly and decisively transforming our organisations. Never before have our challenges been so great and the need for responsible leaders so profound. Successful enterprises know how to excel and compete. They make the most of their resources-their financial, marketing, and technological capabilities-but it is their people who make the deciding difference they are the engine for growth and productivity. Mature-wise leaders make it happen. He should promote the culture of "I AM OK", YOU ARE OK."

12. Creativity to see work as a potential for creating joy and to experience the happiness of creating something totally new

It is immensely satisfying to do work, which contributes to the lives of others and creates radical transformation in the quality of life of those around us. Creative work, which creates a new form, which is original, is very satisfying. Work which is without an effect, or which can be done equally well by anyone else, never inspires us. We all like to give our special touch to whatever we do. This creates an interesting paradox; whether our responses influence the quality of work or does work influence the quality of our responses? The answer is to go beyond the dichotomy?[25]

13. Leadership

Leadership-medical Superintendent/Directors must provide leadership to technical and non-technical workers working under him. Leadership is the process to direct and co-ordinate the activities of members of an organisation towards the achievement of goals, honestly and efficiently.

A leader is a person who plans, organizes, makes decisions and influences people. Leaders have a positive attitude towards people and towards their work. Leaders are always hopeful; they expect their efforts to lead to success. A number of factors are involved in the ability to lead, including the following:

(a) Insight into human behaviour;
(b) Ability to plan, organize and direct efforts of others;
(c) Decision-making ability on a practical and realistic basis;

(d) Ability to co-ordinate the efforts of others; and
(e) Keep the environment of work place stimulating.[26]

Hospital Administrator can function effectively provided he gets all the facilities like adequate and qualified manpower, adequate building (space), adequate equipment and drugs and sufficient resources to run the hospital. The hospital administrator must also optimize the use of resources and discourage wastages. Hospital Administrator must keep in mind that hospital administration is an art and science, which can make the maximum use of resources for the welfare of the patient. The hospital administration is to achieve results at a given point of time with whatever resources are available to him. That is why it has been said that put a good man in a bad set-up he will make things go through; put a bad man in a good set-up, he will create a mess of the whole situation. Therefore, right selection of the hospital administrator is the *sine-quo-non* for the success of hospital administration.

Let us support with the help of an Article by Attar Singh, "Rajendra Hospital Chronically ill" in *The Tribute,* dated September 2007.

The Government Rajendra Hospital Patiala, once a premier health care institution of Punjab that attracted patients from all over the region, is now in a state of neglect. Lack of funds, government apathy and shortage of specialists are some of the factors that have contributed to the slump in its reputation.

Several specialty departments, including cardiology, urology, and nephrology, are running only for academic purposes. These departments are woefully short of staff, particularly senior faculty, which has resulted in a sharp fall in the number of patients visiting the hospital. Masters courses in paediatrics surgery and plastic surgery have been dropped for the want of senior faculty to teach students. The fate of another course in the department of urology, which had been planned to be introduced, hangs in the balance.

Several senior faculty members of the hospital have left the hospital in the past one decade and started their own practice. The patients that were once treated at the hospital by the doctors are now spotted at the latter's private nursing homes.

The government has done precious little to stem this and there has been no concerted effort to check the exodus of doctors from the hospital.

The facilities at the hospital have also been at the receiving end of the government apathy. This 1,000-bed hospital is faced with a fiscal crisis due to lack of funds. The emergency wing has virtually no medicines at its disposal. The hospital, which is attached to the Government Medical College, is the oldest referral hospital in the State. However, the situation has come to such a pass the doctors struggle to run even emergency procedures without outside support. The emergency department does not get any funds separately and has limited medicines at its disposal. These medicines too are used in extreme emergency situations. The incinerator at the hospital has been out of order ever since its installation over 10 years ago. Hazardous biomedical waste is dumped outside in a corner near the main building of the hospital. The waste, which is carted off by the municipal corporation, has been a constant source of infection at the hospital.

Also, the incinerator, which was purchased in 1991, has never been in operation. Initially, the incinerator could not be used due to a dispute between the private firm that supplied it and the public works department.

Later, the high cost of operation went against its use.

The incinerator room, which is situated near the doctors' hostel, is a picture of neglect with wild overgrowth all around it. The health administrators should possess the following qualities.

Intelligence, Alertness, Verbal, Facility, Originality, Judgment, Dependability, Initiative, Persistence, Aggressiveness, Self-confidence, Desire to excel, Activity, Sociability, Cooperation, Adaptability, Humour, Mental Level, Status, Skill needs and Interest of followers, objectives to be achieved, etc.

If the ideal of health administration is to provide better medical care to the people then we shall have to see that in a given situation we make the best possible use of our resources in terms of personnel and finance to achieve optimum results.

Administrative Functions

1. Administrative Functions constitute one of the major activities of the Chief Executives. This involves management of men, money and material. His administrative functions are summed up by Gullick in the word 'POSDCORB'. Let us mention these briefly:

(a) Planning, that is, working out an outline of the things that need to be done and the methods for doing them to accomplish the purpose set for the enterprise.
(b) Organizing, that is, the establishment of the formal structure of authority through which work sub-divisions are arranged, defined and coordinated for the defined objective.
(c) Staffing, that is the whole personnel function of bringing in and training the staff and maintaining favourable conditions of work.
(d) Directing, that is, the continuous task of making decisions and embodying them in specific and general orders and instructions, and serving as the leader of the enterprise.
(e) Coordinating, that is, the all-important duty of interrelating various parts of the work.
(f) Reporting, that is, keeping those to whom the executive is responsible, informed as to what is going on, which, thus, includes keeping himself and his subordinates informed through records, research and inspection.
(g) Budgeting with all that goes with budgeting in the form of planning, accounting and control.[27]

These elementary functions have become highly complex and developed. The Medical Superintendent/Doctor must understand this complexity with the help of advanced techniques and use them to discharge administrative functions.

2. Understanding and Directing Change

New millennium is going to be different and the new millennium needs leaders who can understand and redirect this change into fruitful changes. Leadership and change are closely linked. An awareness of the changing atmosphere at the workplace calls for leaders who can understand and deal with the changing paradigms of corporate culture. No longer is it enough for a manager to limit his job to doing things on time, within budget and the way they were done yesterday, only five percent better. Leaders are today treading on completely unfamiliar territory where yesterday's rules no longer apply. Uncertainty is now an inescapable fact and things no longer happen in a predictable manner. Innovation is the new mantra for the leaders of today. They make new rules almost as fast as the old ones become redundant. Under these circumstances, it is imperative for a leader to have a clear vision of where his organisation is headed. In the absence of such vision, it is all too easy for organisation, both old and new, to flounder and fail.

3. Emotional Intelligence (EI)

Emotional intelligence is concerned with achieving one's goals through the ability to manage one's own feelings and emotions, to be sensitive to, and influence other key people, and to balance one's motives and drives with conscientious and ethical behaviours. The following are the characteristics of EI:

(a) Inter-personal sensitivity covering competencies like listening and sensitivity.
(b) Motivating, including impact and energy;
(c) Emotional Resilience;
(d) Influence and Adaptability covering both influencing and negotiating ability and being adaptable in various types of situations and cultures.
(e) Decisiveness and assertiveness.
(f) Leadership including motivating other people.

4. Code of Ethics for the Medial Personnel in India

The document prepared by Department of Administrative Reforms and public grievances has chalked out a Code of Ethics, which need implementation. The objective of Code is to prescribe standards of integrity and conduct that are to apply in the medical and health services. The principles stated below underlie and supplement the rules and laws to regulate the public and private conduct of various health and medical services.

Selflessness: Holders of public office should take decisions solely in terms of the public interest. They should not do so in order to gain financial or other material benefits for themselves, their family, or their friends.

Integrity: Holders of public office should not place themselves under any financial or other obligation to outside individuals or organisations that might influence them in the performance of their official duties.

Objective: In carrying out public business, including making public appointments, awarding contracts, or recommending individuals for rewards and benefits, holders of public office should make choice on merit.

Accountability: Holders of public office are accountable for their decisions and actions to the public and must submit themselves to whatever scrutiny is appropriate to their office.

Openness: Holders of public office should be as open as possible about all the decisions and action that they take. They should give reasons for their decisions and restrict information only when the wider public interest clearly demands.

Honesty: Holders of public office have a duty to declare any private interest relating to their public duties and to take steps to resolve any conflicts arising in a way that protects the public interest.

Leadership: Holders of public office should promote and support these principles by leadership and example.

These principles apply to all aspects of public life. The Committee has set them out here for the benefits of all who serve the public in any way. Medical Profession needs to follow the following:

- Health and Medical Professionals must maintain highest standards of behaviour so that their actions and decisions result in the benefits for industry, employees, customers, shareholders and society.
- Health and service must conform to the commitment promised to patients.
- Patients must be given best possible service and treated with respect and fairness.
- Best way of promoting high standards of medical practices is through self-regulation. The Code has been designed as an instrument of self-regulation to serve as voluntary guideline towards better quality of life and higher standards of medical practices.

Health Leaders have to work hard to remove callousness, negligence, non-punctuality among doctors working in hospitals under their charge. The doctors are deteriorating in their efficiency, as they remain busy in their private practice. The Hospital Leaders must act decisively to solve existing and emerging problems.

Records Management in a Hospital

Records Management is a programme that involves the functions of creating, administering, retaining, submitting and destroying records. Herbert Hoover has rightly mentioned the advantages of proper record-keeping when he says: "A decision is only as good as the facts on which it is based." Records are the memory of the internal and external transactions of an organisation. By external transaction we mean the correspondence between the organisation and its client-beneficiaries as well as supporters. By internal transaction is meant the dealings on external transactions by persons in the organisations at all levels. Records contain a written evidence of the activities of an organisation in the form of letters, circulars, reports, contracts, invoices, vouchers, minutes of meeting, books of accounts, etc. Thus, the records management is concerned with the retaining, submitting and destroying of records. The proper maintenance of these records in right quantity and quality is the essence of records management. The success of this record-keeping would be reflected in the timely availability of all the records. In the context of Medical Records, Dr. McGibony had said: "A chronicle of the pageantry of medical and scientific progress is found in the hospital records."

The medical record is a clinical, scientific, administrative and legal document relating to patient care in which is recorded sufficient data, written in sequence of vents to justify the diagnosis and warrant the treatment and end results.

Essential of Records Management

1. Comprehensive

The records should be such as can be easily understood when retrieved back for planning, policy-making and decision-making. The language used should be simple and understandable.

2. Properly Planned

The records be screened at regular intervals of time to weed out the information not required for future. In this way, we can reduce the paper work to twenty-five per cent. This would indirectly help us in locating the desired information quickly.

3. Economical

We should manage the records economically so that we may achieve more with minimum efforts.

4. Accurate

The records should be accurate otherwise its utility would be doubtful.

5. Timely

The time taken in retrieving the information should be as short as possible. Reducing retrieval time is essential for effective materials management.

6. Classification

Records must be classified to be of practical use. The classification be done either on the basis of subjects or chronology.

According to Dr. K. Pennathur, records should:

1. Serve specific needs.
2. Have specific objectives and purposes.
3. Be kept to a minimum with respects to number, scope and content
4. Be designed for least expensive handling.
5. Be up-to-date.
6. Be worth their cost.
7. Be related directly to tabulations and reports that will stem from them.
8. Be available when needed.
9. Be considered valuable by supervisors and lines management.

Contents of Medical Records

Broadly medical records at lower level include:

1. The information regarding the characteristics of population collected through baseline survey of villages which provides details about health problems and the health needs in the community. This is useful for preparing a program of health services, education for the area and priorities for health activities.
2. Facts about births and deaths, besides serving as an indicator of population growth, can help to focus attention on target groups for specific health services.
3. The records of pregnant mothers can help to sort out high-risk cases needing institutional delivery, normal pregnancy, cases which can be attended by trained Dai or by female health worker at home for post-natal and infant care at a later stage.
4. Morbidity data about various illnesses occurring in the area can serve as an index of the state of health of the population and prevalent diseases in the area and if any epidemic occurs.
5. Information about reproductive couples, especially together with data on number of living children of each couple, is invaluable for carrying out an effective programme for family planning education and motivation.

6. Records are also most helpful in planning for health education programmes.
7. A carefully kept record of stock of drugs, dressings and other equipment received and issued will help in knowing when and how to indent the items required for sub-centre.[28]

The medical record is clear, concise and accurate history of the patient's life and illness, written from the health and medical point of view. The story of the patients illness narrated by the patient, observations made by nurses and the comments and treatment given by the doctors are recorded in the medical record. Thus, the medical record comprises three general sections:

(i) a general section covering administrative and personal data. The socio-economic record of the patient includes: The name of the Patient, Father's or Husband's Name, Age, Sex, Religion, Income, Patient's Address and the Address of nearest relative. Other administrative information which are included are—The data of admission, The in-patient number, The name of the nursing unit and bed number. This sheet is prepared in the Central Admitting Office;

(ii) a nurses section wherein are noted the observations of the trained nurses and the details of treatment administered. This part of the medical record consists of graphic charts relating to Temperature, Pulse, Respiration, Blood Pressure and any other observations maintained, intake output chart and medicine administered; and

(iii) a medical section containing statements on the studies, observations, conclusions and activities of the attending doctors or of the intern or the resident working under him. The medical section of the record consists of the entire medical history of the patient. It contains:

- History sheet
- Physical examination sheet
- Provisional diagnosis
- All the investigation reports
- Physicians order sheet
- Treatment, medical or surgical
- Anesthesia record
- Operation record
- Obstetric record
- Consultancy report
- Progress report
- Final diagnosis
- Discharge summary

- If death—Cause of death
- Autopsy report.

Men, Money and Materials are the keys to development. We generally find that senior functionaries of health do not pay the desired attention to the materials management resulting in inefficiency. They even forget that 40 per cent of resources are spent on expendable and non-expendable equipment. "Materials management is one of the key factors for improving performance of any health unit. Higher inventories like medicines saddle an organisation with avoidable costs besides blocking scarce funds which might be required by the health institution for its own operations for some other essential development programmes. Proper Management of materials, therefore, assumes considerable importance in functioning of health services as well as in national economy." There are eight primary and seven secondary objectives, which can ensure the best performance and use of materials (Equipment and Drugs). Many of these objectives conflict with each other. Balancing of these various conflicting objectives is one of the main tasks before the materials manager. The better this balance is done, the better the efficiency of the materials management.

Essential Principles

Broadly, we can say that there are seven principles of materials management, which must be kept in mind to ensure good results. Health managers must follow these principles or rights. We can decide about these rights by using the Management Techniques mentioned later:

(a) Right items;
(b) Right quantity;
(c) Right price;
(d) Right source;
(e) Right delivery;
(f) Right method, and
(g) Right people.

Essentials

Materials management must ensure the fulfilment of the following objectives:

(a) To develop a system of supplies whereby there will be right quantity of stock of items properly stored, easily retrievable and distribute close to the points of usage, whenever required, at a given time. In case, there is not enough stock, the work in the organisation may have to be stopped and the men and equipment will remain idle. On the other hand, if there is overstocking of materials, it will unnecessary block capital in inventories.

(b) The reduction in inventory costs- both carrying cost and ordering cost.
(c) To ensure that the resources available are used most effectively and the stores are purchased at the most economical price consistent with the quality.
(d) To bring about co-ordination among the various sections in the organisation, i.e. in a hospital to bring co-ordination among the Doctor, Nurse, Storekeeper and the Medical Superintendent.
(e) To ensure that the formulations do not suffer.

A thorough understanding and use of the techniques of materials management would help in ordering supplies when needed, controlling their use, keeping them safely and in working order, and also motivating the personnel in the best use of equipment and drugs. This also prevents the chance of non-availability of equipment and drugs as being out of stock of these reduces the usefulness of the hospital system. Since the modern health institutions are becoming complex it is adviseable for the health experts who are managing these institutions to make use of these techniques for better equipment and drugs management.

Human Resource Development, an important operational objective for the 21st century is, therefore, to improve personnel systems, develop manpower planning in health services, and expand the opportunity for education and training of personnel to achieve developmental goals as it is the human capacities, which transform the passive natural resources into active agents of production. Most developing countries confront the immense task of reforming their system of personnel administration so that they will assist rather than hinder development programmes. Thus, the most important task is the development of sound personnel planning and improvement of the policy-making and implementation capabilities of personnel units in health care administration.

Ninth Plan priorities for Human Resources Development for Health include:

- Creation of a district data base on requirement, demand and availability for health manpower in the Government, Private and voluntary sectors.
- Periodic updating of information on:
- Requirement of different categories of health manpower.
- Availability of health manpower.
- Health manpower production based on the needs.
- Improvement in quality of under-graduate/post-graduate education.
- Efforts to promote appropriate health manpower distribution.
- Continuing medical education for skill upgradation and appropriate people and programme orientation.
- Continuing multi-professional education for promoting teamwork and inter-sectoral co-ordination.

Significance of Human Resources

HRD in brief is transformation of Potential Human Resources into Kinetic Human Resources for optimization of the potential capacity of employees. It has been rightly said in a study of the Capacity of United Nations Development System that "Human rather than capital is the key to development."[29] Development is not a mechanical process. It is a human enterprise and its success will depend ultimately on the skill, quality and motivation of the persons associated with it.

We may thus define HRD as a process of the development of employees through training, performance appraisals, potential development exercises, communication policies, job enrichment programmes, etc. and building of an organisational climate which may encourage openness, risk-taking, role clarity, awareness of employee's responsibility, increased communication, improvement of personnel policies, management styles, etc. so that employees may be effective in translating their potential energy into kinetic energy and the organisation may be benefited in terms of better image, higher productivity, better utilization of resources, etc. HRD in a way involves total management and for HRD to be effective, we have to introduce changes in management at all levels.

Drugs Management

The provision of appropriate drugs of good quality at affordable cost is essential for the success of disease control programmes. Equally important is to restrict, and if possible, eliminate, the use of irrational drug formulation, detect and eliminate spurious drugs. The Central Government is responsible for the control over the quality of imported drugs, control over the manufacture and import of new drugs into the country, amendments to the Drugs and Cosmetics (D and C) Act and Rules, coordinate the activities with the State Drug Control Authorities for uniform implementation of D and C Act and Rules, laying down standards for drugs and updating Indian Pharmacopoeia, training of drugs analysts and drugs inspectors and licensing of whole human blood and blood products, large volume parenterals, sera and vaccines. Provisions for strengthening Drug Control Organisation in the States and the Centre were made in the Eighth Plan. However, the implementation of the Scheme has been patchy and tardy.

Supply of essential drugs, vaccines/devices holds the key to success in any disease control programme. Funds for drugs used for primary, secondary and tertiary care centers come partly from the State funds and partly from Central Plan funds. Procedures for procurement and distribution vary and bottlenecks in these at the national and State level have been recurrent problems. Inefficient indenting procedures adversely affect drug procurement. Poor inventory management results in unsatisfactory drug procurement and distribution. Some states such as Tamil Nadu have attempted strengthening drug procurement and distribution through formation of a Medical Service Corporation. This

Corporation has drawn up an essential drug list, improved purchase and storage of drugs and organized efficient drug distribution within the states and has brought about effective drug distribution within the state and has brought about effective inventory control. During the Ninth Plan efforts in improving procurement and inventory control and distribution for drugs at Central and State level are to receive priority.

Drugs are very important in a hospital and, therefore, these must be used with due care, skill, knowledge, and need. The drugs can be dangerous if not administered properly. Wasting of drugs also results in wastage of scarce resources of the hospital. Every state must prepare a list to suggest the quantity and quality of drugs required at different levels of health institutions in the country. A World Health Publication has rightly summed up the purpose of Drug Management from different angles, which are mentioned below.

> "The purpose of management of drugs is to use drugs wisely and avoid wasting drugs, and therefore to have enough for patients needs."[30]

CONCLUSION

Time management would not only be beneficial to the executives but would also provide more opportunities to the people to share their ideas and views with the administration and thus we would be able to lay the solid foundation for People's Participation, Development and Modernization.

Prabhat Kumar in his Article, "A Responsive and Effective Government" rightly suggests that "we forget that time is our most valuable resource, the only one that is absolutely non-renewable. No one has the right to waste it, every one should control his own time. It can be given but never should be taken away by another. Unfortunately, lateness is the rule in Government and waiting is a national past time."[31]

The development and modernization of developing countries can be accelerated by an efficient time management. It has been observed that Personnel in Administration are not utilizing their time for the assigned job. They are wasting a lot of time in unnecessary and trivial activities which are non-productive. We must manage our time purposefully to build Modern India, otherwise we would remain and under-developed country as time and tide wait for none.

The management requires a high degree of self-discipline. The habit of entertaining casual visitors during office hours must be shunned ruthlessly. Designate a prime time may be an hour or so, during the working hours, which is strictly your own time and distractions should never be permitted to interfere. It is for us to manage time and not the other way round.

Top personnel in health administration must be the persons with vision, initiative and desire to achieve the operational goals with dedication and perseverance. In the words of Jawaharlal Nehru, "No administrator, I suppose, or anyone else for the matter of that, can really do first class work without a sense of function, without some measures of a crusading spirit. I am doing this, I have to achieve this, as a part of great movement in a big cause. That gives a sense of function, not the sense of individual's narrow approach of doing a job in an office for a salary or wage, something connected with your life's outlook or anything, perhaps being interested, as people inevitably are, one's personal preferment in that particular work."[32]

The greatest efficiency and productivity will flow from the efforts of those who find satisfaction in their work and conditions of service, who sense an awareness of usefulness of their functions, who feel encouraged to move ahead and to meet new challenges, who perceive their working environment as one in which high standards of performance are maintained and rewarded and not one in which indolence and incompetence can be ignored or even protected and rewarded. Motivation can do miracles, as a motivated worker can achieve more than an expert with no motivation. Leaders must, therefore, devote considerable time and effort in planning for, and achieving, high levels of motivation and morale. In such a situation, we would achieve goal congruence, i.e. identity between the individual goals and the organisational goals.

Dr. H. Mahler is very critical about the inability of health workers in contemporary society to influence those social and environmental factors which truly determine public health. He states:

> "There persist widespread negative attitudes among health professionals towards the health care of the poorest strata in the rural and urban population in the developing countries. Most of these attitudes imply—with a repetitiveness of an old gramophones records caught in a narrow, arrogant, condescending and indifferent groove—that these poor people are too apathetic, too superstitious, too illiterate to benefit from the health care potentially availability to them. Health professionals and those who train them should be much more radicals in accepting a social responsibility for the health needs of the people in these poor rural-urban communities so that they can act as agents for change."[33]

Thus, we can say that there is a need to train health administrators and workers in the new art of Public Health Administration so that they can take the benefits of the modern science to the common man and maintain the spirit of Geneva Declaration."[34]

Now being admitted to the profession of Medicine, I solemnly pledge to concentrate my life to the service of humanity. I will give respect and gratitude to my deserving teacher. I will practice medicine with conscience and dignity. The health and life of my patients will be my first consideration. I will hold in confidence all that my patients confides in me.

I will maintain the honour and noble traditions of the medical profession. My colleagues will be my brothers. I will not permit considerations of race, religion, nationality, party politics or social standing to intervene between my duty and my patient. I will maintain the utmost respect of human life. Even under threat I will not use my knowledge contrary to the laws of humanity. These promises I make freely and upon my honour."

The same feelings has been expressed in the Tokyo Declaration. To quote the preamble to the Declaration of Tokyo:

> "It is the privilege of the medical doctor to practice medicine in the service of humanity, to preserve and restore bodily and mental health without distinction as to the persons to comforts and to ease the sufferings of his or her patients."[35]

Prof. J.S. Neki has rightly said in this connection that "to help, to heal, to reconstruct, to comfort-and all along the line to act with compassion-all these bear testimony to the moral consciousness of the doctor. Whatever the new strains imposed upon medical ethics, this structure will survive and continue to guide doctors in their professional conduct. Legal and juridical obligations they have, of necessity, to fulfil. But these are not genuine ethics. Genuine ethics has to be ingrained into character and does not have to depend upon external controls.[36]

- Excellent Hospital Services
- Medical Treatment
- Motivation
- To ensure care of the Patients
- Competence
- Decisiveness
- Physical and Nero's Energy
- Enthusian
- Intelligence
- Faith
- Essential
- Administrative Competence
- Direction
- Staffing
- Work Culture
- Care of the Patients
- Control
- Co-ordination
- Good Rapport with Colleagues
- Chief Executive in a Hospital
- Planning Budgeting Organisation

Notes and References

1. Haiman, Professional Management, Eurasia Publishing House, New Delhi, 1966, p. 440.
2. Keith Davis, Human Relations at Work, McGraw-Hill, New York, 1967, pp. 96-97.
3. Remarks by Richard A. Shelling, Governor of Vermont, Conference Report, Recapturing Confidence in Government, Public Personnel Management Reform, February 1979.
4. Management Techniques: Principles and Practices, "Ecology of Management Techniques, 2001, p. 29
5. M.R. Pinto, Values in Public Services, *IJPA*, January-March, 1989.
6. Bata K. Dey, *IJPA*, April-June 1989, p. 175.
7. Robert H. Rosen, Learning to lead, in Frances Hassellein *et al.* "The Peter Drucker Foundation," 1997, p. 302.
8. Tead Ordway, The Art of Leadership, McGraw Hill, New York, 1935, p. 83
9. Cheser Barnard, The Functions of Executive, Harvard University Press, Cambridge, 1938, p. 260.
10. Dilip Thakor, "Successive Planning in India Industry, in *Business World*, August 31-Sept. 13, 1981.
11. Moddie, A.D., The Brahmanical Culture and Modernity, Asia Publishing House, New York, pp. 106-14.
12. S.L. Goel, Advanced Public Administration, New Delhi, Sterling, 1994, p. 88.
13. Henri Fayol, in Gullik and Urwick (eds.), Papers in the Science of Administration, p. 86.
14. Pfiffner and Presthus, *op. cit.*, p. 86.
15. S.L. Goel, *op. cit.*, p. 88.
16. S.D. Mooney, Principles of Organisation, p. 41.
17. S.L. Goel, *op. cit.*, p. 91.
18. Ernest Dale, Management—Theory and Practice, 1973, Tokyo, McGraw Hill, p. 149.
19. Henri Foyal, General and International Management, London, Pitman, 1956, p. 26.
20. L.D. White, Encyclopaedia of the Social Science, The Macmillian, 1951, Vol. V, p. 43.
21. H.A. Goddard, Principles of Administration Applied to Nursing Services, WHO, Geneva, 1958, p. 85.
22. Gulick, Luther, 'Notes on the Theory of Organisation', in Luther Gulick and L. Urwick, Papers on the Science of Administration, New York, Institute of Public Administration, 1937, p. 13.
23. Gibran Khalid, Between Night and Morn, The Philosophical Library, New York, 1971, pp. 8-9.
24. Moddie, A.D., The Brahmanical Culture and Modernity, Asia Publishing House, New York, pp. 106-14.
25. S.L. Goel, Management Techniques: Principles and Practices, Leadership, p. 265.
26. *Ibid.*, *op. cit.*, p. 256.
27. Gullick, Luther, 'Notes on the Theory of Organisation in Luther Gullick and L. Urwick, Papers on the Science of Administration, New York, Institute of Public Administration, 1937, p. 13.
28. NIHFW, Management Training Modules For Health Assistants (Male and Female), New Delhi; 1987, p. 7.
29. UN: A Study of the Capacity of the UN Development System, Vol. I, Geneva, 1969.

30. WHO: On Being Incharge, Geneva, 1980, pp. 160-61 and 174-75.
31. Prabhat Kumar, A Responsive and Effective Government, in Management in Government, January-March, 2000, p. 3.
32. Jawaharlal Nehru and Public Administration, *IJPA*, New Delhi, 1975, p. 88.
33. Text of Address by Dr. H. Mahler, to the Thirteenths Session of Regional Committee of South-East Asia.
34. Geneva Declaration.
35. I swear by Apollo by Christian Viedma, *World Health*, July 1979, p. 28.
36. J.S. Niki, Medical Ethics, *World Health*, July, 1979.

10

CHAPTER

Functions and Role of Health Professionals in Secondary and Tertiary Hospitals

The profession of medicine is highly respected in the society and that is why doctor is considered as the image of God. Doctors are angels to the suffering humanity. Doctors whether they are only Graduate or postgraduates or possess other high qualifications need some qualities to serve the humanity as well as get job satisfaction. It is difficult to mention all the qualities. We mention here some of the important qualities which are basis for the efficient functioning of doctors.

Human development and improving the quality of life of people are the ultimate goals of all activities of any government. Quality of life and development can be achieved only with healthy mind and body. Health is the vital ingredient of all development activities.[1]

That poor socio-economic conditions worsen the health of the people is well known and accepted by all. Neither wealth nor technological progress will ensure the health of any nation unless they are equitably distributed among its entire population. The United States, arguably the wealthiest, the most powerful and the most technologically advanced among the nations of the world ranks 46th in the human index—behind even economically weaker countries such as Cuba—precisely because the bonanzas of progress have not reached as many as 45 million (More than 15%) of her citizens who do not have health insurance. No country can shine if it is blinded by the glare of glittering wealth and media hype to take notice of the poor and deprived masses existing beyond the arc lights of rightist elitism.

Social inequalities similarly have a profound adverse effect on health and health care delivery. Perhaps the most neglected and least understood among them, and one that is prevalent universally, is the differential impact of gender on disease and health care seeking behaviour. Admittedly the impact is more on women; but men are also not immune to it. Unfortunately little or no attention is paid to the gender dimensions of health by teaching institutions and medical curricula anywhere in the world.[2]

Health Care has long ceased to be the exclusive preserve of the doctors. We, as doctors, know that effective and efficient health care can only be delivered if all members of the team work in a concerted fashion. No matter who we are or what is our particular field of specialization, no matter whether we are physicians, surgeons, anesthesiologists, dental specialists, nurses, physiotherapists, laboratory technologists or any of the several allied health scientists, our common goal is to help heal the sick through our areas of expertise.[3]

1. Competence

The education and training to medical personnel must be thorough so that they can face the challenges of health faced by patients and society. The Doctor who is competent in his field can help the patients with confidence and faith. Competence of a doctor is lifting of his performance to higher standard, the building of he is personality beyond to normal limitations. However, competence acquired in a medical college is not sufficient as science and technology is developing fast, therefore, there is a need to keep in time with the latest developments in his area. This would muster a lot of strength to him and he would be motivated to move in medical field higher and higher. This is called getting continuous medical education. Medical knowledge is not static but dynamic. If we wish to safeguard the future, it is high that all those who are engaged in medical profession should get concerned with creativity and change that is take a second look at their work system and style as well as contour of advanced medical technology to promote creativity and total change if not a revolution.

You are poised on the threshold of a world of opportunities. Some of you will choose to be scientists, discoverers and inventors; some will opt for teaching; but most of you, I am sure, will prosper in professional practice. Whichever fields you may choose, or find yourself in, I wish you a glorious future. But please do remember always that our fellow human being—their health, happiness and meaningful life—are the ultimate reason for our existence. Treat them with care, compassion and empathy. Treat them, as we would like to be treated. Nothing more is required; nothing less is acceptable. Go out and conquer the world by winning the hearts and minds of the people through professional competence, dedicated service and humane treatment.[4]

Unquestionably a physician (and by the word 'physician', I include a doctor practicing any specialty he or she chooses), must need be competent. It is the university and its teachers, which provide and equip you with this competence. However, the acquisition of a degree in my opinion is merely a license to practice medicine is your chosen specialty your consummation as a physician can only come after you have gone out into the world of sickness and suffering and grappled long with death and disease. Unless the unfortunate values of present-day living have poisoned your mind, dulled your sensibilities and blunted your sympathies, you will learn that there is more to a true physician than the mere knowledge of the science of medicine. It is only when the art and philosophy of medicine have encrusted science, and have permeated into its very core that you will have blossomed into a true physician. Bear in mind that competence needs to be perpetually reinforced and renewed. A physician is first and foremost a student for life. Young and old, we are all undergraduates in the school of experience.

I will not detail what constitutes competence. But I would urge you in this machine-age not to forget the use of your eyes, ears and hands. None are so blind as those who have eyes and yet not see, or so deaf as those who have ears and yet not hear, or so unfeeling as those who can touch and yet not feel. The art and science of medicine is not taught by books; it is acquired only if you have lived with disease and made your home at the bedside of patients.

Competence however is not enough. Competence must be associated in even greater measure with what is best termed 'humanity'. Humanity is the sensibility, which enables a physician to feel for the distress and suffering of a patient, prompting him to provide relief. Humanity embraces both care and compassion; it forms the core of a doctor-patient relationship, a relationship which has been increasingly eroded in our present age.[5]

Medical sciences is becoming more knowledge-oriented, integrating inputs from many allied fields, and advances are taking place in all these fields. The common saying that 'education is a lifelong process' is more true in the case of medical experts. Keeping track of the advances elsewhere in the world and fetching those advances to the teeming millions in the rural areas in the country using a cost effective, timely delivery system calls for updated knowledge and continuing efforts. Yet another challenge, the doctors must be cognizant is that the society is increasingly becoming educated and demanding, and thus, have rising expectations. The future knowledge society needs constant updating of skills and extraordinary teamwork across multi-disciplinary fields. I always remind the youngsters that being best in the country is not just enough; one has to be best in the world.

Let me leave with you a word of advice given more than 100 years back by Sir William Osier, the first physician-in-chief of John Hopkins Hospital, and the author of many books including the one titled, "The Principles and practice of Medicine":

> ". . . . Learn to see, learn to hear, learn to feel, learn to smell, and know that by practice alone can you become experts.[6]

Medical and Health Education must equip the medical personnel to pay more attentions to preventive care.

It is also necessary to appreciate that the effective delivery of health care services would depend very largely on the nature of education, training and appropriate orientation towards community health of all categories of medical and health personnel and their capacity to function as an integrated team, each of its members performing given tasks within a coordinated action programme. It is, therefore, of crucial importance that the entire basis and approach towards medical and health education, at all levels, is reviewed in terms of national needs and priorities and the curricular programmes restructured to produce personnel of various grades of skill and competence, who are professionally equipped and socially motivated to effectively deal with day-to-day problems, within the existing constraints. Towards this end, it is necessary to formulate, separately, a National Medical and Health Education Policy which (i) sets out the changes required to be brought about in the curricular contents and training programme of medical and health personnel, at various levels of functioning; (ii) takes into account the need for establishing the extremely essential inter-relations between functionaries of various grades; (iii) provides guidelines for the production of health personnel on the basis of realistically assessed manpower requirements; (iv) seeks to resolve the existing sharp regional imbalances in their availability; and (v) ensures that personnel at all levels are socially towards the rendering of community health services.

2. Work with dedication and commitment to promote individual and community health care

In the patient care scenario you dedicate your life to the care of the individual patient. I recall not long ago in middle of the night a patient who was transferred to our hospital, had a complication during a delivery of her third child. She had severe lung disease following abruptio placenta, 10 year ago she would have died, but for the combination of the dedication of the staff with physicians, nurses, pharmacists and respiratory therapist who stayed at this woman's bedside throughout the night.

Within a weeks' time she left the hospital to go back to care for her other children. So, these children now have a mother because of the efforts of this team that individual care could not have saved a decade ago. Someone's life is being saved because of your efforts. Unfortunately, there are many diseases such as diabetes, chronic lung disease, and some forms of cancer that we can't cure. There you work with your patients to help with the illness, you understand how the illness has influenced their life. You do what you can, to make it easier for them. This may be your life calling. In this patient care approached medicine you take care of one patient at a time. You do the best you can for that patient and for the records of the lifetime you will make a difference in thousands, if not hundreds, of thousand of lives.[7]

I qualified as a doctor a little over 25 years ago and was sworn into medical practice by a modernized version of the Hippocratic oath, devised by the Dean of Medicine at Tufts University in the USA. It may be pertinent to recount that to you now.

I swear to fulfil, to the best of my ability and judgment, this covenant:

- I will respect the hard-won scientific gains of those physicians/ health care workers in whose steps I walk, and gladly share such knowledge as is mine with those who are to follow.
- I will apply, for the benefit of the sick, all measures, which are required, avoiding those twin traps of over treatment and therapeutic nihilism.
- I will remember that there is art to medicine as well as science, and that warmth, sympathy, and understanding may outweigh the surgeon's knife or the chemist's drug.
- I will not be ashamed to say, "I know not," nor will fail to call in my colleagues when the skills of another are needed for a patient's recovery.
- I will respect the privacy of my patients, for their problems are not disclosed to me that the world may know. Most especially must I tread with care in matters of life and death. If it is given me to save a life, all thanks. But it may also be within my power to take a life; this awesome responsibility must be faced with great humbleness and awareness of my own frailty. Above all, I must not play at God.
- I will remember that I do not treat a fever chart, a cancerous growth, but a sick human being, whose illness may affect the person's family and economic stability. My responsibility includes these related problems, if I am to care adequately for the sick.
- I will prevent disease whenever I can, for prevention is preferable to cure.
- I will remember that I remain a member of society, with special obligation to all my fellow human beings, those sound of mind and body as well as the infirm.

If I do not violate this oath, may I enjoy life and art, respected while I live and remembered with affection thereafter. May I always act so as to preserve the finest traditions of my calling and may I long experience the joy of healing those who seek my help. Adapted from that Written in 1964 by Louis Lasagna, Academic Dean of the School of Medicine at Tufts University, and used in many medical schools today.

There is a sentence in the oath there that is very poignant—that you will remain a member of society. So when you are at work, don't forget that patient in front of you is someone's mother, father, brother, sister, or child and how would you want that relative of yours treated. Take pride in what you have achieved so far in graduating and what you will do now.[8]

The late Bertrand Russell also expressed the view that mere knowledge does not have any motivation within it; that comes from a different source, namely, the field of emotions and sentiments in man. Something must stimulate knowledge; otherwise, it remains static and unable to influence human action. Our knowledge, said Russell, that any two sides of a triangle together are greater than the third side, does not motivate us, while walking, that we should go by the short side and not by the long sides, That motivation comes from some other inner source in man. Mere knowledge that obtains in our schools and colleges and universities, even at its best—and it is rarely that it rises to that level—contains no energy of emotion and sentiment relating to ideals of human excellence or to patriotism and national dedication, which alone can stimulate relating to ideals of human excellence or to patriotism and national dedication, which alone can stimulate that knowledge to develop into character-excellence and to make it dynamic, make it into a 'man-making education' leading to a 'nation-building' resolve, in the luminous words of Swami Vivekananda.[9]

A spirit of service and dedication must pervade among the providers of the health care as they are considered second God on earth by the receivers of health care. In the new millennium, we must empower the patients by the looking after them carefully and making them feel important.

The progress and achievements of the past 50 years are solid foundations for a healthier and better world. It is already time to build on them. Life in the 21st century could and should be better for all. We can pass no greater gift to the next generation than a healthier future. That is our vision. Together, the people of the world can make it a reality.

3. Ethical Values

On graduation, the doctor took the oath of honesty, purity, etc. which stressed all the ethical values. Later, with Western medicine becoming popular in the country, the medical students were asked to take the Hippocratic oath, which originated in Greece. The Hindu version of such an oath has been in existence long before the Hippocratic oath. But most Indians have not heard about it or have forgotten it. Since independence, this practice of Oath-taking has been given up in most places.

The training of the medical students and the oath that they took on graduation fully reflected the great ethical values that were instilled into all medical students and doctors. Thus medical ethics became the bedrock of medical practice and dharmic ideals prevailed. As regards remuneration for services rendered, this always took a secondary place. The medical students and the medical profession were indoctrinated with the principle that medical treatment is based on compassion towards all beings and it is not primarily meant for earning money or for fulfiling other desires.

In Vedic India and even later for many centuries, physicians were told that medical practice was never fruitless; it always gave some benefit or other for the doctor, not necessarily material or monetary. A Sanskrit-verse described this idea as follows:

- Sometimes punya, sometimes friendship,
- Somewhere money, somewhere else fame,
- Often knowledge and experience,
- Never is treatment without its fruit.[10]

Ethical or dharmic values are essential for the existence and for the progress of any Society and have to be preserved and practiced if human civilization has to progress. Of these values, ethics in medicine is of the greatest importance, as medicine deals with problems of life and death. To argue that the practice of values in medicine will depend on the condition of society is untenable, as the members of the medical profession belong to the elite in society and must shoulder greater responsibilities. They must have much greater concern about values than any other section of society. The doctor and the teacher—the Vaidya and the Upadhyaya—have to set a noble example to others in any civilized society.[11]

Doctors should not be influenced by pharmacy. They must see that pharmacy suits their requirement and is affordable. Doctors can play a great role in bettering services.

A well informed society expects for accountability, transparency and sound professional services from the health care providers. This requirement is fulfiled by professionalism and ethical practice of profession. The core element of profession is a specialized body of knowledge and commitment to service. Integrity of knowledge base and its expansion through research and ensuring the highest ethical standards in its use in the best advantage of the patient is a professional commitment of a pharmacist. Any failure in his duty is an indicator of falling standards of the profession. Licensing bodies and professional associations have the responsibility and social obligation to discipline unprofessional and incompetent pharmacists. Society believes the profession places the welfare of society above that of the profession. The education institutions have an important obligation to inculcate these values in their graduates.[12]

4. Modern Knowledge of Informatics

All hospital personnel directly involved in looking after patients are obliged to process a large amount of information, so as to provide good care. Physicians, for instance, must obtain each patient's demographic data and a history of the illness, note the signs and symptoms manifested, and compile a past treatment history and associated diagnosis for treatment. Nurses, in turn, need much of this information to formulate a proper care plan, after which they must note the patient's daily progress. Laboratory technicians require details as well, to conduct tests that the doctor has ordered, the results of which are sent back to physicians. Pharmacists too need certain data, to supply the necessary medication. All these examples show that a large part of the daily work of doctors, nurses, laboratory technicians, and pharmacists consists of information handling, perhaps up to 40 per cent of their hospital working day.

5. Time-savers

Fortunately, new technologists are now emerging which help to process this information far more accurately and efficiently. To the computer are now added allied machines that can undertake, for instance, imaging in the audio-visual field and rapid data transmission. Gradually, all these time-servers have been brought into hospitals to solve the problems created by the information explosion. Such technologies have been melded into a uniform system which is designed to meet hospital needs and is generally called a hospital information system.

The basic concept of such a system is to create a cumulative file of each patient's data, which can be quickly updated on a continuing basis. This type of data file in computer terminology is called a database.

Once each patient's database is created and regularly updated, data handling at the hospital improves tremendously, enabling a section requiring specific information on a patient to obtain it rapidly from the database. The information is delivered by a printout from a computer terminal in a standardized form. Or the physician may type an order into the computer database, which the computer then transmits to the laboratory as an instruction to perform clinical tests for a certain patient, the laboratory also receiving pertinent data that is stored in the patient's database. Similarly, when a physician uses his or her computer terminal to write a prescription into the patient's database, the computer transmits the prescription immediately to the pharmacy, while the prescription information is kept and accumulated in the database, which provides this information to the administrator in the form of hospital supply statistics.

However, technological progress will make it possible to transmit the data contained in hospital information systems through a telephone line to the clinics. Once this computer networking is established, the health care provided to the patient at either the clinic or the hospital will be more accurate. And while the privacy of each patient must always be protected, the accumulation of accurate data concerning matters of health that can be achieved through computer linkage with other health care facilities within a district and, ultimately, throughout the country will contribute to better health research and planning for the benefit of all.[13]

6. Data files

Health professionals are increasingly interested in the use of computers and especially micro-computers, for health statistics and epidemiology, not least because the price of today's microcomputer hardware now makes these machines affordable to them and, in some cases, to students. Microcomputers can now be found on the office desks of doctors and in the research laboratories of health scientists. These individuals have been asking about microcomputer-based statistical software that they could use with their desk-top machines to carry out data handling and management functions.[14]

7. Effective Communication

A basic doctor, to effectively deliver health care to the country must be an astute clinician, a good communicator, and a sound administrator, so as to effectively lead an ever-expanding health team for a positive health action. Work and action domain of the doctor has crossed the boundaries to drugs and dispensaries and presently extends to a large extent to the families and to the communities—hence the need for the basic doctor to be a community physician. Thus, has emerged the need for developing a well-designed and structured programme of education for basic doctors with general applicability, departing from the present MBBS curriculum, and with emphasis on the primary health needs of the country. In addition, human values and medical ethics need to be incorporated as a part of the curriculum. In essence, the National Education Policy in Health Sciences aims at, and strives towards the production of basic doctors equipped with adequate knowledge, requisite skills and appropriate behavioural attributes to meet the health needs of the country.[15]

All the health experts from top to both including auxiliary health services need be taught as to how preventive health services through health education can be developed to avoid opening of more and more hospitals and assuring an effective and efficient health services.

Essential of Communication

The essentials of communication are:

(a) Clarity of Thought

The first *sine qua non* of good health communication is that the idea to be transmitted must be absolutely clear in the mind of the communicator. It must spring out form a 'clear' head. It should be understood by the personnel so that it may be fully appreciated and acted upon.

(b) Importance of Action Rather than Words

In all communication, actions are more significant than words. Example is better than precept. A health officer who is not punctual cannot succeed in enforcing the time-rules on the subordinates.

(c) Participation

In this connection it is essential that both the parties (the communicator and the recipient) should participate in the communication. It is the only way to make the communication effective and made health programmes successful.

(d) Transmission

The communicator must plan carefully what to communicate, with whom to communicate and how to communicate. How can the top personnel communicate with the workers when they themselves do not know or cannot understand all the facts about the new plans? Further, delegation of authority without responsibility breaks down the spirit of communication.

(e) Keep the System Always Alive

The system of communication should be kept open and alive all the year round. It is only by honest attempts that good communicative relations can be developed.

(f) Cordial Employer-employee Relations

Effective communication requires good employer-employee relations, which enable mutual appreciation of different viewpoints.

According to Terry, eight factors are essential in making communication effective:

(a) Inform yourself fully;
(b) Establish a mutual trust in others;
(c) Find a common ground of experience;
(d) Use mutually known words;
(e) Have regard for context;
(f) Secure and hold the receiver's attention;
(g) Employ examples and visual aids; and
(h) Practice delaying relations.

According to Millet, seven factors make communication effective, it should be clear, consistent with the expectation of the recipient, adequate, timely, uniform, flexible and acceptable.

8. Need of Effective and Efficient: Good Public Relations to Promote Health Education

The creation of awareness is integral to social and economic development. The possibility for the power of communication to liberate the minds and essential qualities for health professionals, potential of people to critical awareness is real in every field linked to human development, and the generation of public will hinges on effective communication of information and ideas that relate to people's needs, aspirations and capacities for progress in thought the action. In this sense, getting and development process started is largely the task of information, education and communication through public relations. Health Education through public relations is of cardinal importance.

Public relations is the establishment of a climate of understanding. It means interpreting the programme of an organisation to the public and *vice-versa*. "Public relations in health is the composite of all the primary and secondary contacts between the health education and the citizens and all the interaction of influences and attitudes established in these contacts."

According to Harwood: "Public relations may be defined as those aspects of our personal and corporate behaviour which have a social rather than private and personal significance."

The purpose of public relations is not only to supply information, but also to encourage an understanding and cooperation between to citizens and the health professionals. The objectives of public relations should be to increase prestige and goodwill and to protect the life of the health organisation by safeguarding it against unwarranted attacks as well as to remove the genuine complaints and grievances of the people.[16]

9. Relationship with Patients and Relatives

The hospital today is more than the combination of medical and therapeutic treatment by specialists, greater and refined medical and surgical knowledge and even better and more effective facilities and equipment. It includes these factors as the core of its efficient operation but an additional dimension—one, which is too often ignored or at least minimized—is the human and social element in the structure of the organisation.[17]

The ideal of service must be encouraged among the personnel responsible for health care. It is the responsibility of the Health authorities to set the pattern for the philosophy of patient care. It was rightly mentioned by Gardner that:

No society can reach heights of greatness unless in all fields critical to its growth and creativity there is an ample supply of dedicated men and women.[18]

All the personnel engaged in patient care must keep the following definitions of the "patient" in their minds:[19]

- The patient is the most important in the Hospital.
- The patient is not dependant upon us—we are dependent on him.
- The patient is an interruption of our work—he is the purpose of it.
- The patient is not an outsider to our business—he is our business.
- The patient is a person and not a statistic. He has feelings, emotions, biases, and wants.
- It is our business to satisfy him.

10. Holistic Medicine

Medicine for very long time unfortunately differentiated the body-mind binomial. Traditionally, it also separated the disease from the afflicted person, making doctors "specialists in the disease" and "not in the cure as a whole." This attitude was also reflected in medical institutions and in their relationship with their patients. Most institutions have tended to adopt the same attitude in their structure and in their sense of the problems

CHART 10.1

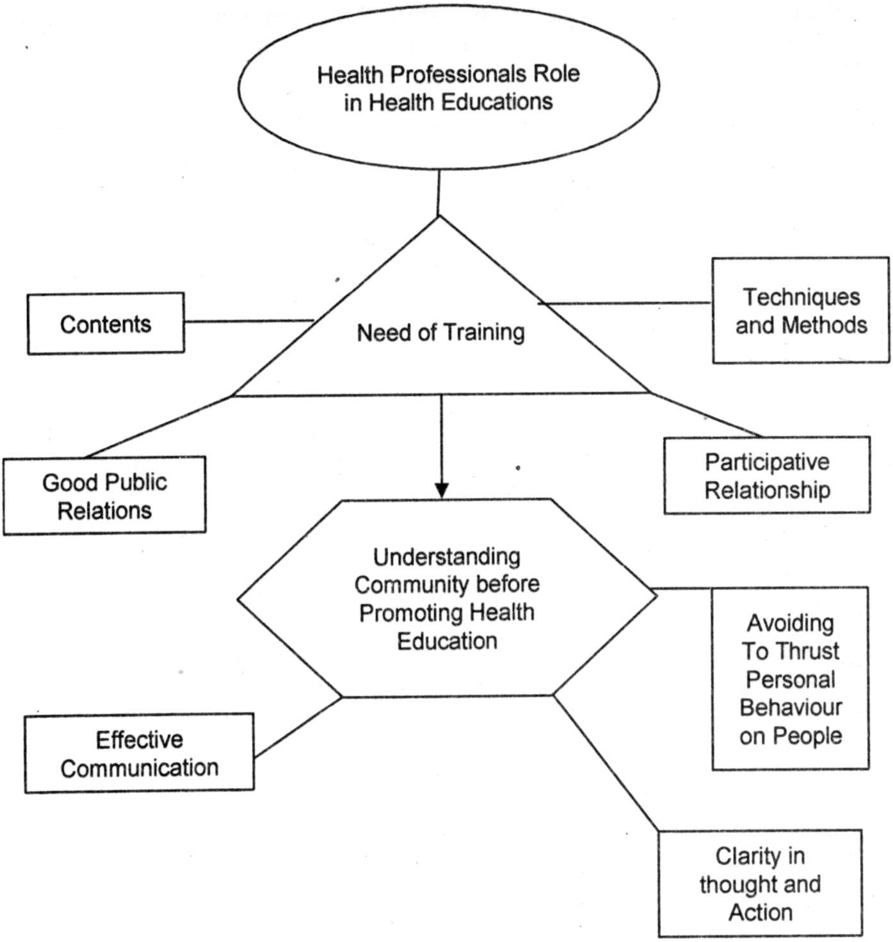

that they faced. You will agree with me that the dissociation of mind and body that permeates the relationship with the patient, rules the institution. However, time has come for all of us to try and help today's medicine to become more humane and complete. This goal-expression effectively informs several professional practices in the treatment of people in hospitals and institutions to adopt "Quality" as a never-ending process.

The modern physician must also be a soul, which strives to attain a moral ideal and to establish equanimity with fellow souls. He should have intense urge to search for a light in the ignorance and the darkness of this world. While treating patients our action must blend with their physiological processes. We should learn to respect their personal rhythm, unique composition and socio-economic individuality.

The distrust, which the public feels towards medicine, the inefficiency, and sometimes the ridicule, of therapeutics are perhaps due to the fact that the patients are seen as diseases described in medicine. Obviously, the remaking of a physician should be inspired by the precise knowledge of his body and of his soul. This remaking would require development of institutions wherein body and mind can be shaped according to the natural laws. One would have to learn to control the mind rather than be controlled by it.[20]

11. Equanimity

Last but not the least we come to an important attribute of every good physician or surgeon, Equanimity or Aequanimitas as Sir William Osler termed it. Equanimity means imperturbability, the ability to be unruffled, to be cool, calm amid stress and storm, to be clear in thinking and judgment, during an emergency, or during grave crisis or peril. It is the ability not to betray the emotions of worry, anxiety and above all of fear when treating critically ill-patients. Some physicians are born with the gift of aequanimitas, some cultivate it with practice and experience. To be possessed of true equanimity within the without is a divine gift. But even if you cannot help the storm that rages within you, train yourself to hide this, so that you present a picture of fortitude and calm from which your patient imbibes sustenance and strength.[21]

Peaceful Mind

From anger arises infatuation; from infatuation confusin of memory; from confusion of memory, loss of reason; and from loss of reason one goes to complete ruin.

When anger is aroused in the heart of man, it deprives him of his power of discrimination. He is unable to weigh the pros and cons of a question. He will not heed the consequences of whatever he does in a fit of anger. Such is the nature of infatuation caused by anger.

Emotional intelligence is concerned with achieving one's goals through the ability to manage one's own feelings and emotions, to be sensitive to, and influence other key people, and to balance one's motives and drives with conscientious and ethical behaviours. The following are the characteristics of Emotional Intelligence:

(a) Inter-personal sensitivity covering competencies like listening and sensitivity.
(b) Motivating, including impact and energy.
(c) Emotional Resilience.
(d) Influence and Adaptability covering both influencing and negotiating ability and being adaptable in various types of situations and cultures.
(e) Decisiveness and assertiveness.
(f) Integrity.
(g) Leadership including motivating other people.[22]

For medical profession, peaceful mind is of utmost significance as a minor wrong decision taken during a disturbed mind can ruin the life of patients. Doctor is dealing with patients and not some statistical data.

12. Action Oriented

Don't wait for your ideas to happen, make them happen. As Adman Carl Ally puts it, "Either you let your life slip away by not doing the things you want to do or you get up and do them." Passion for doing something should be matched with your core capability. It starts with you. You have to be in control to create control. If you can't control yourself you can't control the situation. Once you have control inside you will have control outside. Control doesn't mean suppression. It means regulation. It means channelization. Control adds tempo to performance, daring to vision, and brilliance in performance.[23] The more a doctor would work with patients, the more he would enjoy life. A doctor can be rusted by not acting.

Love and Affection towards all these who are seeking the help of medical personnel—Administration is manned by and meant for people. We must attend to their problems with love and affection, which would in return give strength and bliss.

Happiness on earth and bliss above are certainly the fruits of living the life of love. The changeless abode of the soul is reached by the path of love. Those that are devoid of love are just the skeleton covered with skin.

The journey of this world is delightful to one, who after the removal of his errors and dispersion of the cloud of his ignorance, has come to the knowledge of truth.[24]

13. Honesty and Integrity

> "Some say Knowledge is Powers,
> Others say the above is not True,
> Character is Power and Wealth."
>
> —*Sri Satya Sai Baba*

Integrity is one of the essentials for Character-building and personality development. Integrity means to be pure in thought and action. Integrity is very easy to accept but very difficult to put in practice. A man or woman of integrity is never influenced by temptations and pressures from outside as he or she would only respond to one's conscience. In today's world, it is very difficult to adhere to integrity as every one is in material race.

Honesty and integrity are other attributes integral to a physician. The need for honesty and integrity in all matters pertaining to patients and to the outside world is obvious enough. I however, refer specially to intellectual honesty. Self-delusion comes easy to one and all in medicine and I too admit to the crime of Procrustes was a robber who had become an inn-keeper. When a traveler stopped for the night at his inn, Procerustes would show him to his bed. When the guest was asleep the robber would determine how the guest fitted the bed. If he was short, he would bind him and stretch him so as to fit the bed; if he was too long he would chop off his legs so that he fitted the bed. In medicine it is common to jump to a preformed diagnosis and then delude yourself by making the clinical features fit this diagnosis. You add to what is not or subtract from what is, in order to justify a hasty preformed conclusion.

To err is human, and there is no physician on earth who has not made mistakes. The best-trained faculties may falter in observation, and even in the most experienced, errors in judgment must inevitably occur in an art and science, which often consists in the balancing of probabilities. Cultivate an honesty of mind, which recognizes, regrets and proclaims these mistakes. Only then will you learn from them and perhaps not repeat them. Do not hide your mistakes under a bushel or pretend that they never existed. It you do so, you will be increasingly unable to recognize truth; you will tread the unfortunate path of self-deception and delusion and your mistakes will multiply.

Can there be a true doctor who does not practice charity? Unquestionably not. Never refuse a patient who seeks your help but cannot afford your fees. You will be twice blessed—both by the patient and by the Lord who values the poor more than the rich. You have the right to live in reasonable comfort but let me quote you a pertinent saying—"No one should approach the temple of science with the soul of a money-changer."[25]

14. Humility and Selfless Services

Humility is the hall-mark of a true physician. The grace of humility is a precious gift. "Knowledge is proud that he knows so much, Wisdom is humble that he knows no more." Extend you charity, humility and consideration not only to your patients, but also to you colleagues, so that you do unto them as you would have them do unto you.

In my opinion, what distinguishes a great physician from an ordinary one is the power of judgment. Hippocrates said, "Judgment is difficult, and indeed medicine has been defined as the art of coming to a conclusion on insufficient evidence." We can increase our power of observation by constant practice. We can become more knowing and more wise through study and experience, but can we improve on our judgment? To an extent judgment is an inborn faculty; "the result of a union of mind and character, which a man either has or has not, and it is almost a difficult for him to increase it as to add a cubit to his stature."

Perhaps the only way to help improve judgment is to improve our mind, not by scientific training alone, but by an exposure to art, culture, literature, history, philosophy-the other great fields of human endeavour. A broader study of the humanities will enable you to understand Man and his afflictions far better than the detailed study of medicine alone. Dip therefore into the treasures of the world around you. Medicine is the study of Man. Study mankind and you will have enhanced your study of Man.[26]

The essence of the spirit of service is contained in the following words of Vivekananda: "This is the gist of all worship—to be pure and to do good to others. He who sees Shiva in the poor, in the weak, and in the diseased, really worships Shiva; and if he sees Shiva only in the image, his worship is but preliminary. He who has served and helped one poor man seeing Shiva in him, without thinking of his caste, or creed, or race, or anything, with him Shiva is more pleased than with the man who sees Him only in the temples. He who wants to serve the father must serve the children first. He who wants to serve Shiva must serve His children and all creatures in the world first."[27]

Swami Chinmayananda rightly observes that in order to live and to bring out the maximum happiness from ourselves, to work out the best for ourselves, everyone of us must have a goal in life, a mission, an inspiring ideal; looking up to that ideal and hitching our eyes to it, we must work on in the world outside. Thereby, the work becomes chastened; the work itself become its own reward for the individual and a great joy wells up in his mind, not in terms of what he gets on the first of the month, but what he gives to the society as best as he can, from the place where he is.[28]

Let us explain the role of serving others with the help of medical profession.

Dr. H. Mahler is very critical about the inability of health workers in contemporary society to influence those social and environmental factors which truly determine public health. He states:

> "There persist widespread negative attitudes among health professionals towards the health care of the poorest strata in the rural and urban population in the developing countries. Most of these attitudes imply—with a repetitiveness of an old gramophones records caught in a narrow, arrogant, condescending and indifferent groove—that these poor people are too apathetic, too superstitious, too illiterate to benefit from the health care potentially availability to them. Health professionals and those who train them should be much more radicals in accepting a social responsibility for the health needs of the people in these poor rural-urban communities so that they can act as agents for change."[29]

In the words of Swami Ranganathananda, "The subject of the philosophy of service, therefore, is not meant for academic discussion in the dull philosophy course of our universities; it should stir the minds and hearts of every section of the population. It is thus, that the nation will get the necessary strength to meet the recurring challenges that this age of revolutionary transition will throw at it. If India succeeds in responding to these challenges adequately, she will become a beacon of hope not only to herself but also to the whole of humanity. We have responded successfully to many a challenge to our national existence and integrity in our long history. And we shall face and overcome this challenge as well. With this faith in ourselves and in our national destiny, let us, from this day onwards, enter our respective fields of life and activity with hope and courage."[30]

To the mechanization of medicine is added the sin of commercialization. This is an age of consumerism where the lure of money—which brings with it power, luxury, comfort and enjoyment of life in all its varied physical forms is paramount. Dreadful as it may sound, medicine is fast becoming a business rather than a profession, and that too, not uncommonly a nefarious, corrupt business. What could be more nefarious than charging exorbitant fees from those who cannot afford them? What could be more corrupt than the practice of doctors who on purpose refer unsuspecting vulnerable patients from one specialist to another for no reason other than profit? What could be more corrupt than the unethical practice of commissions demanded by general practitioners from a specialist to whom a patient is referred?

Another major drawback of contemporary medicine is the crippling expense an ill-patient often incurs—an expense that is often ruinous to the family. This is partly due to the fact that the physician of today has forgotten the art of medicine and remains solely pre-occupied with its science. His rapport is with machines and not with patients; it is technology that dictates his course of action and not his clinical judgment. History taking is a neglected art; he forgets to use his sense—his eyes, ears and hands, but remember numbers, equations and formulae. Expensive investigations and expensive modes of treatment result, when simple tests and simpler measures would have sufficed.

Institutionalized medicine has also led to malpractice. Expensive glittering machines and foyers resembling five star hotels are the landmarks of modern institutions. To meet the cost, and, hopefully, make profit, machines have to be fed, and patients become the fodder for these machines. If an audit were to be carried out on the cost-effectiveness of modern day investigations, the result would indeed be shocking.

Why has there been such a decline in the ethics of contemporary medicine? It is almost certainly related to the decline in the sense of values in our present-day world. This decline is observed in all professions and in the whole of society, perhaps even to a greater extent than that observed in medicine. A burning desire for material gain and wealth dominates life today. It is indeed difficult for a profession to remain an island of virtue when surrounded by a sea of filth and corruption. The island is first eroded and then gradually swamped. But please remember what we have an ancient heritage to cherish and maintain. We must therefore combine and rise to root out the canker eating into the heart of medicine.[31]

Mahatma Gandhi nicely observed, "Living the Gandhian life is supremely hard, for it means stripping oneself of all wants. The people at Sewagram and Sabarmati have made their own uneasy compromises with modernity, but what gives their lives meaning and purpose is that they continue along the Gandhian path. In doing so they remind us that there are higher goals than earning a livelihood, and that in seving our fellowmen, we may best serve ourselves."

15. Keep Abreast with Latest Changes through Readings

Rapid advances in our understanding of the structure and function of the human body, the aetiopathology of diseases and their path physiological consequences have enabled us to help our fellow human beings to overcome disease and disability to a considerable extent. Concomitant technological developments have furthered our ability to devise more precise management strategies to successfully deal with an ever-expanding spectrum of congenital and acquired anomalies. The frontiers of medicine are in fact advancing at an accelerating pace and are destined to continue so in the coming years. Mapping of the human genome, the steady unraveling of the genetic basis of health and ill-health and the resultant progress in gene therapy and gene modification are opening up new vistas of diagnosis and therapy. The merging fields of stem cells, tissue engineering and Nan technology hold forth fascinating possibilities in the not too distant future. And the prospective marriage between molecular biology and powerful computational technology could transform the process of the designing and delivery of drugs. These and several other avenues of research have the potential to bring about a major paradigm shift in our understanding and approach to human health during your professional lifetime. And this possibility of medicine moving from the species level to the level of the individual—that is, moving from the current assumption that drugs and diseases work the same way in all human beings to the realization that there are subtle but significant individual variations—may become a reality as you progress in your practice of medicine.[32]

The human body is undoubtedly the most wonderful, the most intricately designed and the most functionally efficient machine—a machine that was perfected through billions of years of experiment and evolution of life by Nature. It has withstood the ravages of disease, famine and other hostile environmental conditions—and survived. A true gift of Nature. Preservation and promotion of health of the Nature's gift, I believe, is the *raison d'etre* of our profession. While we do have to treat the sick, it should always be our endeavour to prevent sickness in the first place. For, despite all the scientific and technological advances—past, present and future—the old adage, 'prevention is better than cure,' I believe, will always hold true.

16. Team Work

Health Care has long ceased to be the exclusive preserve of the doctors. We, as doctors, know that effective and efficient health care can only be delivered if all members of the team work in a concerted fashion. No matter who we are or what is our particular field of specialization, no matter whether we are physicians, surgeons, anaesthesiologists, dental socialists, nurses, physiotherapists, laboratory technologists or any of the several allied health scientists, our common goal is to help heal the sick through our areas of expertise.[33]

17. Treat the Patients with Dedication

Ever increasing population and lack of adequate, affordable health care facilities, particularly for the rural masses, is a matter of serious concern for India. A large proportion of our population has no access to even safe drinking water. The continued practice of open drainage system, indiscriminate disposal of waste and industrial effluents into water bodies, and added to this, increased migration from rural areas to cities resulting in uncontrolled growth of large slums in the urban centers without any sanitation facilities, etc. have created an environment unsuitable for healthy living. It has aggravated the spread of water-borne diseases like cholera, typhoid, tuberculosis, dysentery, and gastroenteritis. Yet another area of concern to the country is the spread of vector-borne diseases such as malaria, filariasis, Japanese encephalitis, and dengue to newer areas with mosquitoes, the vectors carrying these diseases, breeding in stagnated water bodies. It is said that in India alone, over two million cases of malaria are reported every year. Vector Borne Diseases are spreading to newer areas due to increased risk of transmission fuelled by developmental activities, demographic changes and introduction of new chemicals, to name a few possible causes.

Health Care for our rural populace has become a nightmare with no facilities nearby, and forcing the rural poor to travel long distances for medical help. While specialist medical practitioners are particularly scarce in rural areas, those few who chose to serve in rural areas suffer from lack of infrastructure facilities and technological advances including missing the essential professional interactions found in larger medical centers in the cities. Hardly 2% of the doctors go to villages to practice and more than 70% of our population lives in those villages, and they do not have access to better facilities compared to their privileged urban brethren. Of the 650 million people dwelling in the rural areas in our country, 360 million people are illiterate and almost 70% of them are below poverty line. For these disadvantaged people, health services are distant dreams. It is one of the major issues, the country is facing today. Even as India is hailed as an upcoming developing country with consistent economic growth wherewithal's in the knowledge society, we have a long way to go in health care and you have a major role to play in that.[34]

18. Health Education

Education must create a true health mentality, so that the application of rules for a healthy life becomes part and parcel of the daily round.

For thousands of years, disease and death have been accepted with resignation as normal ingredients of daily life-aspects of a tragic destiny, which strikes some and spares others without rhyme or reason. Today this resignation is unacceptable. We are aware that the dangers that threaten our health are often caused by imperfections in our social structures or in our own behaviour. We can afford to scoff at some of these threats, now that a correct application of new discoveries in medicine enables us to reduce them to reasonable proportions.

The task of education is to apprise people of their responsibilities, since diseases and accidents are so often linked with ignorance, carelessness, and inadequate precautions on the part of national authorities.

Studies made in different countries of the world have shown that fluctuations in the toll of disease and death depend even more on the level of education than on the social and economic conditions in which people live. Ignorance can be just as much a killer as poverty, and these two often go hand in hand.

Informing people is not enough; they have to be motivated. Education must create a true health mentality, so that the application of rules for a healthy life becomes part and parcel of the daily round; it must not limit itself to the domain of ideas. So in the field of education, we have to draw a distinction between real needs and felt needs. Providing water in a desert area is a powerful felt need. But pure water that is not contaminated by microbes or parasites is a real need rather than a felt need, and one which only education can make apparent.[35]

19. Personal-relathionship

It is the fallacy of modernity that we believe we communicate better through machines. Human beings communicate through bonds of mutual confidence. It is the prime task of the health communicator to facilitate a state of communal trust. Unfortunately, the staff of the public health services belongs to the educated elite. Therefore, typical bourgeois values permeate the hierarchy from the top to the level of the field-worker. Reality is seen through the reports of the latter, who knows that his superiors only welcome "facts" which are consistent with their social values and views. Large amounts of pseudo-information are concentrated around the false fact that poverty and ill-health are caused by ignorance. This allows the establishment to launch masses of educational programmes, the purpose and result of which only distract attention from the need for a structural change in society and a redistribution of wealth. In the process, the livelihood of the health education establishment is sustained.

Health and nutrition messages processed by the system have been devised and meted out according to the measure stick of the middle-class bureaucrat behind a desk. With their frequent characterizations of rural or village people's actions as mistakes, habits as bad and attitudes as wrong, they reflect a feudalistic lack of trust in the ability of common people to cope with their lives. There is little doubt that the pattern of working life in an organisational bureaucracy of which health services are a part tends to retard emerging moves towards change.[36]

20. Need of Vision among Medical Professionals to Inject Quality

Medical profession through, Indian Council of Medical Research, Medical Council of India and other organisations should define the role of the medical profession in the new millennium in the context of social development and improvement of the quality of life of the people.

A nation without a 'Vision' perishes. It is the vision that drives the progress of the nation. More than 500 experts drawn from various fields have prepared the "Technology Vision 2020" document for the country, which was released by the Prime Minister in August 1996. This vision document consists of 17 major technology packages. It deals with agricultural infrastructure and production, food-processing, health care, electric power, water-ways, life sciences and bio-technology, inland transportation, civil aviation, engineering industries, electronics, information and communication technology, material technologies and strategic industries, etc.

The Technology Vision Report aims to develop variety of indigenous technologies to transform India into a developed nation by the year 2020. With effective use of indigenously developed technologies in the next quarter century some of the visible results by the year 2020 will be, enhanced wealth of the nation, abundant production in various areas, well being of the people and national security.[37]

ICMR should prepare a document for the new millennium to ensure quality health care which should not be second to developed countries so that our people do not rush to the health institutions of advanced countries and waste financial resources and bring discredit to the country. We should develop our own health system which should possess all quality standards.

CONCLUSION

The success of medical profession that is delivery of health services to the people depends upon the sincerity, dignity, honesty, integrity, perfection, etc. of medical professionals. The medical professionals can create confidence and credibility among patients and usher an era of best health services.

Medical professional can promote health and make India healthy and strong.

India has its own well developed indigenous systems of health care like ayurveda, yoga, siddha, unani, etc. along with diverse ecosystem specific, local health traditions. These systems could be used to complement the allopathic system, as they could be more useful in certain areas of curative/preventive health care. This would enhance the quality and outreach of public health services, which are currently unable to meet the health needs of our people. However, care would have to be taken to ensure that we do not substitute the allopathic system of health care in areas like immunization, etc. where it has not alternative.

At present, our health care system suffers from a severe shortage of trained personnel. Across states, 6.30% posts of doctors remain vacant and random checks show that 29-67% doctors are absent. One way of overcoming the difficulty in recruiting qualified doctors to serve in rural areas is to make greater use of trained paramedical personnel. There is a strong case for reintroducing the 2-year licentiate course in medicine, which existed earlier but was abolished. We also need to devise ways of training and accrediting the rural health providers (popularly called RMPs) and permitting them to provide select services under the supervision of a licensed medical practitioner.[38]

Health is of great significance for the overall development of the country. Until and unless people of a country are not healthy, they cannot contribute their potential energy to socio-economic development, nation-building and modernization.

Dr. E.J. Thierry in his article, "Laying the Foundations", succinctly remarked that,

> "Health is man's most precious possession; it influences all his activities; it shapes the destinies of people. Without it, there can be no solid foundation for man's happiness. Nevertheless, all too often, social planners forget this simple truth and leave health out of account. Integration of health schemes in overall development plans are of paramount importance."

Health is fundamental to the national progress in any sphere. In terms of resources for economic development, nothing can be considered of higher importance than the health of the people which is a measure of their energy and capacity as well as of the potential man-hours for productive work in relation to the total number of persons maintained by the nation. For the efficiency of industry and of agriculture, the health of the worker is an essential consideration.

To improve understanding between the citizens and the hospital personnel, public relations need to be developed in an effective manner to create favourable community opinion towards the hospital services. This would create confidence in the minds of the people towards the competence, fairness, honesty, impartiality and sincerity of the hospital personnel. The following do's and don't may always be kept in mind for better public relations:

1. The patient is never interruption to work: the patient is our work. Everything else can wait!
2. Greet every patient with a friendly smile. Patients are people and they like friendly contact. They usually return it.
3. Call patients by name. Make a game of learning patients' names, and see how many you can remember.
4. Teach your staff members that for patients, all staff members are as important as the doctor.

5. Never argue with a patient. The patient is always right (in his or her own eyes). Be a good listener, agree with them where you can, and do what you can to make them happy.
6. Never say, "I don't know." If you don't known the answer to a patient's question, say, "That is a good question. Let me see it can find out for you."
7. Remember that the patient pays your salary: treat him like your boss!
8. Choose positive words when speaking to a patient. This is a valuable habit that will help you become an effective communicator.
9. Brighten every patient's day, and you'll soon discover that your own life is happier and brighter.
10. Always go the extra mile, do just a little more than the patient expects you to do. For example, make it a habit to phone the patient after discharge from the hospital, to ensure he is doing well. Exceeding patient expectations is the best way to keep your patients happy and keep them as your patients for life.

WHO in its Report of WHO Inter-country meeting on quality assurance in health care from 16-20 December 1996 at Indonesia suggested the following for South-East Asian countries:

(1) Ensure that quality of health care is an integral part of health services delivery at all levels of health care covering public and private sectors;
(2) Organize advocacy/awareness workshops on quality assurance for policy-makers, administrators and the leadership of health care to get their commitment for quality assurance;
(3) Establish a coordinating mechanism for quality assurance activities at national level through the nomination of focal point(s) and constitute a multi-disciplinary task force of national experts to provide advice on technical aspects of quality assurance;
(4) Initiate quality assurance of health care in selected hospitals and in primary health care through the district health system approach, document the experiences and expand gradually to more health care facilities;
(5) Organize national strategic planning workshops with technical assistance from WHO;
(6) Formulate guidelines to set standards and select national key indicators on quality assurance to monitor compliance and measure performance;
(7) Invest on building local capacity in health care quality through the creation of a critical mass of expertise within the country;

(8) Mobilize potential resources from within the country including support from international agencies; and
(9) Ensure that orientation on quality assurance be integrated in both basic and in-service training programmes of all health care professionals.

Implementation of TQM in health institution calls for a total change in culture in terms of customs, practices and improvement by creating increased sense of caring brought about by improved communication, involvement and training. It involves the integration of all functions, processes and personnel with an organisation in order to achieve continuous improvement in the quality of health care delivery systems.

By following TQM principles we can bring about harmony and quality working style in all the facets of the health institution and help it gain the top position and maintain it.

Finally, TQM consists in doing for the institution what should be done as a matter of course. The fruits of implementation of TQM may not be available instantly, lie magic tree, but it is sure to show improvements in health standards over a period of time.

Notes and References

1. Y.S. Rajasekhran, A Holistic Approach to Achieve the Health Targed, *University News*, 44(16), April 17-23, 2006, p. 15.
2. K. Mohandas, 'Presentation and Promotion of Health', *University News*, 44(33), August 14-20, 2006, p. 20.
3. K. Mohandas, 'Presentation and Promotion of Health', *University News*, 44(33), August 14-20, 2006, p. 20.
4. *Ibid.*, p. 20.
5. *University News*, 42(34), August 23-29, 2004, pp. 13-14.
6. *University News*, 43(15), April 11-17, 2005, p. 20.
7. Jeffrey on Dragen, Care of the individual patient, *University News*, 42(36), September 6-12, 2004, p. 15.
8. Steven Hla Myint, Training For Global Health Care Market, *University News*, 44(21), May 22-28, 2006, p. 21.
9. Swami Ranganathananda, "Democratic Administration in the light of Practical Vedanta," p. 47.
10. Dr. B. Ramamurthi, Values in the Medical Field, in values, p. 171.
11. *Ibid.*, p. 178.
12. Y.C. Simadhri, Societal Relevance of Pharmacy Education, *University News*, 42(26), June 28-July 4, 2004, p. 23.
13. Shigekoto Kailhara, "Information explosion", *World Health*, August/September 1989, pp. 6-7 and 8.
14. *Ibid.*, p. 11.
15. Prof. K.J. Nath, Public Health in India: Five Decades, Vol. 1, pp. 6-7.
16. Harwood, Childs L., An Introduction to Public Opinions, *op. cit.*, p. 2.
17. Mary D. Shanks and Dorothy A. Kennedy, The Theory and Practice of Nursing Service Administration, McGraw-Hill, London, 1965, p. 95.
18. John W. Gardner, Excellence, New York, 1961, Harper and Brothers, p. 154.

19. Edythe Alexander *et. al.*, Nursing Service Administration (ed.), New York, C.V. Mosby Co., 1962, p. 63.
20. Mahendra Bhandari, Holistic Medicine and a Complete Human Physcians, *University News*, 44(08), February 20-26, 2006, pp. 18-19.
21. *University News*, 42(34), August 23-29, 2004, p. 14.
22. Aruna Goel, "Good Governance and Ancient Sanskrit Literature," New Delhi, Deep & Deep, 2003, pp. 59-60.
23. *Ibid.*, p. 60.
24. *Ibid.*, p. 108.
25. *University News* 42(34), August 23-29, 2004, p. 14.
26. *University News*, 42(34), August 23-29, 2004, p. 14.
27. The Complete Works of Swami Vivekananda, Vol. IV, p. 324.
28. Swami Chinmayananda, Kindle Life, *op. cit.*, p. 192.
29. Text of Address by Dr. H. Mahler, to the Thirteenth Session of Regional Committee of South East Asia.
30. Swami Ranganathanand, *op. cit.*, p. 251.
31. *University News*, 42(34), August 23-29, 2004, pp. 15-16.
32. R. Mohandas, Preservation and Promotion of Health, *University News*, 44 (33), August 14-20, 2006, pp. 19-20.
33. *Ibid.*, p. 20.
34. *University News*, 43(15), April 11-17, 2005, p. 17.
35. Etienne Berthet, A New role for teachers, *World Health*, May 1979, pp. 23-24.
36. Andreas Fuglesang, "Folk-wisdom and pseudo-information," *World Health*, January-February, 1989, p. 7.
37. *University News*, March 2, 1998, p. 12.
38. Government of India, Planning Commission, New Delhi, December 2006, Towards Faster and More Inclusive Growth, An Approach to the 11th Five Year Plan (2007-12), p. 68.

11

CHAPTER

Doctor-Patient Relationship

Doctor-patient relationship is of utmost significance in medical science. In this context the first and foremost requirement is that the doctor need to develop a good rapport with the patients, which would enable him to know about him. There are large number of questions in the mind of the patient; which are creating problems and bad health. Doctor can remove many of his doubts through discussion. It is of great significance for the doctor to take the patient in confidence. Doctors and patients are intimately connected as the existence of one without the other is not possible.

In Ancient Universities in India, convocation address to the medical personnel said:

> ". . . . Everyday you should continuously and whole-heartedly try to promote the health of the patients. Even if your own life is in danger, you should not desert your patients. You should not entertain an evil thought about the wealth or wives of others. Your dress should be modest, not foppish. Avoid drinking; do not commit a sin, nor help one who is committing it. Your speech should be smooth, polished, truthful and to the point. Taking all facts into consideration, you should make a deliberate endeavour to increase the stock of your knowledge and instruments . . . When you enter a patient's room, all your attention should be centered on the patients, his expression, movements and medicines, to the exclusion of anything else. . ."

> "Though well grounded in your line you should not praise your knowledge much; for some people get disgusted even with their friends and relatives if they are given to boasting. One can never get a mastery of the entire medical science . . . One should therefore pass one's time in making a constant effort to learn something more. A wise man will indeed gather something from every quarter; a fool

only thinks otherwise, and shows jealously. Taking all things into consideration, a wise physician should listen to and derive benefit from the discoveries or observations even of an enemy, if they are calculated to promote one's fame and prosperity in this world."[1]

The harmonious relationship depends upon the sincerity, earnestness and co-operation between the Doctor and the Patient. The achievement of good relations between the Doctor and the patient is a matter that does not depend by any means solely on the conduct of Doctors. It equally depends on the attitude of patients and thus their relations. People must behave well towards Doctors. If loose and unsubstantiated allegations are made about their incompetence, dishonesty, laziness and indifference to the public interests, it is unlikely that doctors will develop or display qualities of integrity, industry and public spirit. Both the doctors and the public must exhibit harmonious relationship between them. This would promote good rapport between the two, which would promote good relationship. Doctor-Patient relationship means the development of cordial, equitable and therefore mutually profitable relations between the two. Let us now discuss the essential features of their relationship.

Patients are demanding a more substantive, collaborative role in their own health care decision-making. Collaborative healthware is the application of information and communication technologies designed to enhance decision-making and communication between providers, patients, and their families. The emergence of collaborative healthware will play an important role in supporting the relationship between patient and provider and will assist patients in better understanding their illness experience and how their own values affect decision-making. Collaborative healthware is defined as "software for health care, tightly integrated with people systems"[2] and its creative and successful implementation will improve patient care and care management.

Collaborative healtware supports the relationship between health care provider and patient by engaging patients and their families as full partners in the health care process. In a collaborative partnership, patients expect that their clinicians will provide informations and guidance. Patients expect that their clinicians will educate them and their families on illnesses, available therapies, potential outcomes, and complications, so that decisions can be made based on the patient's individual preferences.[3]

More often patients are presented with opportunities to actively participate in decisions that affect their lives and well-being.[4] While patient preferences for participation in clinical decisions vary greatly,[5] the desire for information about their health and health care is high.[6] Patients want information that addresses their individual concerns and conditions as well as interactive tools to manage their health and disease.[7] Providing patients with enhanced health-related information favorably affects their trust in, relationship with, and confidence in their health care providers.[8]

A Framework for Patient-Provider Collaboration

Supporting patient-provider collaboration with technology requires an underlying framework to facilitate participation. Goldberg et al suggest a framework for patient empowerment and the technical realization of that framework. Such a framework is a requirement for properly designed collaborative healthware applications. This framework consists of core elements essential to facilitating patients' active access to personally relevant credible information, ongoing and facilitated communication, clinical data capture, a reporting and feedback mechanism, and community support. In addition to this framework, other issues must be considered prior to the design, implementation, and evaluation of collaborative healthware.

Such consideration should include:

- What do patients need?
- What do providers want?
- How can the patients' "view" be designed into the system?
- How can prescribed, profile-driven knowledge be delivered?
- What are the best methods of information delivery?
- How can credible data be collected from patients?
- How can the system be integrated into the current work flow?

With widespread adoption of collaborative healthware applications, all patients and their families will come to expect improved access to services, greater convenience, and alternative methods of communicating with their health care providers. Since the emphasis is on the partnership between patient and provider, collaborative healthware will be used to promote informed decision-making, improve patient outcomes, increase patient satisfaction, enhance patient education, lower health care costs, and improve the coordination of care. While collaborative healthware applications have intuitive appeal to diverse groups of health care stakeholders, adoption of such systems will likely depend on their ability to demonstrate positive impact on outcomes.[9]

(I) Confidentiality

The doctor must keep all the information shared by the patient with him as confidential. Patient is afraid of family and society if some adverse information about the patient is leaked. This becomes very important for a psychiatric patient as the stigma is attached with the disease in the society. There are members in society who can take advantage of his secret problems. The doctor must not tell to anybody until and unless it is desirable.

Consumers expect change, and they want to be able to interact with their health care provider and their health care system as they do with their stockbroker or their favorite merchants on the Web. Privacy, the credibility of medical information, and the ability to correctly use that information for decision-making will be essential features of the medical Internet. We must create the environment for consumers to feel at least as secure as they do when transacting business or viewing information from stockbrokers, mortgage lenders, and educational institutions. The Medical consumer is a vital part of the supply-and-demand system that drives the world economy today and into the future. We cannot afford to fail to meet the medical consumers' needs and to empower them to assume a greater role in their care. We need to carefully identify the best approach to these challenges and act on them professionally and responsibly. The Internet will have an impact on how health is maintained and how care is delivered. The authors of the chapters in this section suggests that we are at a crossroads in health care, and we must be careful to effectively and responsibly use the tools that are available to improve consumer access, understanding, and quality of life.[10]

(2) Effective Communication

Communication is the touching of mind by mind, of person with person. It can include conversation, interview, dialogue, visual technique carefully used.

Communication is an integral part of every function of health administration "and that is why it is said to be the bloodstream of an organisation." It is a two-way process between people. In communication a message is transmitted and received.

Transmission	→	**Reception**
Message transmitted is the first half of the communication	←	Message received and understood is the second half of is the second half of the communication

Communication can be transmitted through audio, visual and audio-visual means. Communication plays the same role as the nervous system in a body. Norbert Wiener has rightly observed that "communication is the cement that makes an organisation." Communication is central to the exercise of authority in an organisation. In the words of Ordway Tead, "Communication is the touching of mind by mind, of person with person, whether it be one man, or a thousand . . . . it can include conversation, interview, dialogue, visual technique carefully used."[11]

According to Terry, eight factors are essential in making communication effective:

(a) Inform yourself fully;
(b) Establish a mutual trust in others;
(c) Find a common ground of experience;
(d) Use mutually known words;
(e) Have regard for context;
(f) Secure and hold the receiver's attention;
(g) Employ examples and visual aids; and
(h) Practice delaying relations.

Online health consumers are increasingly prevalent and are therefore important to health care providers. Organisations must fulfil their needs for communication, information, convenience, and access to their health records. Patient Site is an excellent way to meet these needs. Both patients and providers have vigorously adopted it, yet the demand on physician time is modest. The system has introduced controversial and interesting issues that we continue to work through. Patient Site is also a useful platform for future projects, such as patient-computer interviewing, disease management, health care quality, and patient safety.[12]

(3) Developing Rapport and Relationships

Building rapport with the client is the first important step as he feels to divulge all his problems frankly and freely. This is also called principle of acceptance.

Sanjay Bhattacharya rightly suggests that the principles of acceptance implies that social workers must perceive, acknowledge, receive and establish a relationship with the individual client as he actually is, not as we wish the individual to be or think he should be. It means that no matter how much our perception of it may differ from his, we must acknowledge and accept him as if we are to help him. In health education one begins from where the client is.

Purpose—to respect, to help, to add, to comfort, therapeutic understanding, acknowledge, receiving, etc. Quality of acceptance—warmth, courtesy, listening, respect, concern, interest, consistent, maturity, fairness, willingness to enter and share life experience, etc. Object—his integrity as a fellow human being, the individual as he is with all his limitation, his real potentiality, etc.

Obstacles to Acceptance

- Insufficient knowledge of human behaviour.
- Non-acceptance of something in self (lack of self-awareness).
- Biases and prejudices.
- Imparting to the client one's own feelings.
- Unwanted assurance.
- Confusion between acceptance and approval.
- Loss of respect for the client.
- Over identification.[13]

Imagine an entire population with access at home to a network that enables people to access information, communicate with providers and other interested parties, and receive some diagnostic and therapeutic services. The home, as a site of health care delivery, is of increasing interest to health care planners and providers. For those individuals whose access to traditional health care delivery is limited by circumstances such as distance and mobility, home-delivered services would be particularly attractive and potentially beneficial. In recent years, major advances in computing and telecommunication technologies, particularly the exponential growth of the Internet, have suggested possible approaches to improving health through the direct provision of services to patients.[14]

(4) Motivating the Patients

Doctors should not discourage the patient about disease. He should rather motivate the patient and create will power, which is basic for any treatment.

They should be motivated to do this job as a part of their medical duties. S.S. Sooch in his Article, "Revamping Health Care," in *the Daily Tribune*, (26th January 2000) rightly remarks that there is a general feeling that most of the health care providers in the government-run hospitals are indifferent, apathetic and insensitive and a few even outrightly arrogant in their behaviour. A sense of compassion and human touch is simply missing. A series of crash courses should be arranged to expose the entire staff to the art of public relations.

Health Education is vital to provide health to all in 21st century. This is the cheapest and most effective tool of health care. The success of health care in 21st century depends upon the identification of community needs through community needs assessment surveys and later on providing health education to the community so that they can solve their problems themselves.[15]

(5) Doctors must devote time and energy to solve patients' problems in collaboration of paramedical personnel

(a) that the patients are treated as close to their homes as possible in the smallest, cheapest and simply equipped unit such as a sub-centre which is capable of looking after them adequately;
(b) that the medical services should be organized and administered in such a way that the quality of medical care improves gradually;
(c) the medical care services should be organized from the bottom-up and not from the top-down;
(d) that the services planned should meet the needs of the people;
(e) that all members of the health and medical personnel function as a well-knit team; and
(f) that new categories of health personnel such as multi-purpose health workers and community health workers should be given suitable training to provide simple medical care and preventive services to large sections of the community.

In the case of virtual epidemic of behavioural disorders, modern health care must place a new emphasis on solving the human side of medicine. As stated by Maureen A. Backy, "The crucial link between the person providing health care and the persons receiving it, is often very weak indeed. Modern medicine tends to emphasize technical solution and to overlook the value of close personal contact and relationship."[16]

(6) Health Education

The most important aim of Health Education is to alter behaviour, which may have directly or indirectly influenced occurrence of spread of diseases in a given cultural setting. A culturally relevant health education programme can be planned only after understanding the behaviour in all its manifestations. One of the best definitions of Health Education was offered by Wood in 1926; "Health Education is the sum of experiences which favourably influences habits, attitudes and knowledge relating to individual, community, and racial health."[17]

Different authorities have differently viewed the aims of health education. According to one source:[18]

> "The aim of health education is to help people achieve health by their own actions and efforts. Health education begins therefore with the interest of people in improving their condition of living, and aims at developing a sense of responsibility for their own health betterment as individuals and as members of families, communities or government."[19]

Another source[20] highlights that, "Health education aims at promoting the greater possible fulfilment of inherited powers of the body and the mind and the happy adjustment of individual to society. It is the educational approach to health problem and as such is concerned with practical measures for the promotion of health and the control and treatment of diseases.

Studies made in different countries of the world have shown that fluctuations in the toll of disease and death depend even more on the level of education than on the social and economic conditions in which people live. Ignorance can be just as much a killer as poverty, and these two often go hand in hand.[21]

An excellent examples of the success of health education can be cited from Egypt. Esmut Mansour in his Article, "Egypt Tackles Polio," rightly suggests the role of health education in polio eradication. To quote:

In fact, women in Egypt represent a considerable proportion of all private and public physicians and health service administrators. As in many other countries, the nursing staff are predominantly women and are therefore engaged in the front-line battle to eradicate polio. The nurse's role here is much boarder than the one she plays during clinic hours, and her value to her community and its welfare should not be underestimated.

Not only does she routinely give the polio vaccine, but she is the primary mechanism for dispensing health care information to each child's careers, thus increasing their awareness about the dangers of disease, the importance of vaccination, and any possible side-effects of the vaccine. Therefore, she acts as the first defence line against the disease, and her understanding of the early effects of polio and her ability to recognize the disease is essential.

Egyptian society is particularly blessed by a culture and history that produces strong family ties. So untimely the success of our programme to eradicate polio must also credit the mothers who have listened to the information provided at the official level of health care and who have been convinced that the health of their children is worth all the expense and effort they make.

Egypt's Expanded Programme on Immunization is one of the most effective in the world. Reaching our goal of eradicating polio will be a worthy tribute to the hard work contributed by all of us—women and men together—to protect out children.

Health education does not mean merely removal of ignorance. On the contrary, it involves three important things:[22]

(i) It provides a person with appropriate knowledge to enjoy decent health and also the knowledge about the occurrence and spread of disease thus enabling him to adopt relevant preventive measures;
(ii) It creates in him an interest for the health of other members of his family as well as of those living in his surrounding; and
(iii) It creates in him a desire to support health education programmes in this area.[23]

Health education is an essential component of any programme to improve the health of a community, and it has a major role in promoting;

(a) good health practices—for example, sanitation, clean drinking water, good hygiene, breast feeding, infant weaning, and oral rehydration;
(b) the use of preventive services—for example, immunization, screening, antenatal and child health clinics;
(c) the correct use of medications and the pursuit of rehabilitation regimens—for example, in tuberculosis and leprosy respectively;
(d) the reorganisation of early symptoms of disease and promoting early referral; and
(e) community support for primary health care and government control measures.

Despite the potential benefits of health education, existing schemes are often inadequate and ineffective. The key decisions that form the basis for any planning are decisions over what the desired change should be, where the health education should take place, who should carry it out, and how it should be done.[24]

We mention here the following points to prove the important role of health education in health delivery system:

(1) Health Education develops a permanent base to support the delivery of health services.
(2) Health Education kindles interest among people about their health.
(3) Health Education, being preventive in nature is cost effective.
(4) Health education promotes Community Participation in the health programmes of the Community.
(5) Health Education can reduce dependence on health system, as 75% diseases are preventive.
(6) Health Education creates a chain effect as it passes on from individual to family to society.
(7) Health Education removes many mis-conceptions entangled into the minds of people.
(8) Health Education can promote partnership among health professionals and health receives.
(9) Health Education can promote individuals to take timely action to avoid complexities.
(10) Health Education can check the rush for secondary and tertiary health care system.
(11) Health Education being a two-way process can help in providing knowledge to health professionals.
(12) Health Education can help professionals in creating right attitudes among people about their health.

(7) Patient is a person and not a statistic

Need of dedication and not an earning machine on the part of Doctor.

To the mechanization of medicine is added the sin of commercialization. This is an age of consumerism where the lure of money—which brings with it power, luxury, comfort and enjoyment of life in all its varied physical forms is paramount. Dreadful as it may sound, medicine is fast becoming a business rather than a profession, and that too, not uncommonly, a nefarious, corrupt business. What could be more nefarious than charging exorbitant fees from those who cannot afford them? What could be more corrupt than the practice of doctors who on purpose refer unsuspecting vulnerable patients from one specialist to another for no reason other than profit? What could be more corrupt than the unethical practice of commissions demanded by general practitioners from a specialist to whom a patient is referred?

Another major drawback of contemporary medicine is the crippling expense an ill-patient often incurs—an expense that is often ruinous to the family. This is partly due to the fact that the physician of today has forgotten the art of medicine and remains solely pre-occupied with its science. His rapport is with machines and not with patients; it is technology that dictates his course of action and not his clinical judgment. History taking is a neglected art; he forgets to use his senses—his eyes, ears and hands, but remember numbers, equations and formulae. Expensive investigations and expensive modes of treatment result, when simple tests and simpler measures would have sufficed.

Institutionalized medicine has also led to malpractice. Expensive glittering machines and foyers resembling five star hotels are the landmarks of modern institutions. To meet the cost, and, hopefully, make profit, machines have to be fed, and patients become the fodder for these machines. If an audit were to be carried out on the cost-effectiveness of modern day investigations, the result would indeed be shocking.[25]

Commercialization of Medical Education

During recent years we have seen mushrooming of private medical colleges in many states. The trend is towards increasing commercialization. The health industry would like to get quick return for their huge investments at the cost of patients who are required to undergo unnecessary investigations and expensive treatment.

Even though charging capitation fees is punishable under the law the practice continue to go unabated with tacit understanding between different agencies. Through the private medical colleges we are creating a large number of affluent medical professionals from the privileged sections of the society. Having spent a fortune to get medical education how do we expect them to serve the rural population? Many of us feel that the medical degree would be awarded only after two years of service in rural areas irrespective of where the candidate comes from-Government or Private Medical colleges.[26]

(8) Faith in Values of Medical Problems (Doctors no longer believes in Values)

Why has there been such a decline in the ethics of contemporary medicine? It is almost certainly related to the decline in the sense of values in our present-day world. This decline is observed in all professions and in the whole of society, perhaps even to a greater extent than that observed in medicine. A burning desire for material gain and wealth dominates life today. It is indeed difficult for a profession to remain an island of virtue when surrounded by a sea of filth and corruption. The island is first eroded and then gradually swamped. But please remember that we have an ancient heritage to cherish and maintain. We must therefore combine and rise to root out the canker eating into the heart of medicine.[27]

(9) Look to the longer welfare of patient

The first is clinical iatrogenesis-diseases produced by physicians, either by treatment or investigations, or by the hospital in which patients are treated. But then iatrogenic disease is as old as medicine; it is an inseparable companion of medicine since antiquity. Contemporary medicine is aware of the epidemic of iatrogenesis resulting from the frequent use of potent drugs, sophisticated gadgetry and invasive procedures used in the diagnosis of management of patients. Far too often, the treatment meted out to patients today may be worse than the disease.

The second form of iatrogenesis is social iatrogenesis by which is meant the creation of an environment, which no longer has the ability to allow people in society to look after themselves. People are hopelessly dependent on the medical system and the medical system operates to ensure that this remains so. Medical help is sought for trivial and unnecessary reasons, to the benefit of the medical profession and to the detriment of people in society.

The third form of iatrogenesis, accordingly to Illich, is cultural iatrogenesis whereby institutionalized medicine has sapped the ability of the people to face the reality of the sufferings in life and the inevitability of death. This may be true in the West but is not so in India and many Eastern countries. A patient's, and for that matter a doctor's attitude to suffering, pain and death is conditioned by socio-cultural and religious factors. Most people in the East accept that life cannot be divorced from suffering and pain, and that each one is apportioned his or her share of pain and suffering in life. It is being increasingly recognized today that modern medicine with its science and technology should relieve suffering but should refrain from prolonging the act of dying. Above all, it should prevent death from being lonely, gruesome, obscene, de-humanized and ruinous to the patient and his family.[28]

(10) Sympathy

'It is necessary to recapture the spirit of humanism and reestablish the special sympathy in doctor patient relationship. To restore the image we need to distance from lure of money, raise the ethical standards and place the welfare and care of patients above all.' It is felt there is decline in values in medical profession. The frustration of patients and relatives is often translated into litigation demanding compensation; to protect himself the doctor falls back on defensive medicine. He over investigates not to miss even a rare disorder. There is need for healthy interaction between medicine and society, which is a two-way reciprocal affair. In India, doctor is often brought before a consumer court for any alleged incompetence or offence. The Judiciary in India considers practice of medicine as "Consumer Industry" and services rendered to a patient like "consumer product." It is unfortunate that the doctor with years of study, knowledge, expertise and experience and above all in spite of the care provided to the patient his services are to be equated as consumer product. In most countries the disputes between doctors and patients are decided by duly constituted professional bodies. Lack of Internal audit and control within the profession is responsible for this sad state of affairs. The medical professionals must develop effective public relations and media management skill. These will help in true projection of our achievements, avoid or dispel rumors, respond to criticism, diffuse controversies and project a positive image.[29]

(11) Trustworthiness

Medical professors are the architects and builders of students' behaviour using a standard program. They are also the curricular developers and thus have pivotal role in shaping the future medicos. Charka Samhita lays down that the teacher should be one "whose doubts have been all cleared in respect of medical scriptures-possessed of experience-clever in the practice in his profession. Conversant with nature-his knowledge of medical science supplemented with a knowledge of other branches of study-without malice-of a peaceful disposition-capable of bearing privation and pain-well affected towards disciples and prone to teach them-capable of communicating his ideas, etc. (Chaudhary, 1994). The professional temperament of the doctor with capability for clinical training/ educational tutelage is as follows:

Every doctor who is appointed afford clinical or educational supervision for a doctor in training, or who undertakes to provide clinical training and supervision for medical students, should demonstrate resolution to our professional guidance in Good Medical Practice. This will encompass:

- Presuming a high standard of professional and personal values in relation to patients and their care.
- Being available and accessible to patients.
- Maintaining a high standard of clinical competence.
- An ability to communicate effectively.
- An assurance to personal, and professional, development as a doctor.
- An assurance to professional audit and peer review.
- An assurance to team working in a multi-professional environment.
- An understanding of the multi-cultural society in which medicine is practiced.
- An enthusiasm for his/her specialty.
- A personal assurance to teaching and learning.
- Impressionability and responsiveness to the educational needs of students and junior doctors.
- The capacity to promote development of the required professional attitudes and values.
- An understanding of the principles of education as applied to medicine.
- An understanding of research method.
- Poetical teaching skills.
- A willingness to develop both as a doctor and as a teacher.
- A commitment to audit and peer review of his/her teaching.

- The ability to use formative assessment for the benefit of the student/trainee.
- The ability to carry out formal appraisal of medical student progress/the performance of the trainee as a practicing doctor.[30]

(12) See the patient as integrated whole

Improvements in the health status of a population cannot be achieved simply by expanding and developing the health services. The prevention and control of disease and the promotion of health require a concerted effort for the improvement of human well-being as a whole. In this task, what has been defined as "health care" has to be supported by improvements in the social and economic infrastructure, and contributions from various sectors other than health.

Certainly there has been a broad understanding of the linkages between health development and development in other sectors. The health experience of the industrialized countries has contributed significantly to this understanding. We know that the major causes of sickness and death arising out of a large cluster of diseases associated with poor sanitation, illiteracy and low levels of income were effectively controlled in these countries well before the discovery of antibiotics and other spectacular curative "break-throughs." The control of diarrhoeal diseases, tuberculosis and a wide range of communicable diseases was primarily achieved through far-reaching improvements in the urban infrastructure, housing and environmental sanitation, through the changes in health behaviour which accompanied higher levels of education and literacy, and through the improvement in nutritional status as incomes and living standards steadily rose. The positive outcome in health was therefore the result of an intersectoral effort.

The more recent experiences of a few developing countries illustrate even more dramatically the way in which health forms part of an integrated process of development. These countries have been able to achieve high level of life expectancy and have shown remarkable progress in reducing infant and maternal mortality at comparatively low levels of income. The state of Kerala, with per capita incomes well below the average for India as a whole, enjoys a health status—as measured by life expectancy, infant mortality and other health indicators—which is well above the rest of India.[31]

(13) Not Exploitative

Doctor must treat the patients with economy and efficiency. It has been seen that Doctor prescribes large number of tests relating to laboratory investigations and Radiology, which are costly and dangerous. These are prescribed only to get 50-60 per cent commission. Doctor is not interested in treating the patient but exploiting this for material benefits. In this way mind of the doctor gets perverted and he looses self-respect in his own mind. This trend is on the increase, which should be curbed by Government through some legislation. If the tests prescribed by the doctor are not needed legal action must be taken against the doctor.

(14) Doctor must treat the patient on the basis of equity

It is well known that Doctor is highly qualified in medicine but this is not sufficient until and unless the doctor treats the patients on the basis of equality and in a dignified way. His diagnosis and treatment would depend upon the information he is able to get from the patient. If the doctor keeps himself on high pedestrian which prevents the disclosure of information and prevents the good rapport between patient and the doctor. Doctor must make the patient feel as equal partner of treatment.[32]

Involving patients in the provision of their own care offers enormous benefits to both the patients and their providers. Physicians recognize that the patient is their primary source of information regarding symptoms and perceived reactions to treatment. They would further assert that the critical factor in the effectiveness of treatments is the patient's compliance with prescribed protocols. So patients already are involved in their own care. "Empowering" patients simply acknowledges their shared responsibility and builds upon the trust that has historically served as the foundation of the provider-patient relationship. The empowerment comes from giving patients greater access to information and from facilitated patient-provider communications. Empowered patients are better equipped to manage their own health, to educate themselves regarding their health condition, and to play an active part in their treatment.

(15) Doctor must be prompt, thorough and patient's friendly

In a poor country like India, there is great rush of patients. How to deal with them? Doctor must be prompt, i.e. not waste time talking to friends, colleagues, etc. He must understand the concept of Time Management, i.e. Time is Money. He must concentrate on patient's treatment with dedication and sincerity. In this way he can deal efficiently both quantitatively and qualitatively. He must also deal with the patients sympathetically. Even a single good word to the patient can help the patients in fast recovery.

(16) Medicines must be prescribed of generic nature which are cheap and patients can afford

People in India are poor and they cannot spend much on health care. It has become a fashion to prescribe costly medicines, which make the patients sicker as he has not the means to purchase them. Doctors prescribe them under the pressure of pharmaceutical companies to get some money from them. Medicine is a noble profession; therefore, doctor must attend to the patients as per his need and affordability.

(17) Doctor should ensure the satisfaction of the patient

Doctor must understand the problems of the patients first. After understanding, he must tell him his diagnosis and satisfying the patient with all the questions in his mind. Many questions in the mind of the patient are unfounded but still the doctor must remove the doubts of the patient. When the patient is satisfied, he develops trust in the doctor and at this stage doctor can suggest him both preventive and curative measures.

(18) Doctor must understand the art and science of counselling patients

Doctor has to change the attitude and behaviour of patients towards positive health. It is highly difficult as it is easier to destroy the mountains than to change the minds of the people. Counselling requires patient listening and better understanding of patients. Doctors should not use harsh language. He must convey in polite and simple language. It has been seen that some doctors start quarreling with the patients when they do not agree with his viewpoint, which is wrong in principle and practice. He must learn that there is and science of counselling, which can create positive change in his mind.

Counselling is one of the effective methods used in health education and social work to help individuals and families to require their health problems solved.

A recent English definition may also be quoted for further clarification: "Case work is professional service offered to those who desire help with their personal and family problems. Its aim is to relieve stress and to help the client to achieve a better personal and social adjustment. It proceeds by the study of the individual in his social milieu, by the establishment of a co-operative relationship with him, and by the mobilizing of both his own resources and those of the community to work towards these goals."[33]

Analysis of case studies suggest the following for effective counselling:

(1) A harmonious rapport between the individual and Doctor is the first most important requirement to make counselling effective.
(2) Doctor must be knowledgeable and competitive so that he can take a firm decision.
(3) Individuals must develop trust and faith in the Doctor.
(4) Doctor must keep the individual's problems confidentially.
(5) Counsellor must learn the art and science of communication to be effective.[34]

We must all learn together to see how we are going to communicate in the future. We are at the advent of a new era in health care and medicine in which users; health care providers and practitioners, directors, and managers work together to make efficient use of new information and communication technologies.[35]

Doctors must also attend these patients who do not shown any sign of physical ailments—Patients generally complain of many problems but physically they are fit and fine: How to deal with them? There is a need of advice to the patient to change lifestyle, etc. Doctors must try other methods to improve him rather than sending the patient to a psychiatric department till he shows severe signs of stress and strain.

(19) Ethical Values

Doctors must follow Ethical Values. It has been reported that few doctors misbehave with the patients and even outrage the modesty of women patients. It is highly deplorable act. That is why primary health centers have been provided a post of woman doctor.

Such acts by few individuals create a poor image of medical profession. It is suggested that strict action must be taken against doctors indulging in such heinous crimes.

We have discussed the duties and responsibilities of Doctors to the patients. Let us discuss the duties of patients toward doctor, which would ensure complete integration between the doctor and the patient. Patient should be as good as he wants doctor to be good. Let us discuss some of important qualities in-patient, which can make the doctor a co-partner in the process of treatment and health care.

1. Patient's faith in the Doctor

Patients must have respect for the doctor as well as have full faith in the capability and capacity of the doctor. It has been rightly said that faith begets faith. It is the duty of the patient to have complete faith in doctor otherwise doubt would emerge in the patient which would make his disease more serious. If he has no faith for reasons known to the patient, then he can approach other doctor of his choice and have faith in him. Faith is the first ingredient for the patient in the Doctor for treatment.

2. Patients need to disclose all problems

Past, Present, i.e. case history—The patient must disclose all the information asked by the doctor correctly without fear as his diagnosis is going to based upon that. There is a tendency among patients not to tell correctly all the information for fear of shame or being let down by the doctor. Even if the doctor does not ask any information; the patient must tell every thing, which is perturbing the mind of the patient. He can get the treatment for all the problems otherwise the treatment can not be effective.

3. Good Behaviour of the Patient

We already discussed that the doctor must have good behaviour with the patient, the same way patients must have good behaviour towards doctor. Patients must understand the limitations of doctors, i.e. number of patients are so large that doctor cannot provide time immediately. Patient must wait for his turn. Good behaviour of patient can make the doctor more careful and attentive to the patient. He should show respect to all medical fraternity who are engaged in a noble profession.

4. Patients need to follow doctor's prescription in letter and spirit

Disease prevention is possible only if the patient acts on the prescription. Even time schedule of taking medicines, etc. must be followed scrupulously. Some patients for one reason or the other do not follow the prescription and start taking something else, they cannot be treated. So follow the prescription of one doctor only religiously.

5. Diet must be taken as prescribed

Patients must take diet as prescribed. Indoor patients are given only the diet suitable for them. Out-patients are however advised to take particular diet at home. Diet and disease are related. Patients must take the prescribed diet.

6. Regular Follow-up

The patients must follow-up his treatment as advised by the doctor otherwise the disease can re-appear with more serious threat. Therefore, till the doctor wants follow-up, the patients must go and see the doctor.

7. Be patient for his turn at every place

Whether it is examination by the doctor or laboratory tests.

8. Respect to Lady Doctor

There have been some cases where patients have misbehaved with the lady doctors and even sometimes harassed them. Exemplary punishment must be given to patients or their relatives who indulge in anti-social activities. The administration must also be strict to take care of lady doctors so that no patient can dare to misbehave with the lady doctors.

9. Patients must bear in mind about

The shortage of staff/non-availability of medicine, etc. Most of the hospitals in our country are starved of funds resulting into shortages of men, money and material. The patients must cope up with such situations rather than creating unnecessary trouble. Patients may contact the Government/Health department which is responsible for all these problems. The problems in AIIMS recently were not due to doctors but because of interference of the ministry of Health and Family Welfare.

A basic doctor, to be effective to deliver health care to the country must be an astute clinician, a good communicator, and a sound administrator, so as to effectively lead an ever-expanding health team for a positive health action. Work and action domain of the doctor has crossed the boundaries to drugs and dispensaries and presently extends to a large extent to the families and to the communities—hence the need for the basic doctor to be a community physician. Thus has emerged the need for developing a well-designed and structured programme of education for basic doctors with general applicability, departing from the present MBBS curriculum, and with emphasis on the primary health needs of the country.

In addition, human values and medical ethics need to be incorporated as a part of the curriculum. In essence, the National Education Policy in Health Sciences aims at, and strives towards, the production of basic doctors equipped with adequate knowledge, requisite skills and appropriate behavioral attributes to meet the health needs of the country.[36]

CONCLUSION

The success of the medical profession depends to a great extent upon the harmonious relationship between the medical team and the patients. Medical team should not function as machinery but in a human and purposeful way. The medical team should have a sense of dedication, responsibility and be responsive and alert to the aspirations and problems of the patients. Patients on the other hand should also provide meaningful co-operation to medical team. Under such an atmosphere, it would be very easy to implement the patient care activities smoothly.

While endorsement of inefficiency or sheer neglect on the part of a hospital or its staff is uncalled for, it would be prudent to understand the constraints under which the hospitals and the medical personnel have to serve the ever increasing number of critical patients, some of which may not respond to a well proven treatment or the nature of affiction may be incurable or the delays in administration of treatment may occur despite the best efforts of the doctors on duty—due to multifarious pressures and bottlenecks, while judging their performance it is imperative to examine, whether the person was adequately skilled to handle the situation, whether there was intention to help to the best of his capability, whether an all out effort was made to render the service promptly and properly. If the answer to the above questions is 'Yes' no charge of negligence can be made out. It goes without saying that the staff has been accessible, humane, commitment . . . sympathetic in the hand of stern and grief, which patients and their attendants face in the hospital situation.

A spirit of service and dedication must pervade among the providers of the health care as they are considered second God on earth by the receivers of health care. In the new millennium, we must empower the patients by looking after them carefully and making them feel important.

The progress and achievements of the past 50 years are solid foundations for a healthier and better world. It is already time to build on them. Life in the 21st Century could and should be better for all. We can pass no greater gift to the next generation than a healthier future. That is our vision. Together, the people of the world can make it a reality.[37]

Dr. H. Mahler is very critical about the inability of health workers in contemporary society to influence those social and environmental factors, which truly determine public health. He states:

> "There persist widespread negative attitudes among health professionals towards the health care of the poorest strata in the rural

CHART 11.1

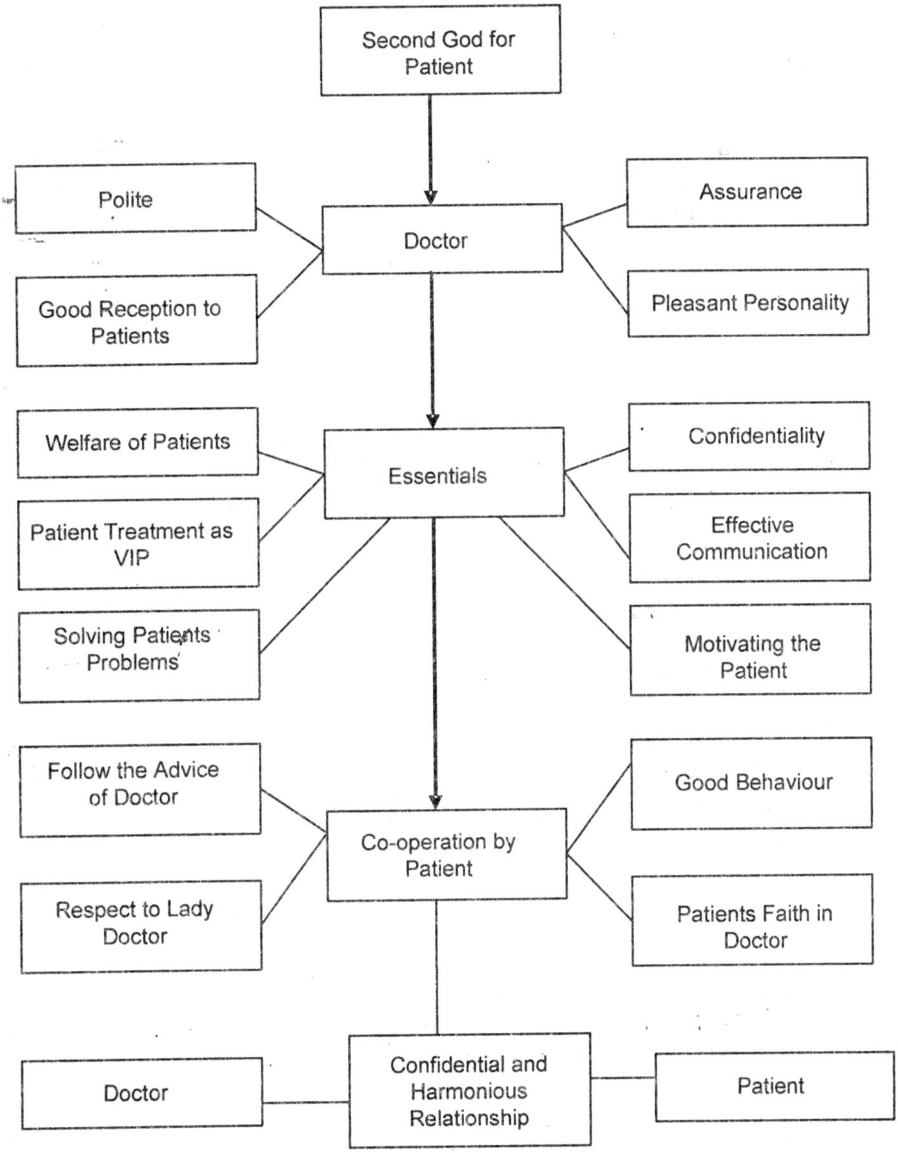

and urban population in the developing countries. Most of these attitudes imply-with a repetitiveness of an old gramophones records caught in a narrow, arrogant, condescending and indifferent groove—that these poor people are too apathetic, too superstitious, too illiterate to benefit from the health care potentially availability to them. Health professionals and those who train them should be much more radicals in accepting a social responsibility for the health needs of the people in these poor rural urban communities so that they can act as agents for change."[38]

"Thus, we can say that there is a need to train health administrators and workers in the new art of Public Health Administration so that they can take the benefits of the modern science to the common man and maintain the spirit of Geneva Declaration."[39]

"Now being admitted to the profession of Medicine, I solemnly pledge to concentrate my life to the service of humanity. I will give respect and gratitude to my deserving teacher. I will practice medicine with conscience and dignity. The health and life of my patients will be my first consideration. I will hold in confidence all that my patients confide in me. I will maintain the honour and noble traditions of the medical profession. My colleagues will be my brothers. I will not permit considerations of race, religion, nationality, party politics or social standing to intervene between my duty and my patient. I will maintain the utmost respect of human life. Even under threat I will not use my knowledge contrary to the laws of humanity. These promises I make freely and upon my honour."

The same feelings has been expressed in the Tokyo Declaration. To quote the preamble to the Declaration of Tokyo:

> "It is the privilege of the medical doctor to practice medicine in the service of humanity, to preserve and restore bodily and mental health without distinction as to the persons to comforts and to ease the sufferings of his or her patients."[40]

Prof. J.S. Neki has rightly said in this connection that "to help, to heal, to reconstruct, to comfort-and all along the line to act with compassion—all these bear testimony to the moral consciousness of the doctor. Whatever the new strains imposed upon medical ethics, this structure will survive and continue to guide doctors in their professional conduct. Legal and juridical obligations they have, no necessity, to fulfil. But these are not genuine ethics. Genuine ethics has to be ingrained into character and does not have to depend upon external controls.[41]

To err is human, and there is no physician on earth who has not made mistakes. The best-trained faculties may falter in observation, and even in the most experience, errors in judgment must inevitably occur in an art and science which often consists in the balancing of probabilities. Cultivate an honesty of mind which recognizes regrets and proclaims these mistakes. Only then will you learn from them and perhaps not repeat them. Do not hide your mistakes. Only then will you learn from them and perhaps not repeat them. Do not hide your mistakes under a bushel or pretend that they never existed. It you do so, you will tread the unfortunate path of self-deception and delusion and your mistakes will multiply.

Humility is the hall-mark of a true physician. The grace of humility is a precious gift. "Knowledge is proud that he knows so much, Wisdom is humble that he knows no more." Extend your charity, humility and consideration not only to your patients, but also to your colleagues, so that you do unto them as you would have them do unto you.

In my opinion, what distinguishes a great physician from an ordinary one is the power of judgment. Hippocrates said, "Judgment is difficult, and indeed medicine has been defined as the art of coming to a conclusion on insufficient evidence." We can increase our power of observation by constant practice. We can become more knowing and more wise through study and experience, but can we improve on our judgment? To an extent judgment is an inborn faculty; "the result of a union of mind and character, which a man either has or has not, and it is almost as difficult for him to increase it as to add a cubit to his stature."

Perhaps the only way to help improve judgment is to improve our mind, not by scientific training alone, but by an exposure to art, culture, literature, history, philosophy—the other great fields of human endeavour. A broader study of the humanities will enable you to understand Man and his afflictions far better than the detailed study of medicine alone. Dip therefore into the treasures of the world around you. Medicine is the study of Man. Study mankind and you will have enhanced your study of Man.[42]

Notes and References

1. Chandni Saxena, Role of Ancient Indian Universities in value orientation to the contemporary society in India, in *University News*, 44(05), January 30-February 5, 2005, p. 30.
2. Safran, C., The collaborative edge: patient empowerment for vulnerable populations, *Int J Med Informatics*, 2002, 1-6.
3. Ferguson, T., Consumer health informatics, Health Care Forum, 1995, 28-23.
4. Brennan, P.F., Ripich, S., Use of a home care computer network by persons with AIDS, *Int J Technol Assess Health Care*, 1994, 10(2): 258-72.
5. Brennan, P.F., Health informatics and community health: support for patients as collaborators in care, *Methods Inform Med*, 1999, 38(4-5): 274-78.
6. Tang, P.C., Newcomb, C., Gorden, S., Kreider, N., Meeting the information needs of patients: results from a patient focus group, *Proc AMIA Annual Fall Symposium*, 1997, 672-76.
7. Kaplan, B., Brennan, P.F., Consumer informatics: supporting patients as co-producers of quality, *JAMIA*, 2001, 8(4): 309-16.
8. Tang, P.C., Newcomb, C., Information patients: a guide for providing patient health information, *JAMIA*, 1998; 5(6): 563-70.
9. D. Goldsmith and C. Safran, Consumer Informatics, pp. 9-11 and 17.
10. *Ibid.*, p. 62.
11. Ordway Tead, The Art of Administration, New York, McGraw-Hill, 1951, p. 45.
12. D. Goldsmith and C. Safran, Consumer Informatics, p. 31.
13. Sanjay Bhattacharya, Social Work, Deep and Deep, New Delhi, 2003, pp. 223-24.
14. D. Goldsmith and C. Safran, Consumer Informatics, p. 40.
15. S.L. Goel, Health Care Policies and Programmes, Deep & Deep Publications, New Delhi, Vol. 2, pp. 23-29.
16. WHO, *World Health*, December 1975, p. 6.

17. John J. Hanlon, Principles of Public Health Administration, St. Louis, 1960, p. 402.
18. WHO: Technical Report Series No. 89, p. 4.
19. S.L. Goel, Health Care Policies and Programmes, Deep & Deep Publications, New Delhi, Vol. 2, p. 6.
20. WHO: Technical Report Series No. 156, p. 3.
21. WHO: Etienne Berthet, A new role for teacher, *World Health*, May 1979, p. 23.
22. WHO, Esmat Mansour, "Towards a World without Polio", January-February 1995, p. 27.
23. Dr. S.L. Goel, Health Education: Theory and Practice, "Nature and Scope", p. 93.
24. K. Mahadevan (Ed.), Health Education for quality of life, Delhi, B.R. Publishing Corporation, 2002.
25. Farokh Erach Udwadia, Emeritus Professor of medicine, "Humanity: The Core of Doctor-Patient Relationship", *University News*, 42(34), August 23-29, 2004, pp. 15-16.
26. A. Rajasebram, Radical Changes required in Medical Education, *University News*, 44(23), June 05-11, 2006, p. 15.
27. Farokh Erach Udwadia, Emeritus Professor of medicine, "Humanity: The Core of Doctor-Patient Relationship", *University News*, 42(34), August 23-29, 2004, p. 16.
28. Farokh Erach Udwadia, Emeritus Professor of medicine, "Humanity: The Core of Doctor-Patient Relationship", *University News*, 42(34), August 23-29, 2004, p. 16.
29. A. Rajasebram, Radial Changes required in Medical Education, *University News*, 44(23), June 05-11, 2006, p. 17.
30. Vijay Pithadia and Vandana Parmar, Appraisal of Medical Education in India, *University News*, 44(44), October 30-November 5, 2006, pp. 11-12.
31. Aleya Ei Bindari Hammad, Intersectoral Cooperation in Primary Health Care, *World Health*, March 1986, p. 3.
32. D.B. Baker and D. Masys, "Research and Development," Consumer Informatics, p. 67.
33. S.L. Goel, "Health Education with Individuals (Counselling)", p. 299.
34. *Ibid.*, p. 315.
35. R.D. Appel and C. Boyer, "Steps Toward Reliable Online Consumer Health Information, Consumer Informatics, p. 89.
36. Public Health in India: Five Decades, 50th Anniversary of India's Independence, Vol. I, p. 7.
37. S.L. Goel, Health Education, Theory and Practice, pp. 82-83.
38. Text of Address by Dr. H. Mahler, to the Thirteenth Session of Regional Committee of South East Asia.
39. Geneva Declaration.
40. I swear by Apollo by Christian Viedma, *World Health*, July 1979, p. 28.
41. J.S. Neki, Medical Ethics, *World Health*, July 1979.
42. Farokh Erach Udwadia, Emeritus Professor of Medicine, *University News*, 42(34), August 23-23, 2004, p. 14.

12

CHAPTER

Referral System

Referral system is an indispensable element of health care to ensure adequate and quality health care to people. Without scientific planning for referral services, we are witnessing huge crowds at secondary and tertiary health care institutions. The cost of treatment at secondary and tertiary levels are very high. If there is a proper referral system it would result into:

(a) Adequate facilities at each level of health care.
(b) Quality services based on standard norms.
(c) Less rush at secondary and tertiary level.
(d) Increased competence of personnel at lower levels.
(e) Less cost.
(f) Develop permanent linkages among Primary, Secondary and tertiary health care.
(g) Create interest among health professionals in identifying rural health problems and their solution.
(h) Optimum use of resources.
(i) Encourage research into local problems.
(j) Keep the health systems effective, efficient, responsive.
(k) Result into the satisfaction of the ailing humanity.

Karnataka Health System Development Project in its report defines ideal referral health system as:

Conceptually a multi-tier system which combines preventive, curative and specialised care is efficient when it provides patients access to levels of care that are appropriate to their health needs with a minimum of inconveniences and delay. It works best when the lowest tier is easily accessible to the community and provides the bulk of the preventive care as well as curative care services for common illnesses. Patients with more complex problems are identified in a timely and systematic manner and referred to the appropriate high level. Each successive level provides

CHART 12.1

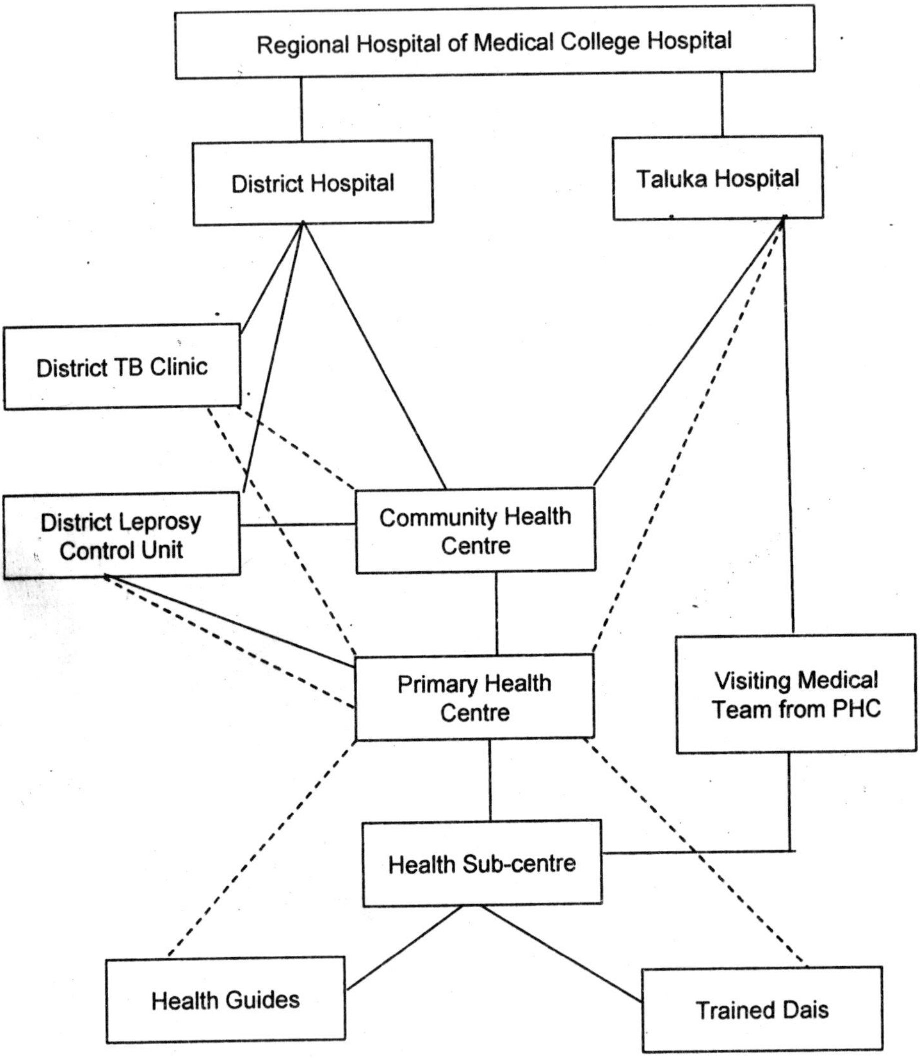

services that are more complex and therefore more expensive. In such a system, the higher tier provides technical leadership and support for the lower tiers, and the community has confidence in the quality of care provided at each tier and the patients understand they will be in accordance with patient needs.[1]

As health services are extended to rural areas, and as more and more responsibility for health care is placed on paramedical staff, a patient referral system becomes the means for ensuring quality health care to all patients. A good patient referral system is an essential component of primary health care. In India, health assistants are the supervisors responsible for maintaining a functioning patient referral system between sub-centres, the primary health centre and community health centre.

A simple patient referral system is shown in Chart 12.1. Patients enter the system at the sub-centre level; if adequate treatment is not available at the sub-centre, they are referred to PHC and CHC where appropriate treatment is available. In certain unusual situations, one or more of the referral levels may be skipped; for example, a patient with a serious head injury may be referred from a PHC directly to a Regional Hospital. But normally, a patient will move up the referral system, step by step, as shown in the diagram.[2]

World Bank appointed working group to establish referral system in the states assisted by it. The work group suggested the following to make effective referral systems:

- services to be provided at each level should be defined,
- services should be of adequate quality to inspire confidence among patients that they will be treated in an effective manner at that level,
- patients and the community must have the confidence that if the need arises, the patients will be properly referred and promptly transported to higher level of health care,
- the public is aware about the type of services available at each level of the health system, and
- procedures should be followed to ensure that patients do not skip the lower levels at which they could be effectively treated.[3]

Besides, the working groups suggested the following administrative directions to streamline the procedure of referral system:

1. ensuring that referrals are made to the nearest properly equipped referral centre to provide treatment at the earliest, rather than the hospital to which the referring hospital is administratively linked;
2. transportation facilities for the referral of critically ill-patient along with results of laboratory investigations, diagnosis and treatment provided by the referring hospital, and for the referral of poor and disadvantaged patients;
3. ensuring that all possible measures are taken to stabilise the patient before referral;
4. avoiding unnecessary delays in the receiving hospitals by, for example, publishing information on clinic hours, laboratory hours, X-Ray hours, giving priority to referred cases, simplifying admission procedures, etc.;
5. maintaining registers or records at both the referring hospitals and the receiving hospitals. This information will facilitate the

monitoring and evaluation of the referral system in terms of the number of cases, purpose of referral, destination or source of referral, etc.;
6. issuing guidelines in respect of referrals from private sector;
7. the District Surgeon will review once a month, the working of referral system and also visit the institutions each quarter for inspection; and
8. the referral hospital will attend to the referred patients on top priority.

Mrs. Indira Gandhi, the then Prime Minister of India, while presiding over a function at Lady Hardinge Medical College at Delhi, had rightly mentioned (quoted by Dr. P.N. Chhuttani, Ex-Director, PCI, in his article, "Decentralisation Needed" published in Medical View Point column of *The Tribune*, dated 4-5-1980) that "The referral system has entirely failed in almost all our larger towns and cities. Consequently, there is growing over-crowding at our major hospitals whose services stand diluted. In the larger cities there is the multiplicity of the controlling authorities—The Government, the Municipal Corporation, the Municipal Committee, Voluntary Organisations, private hospitals, etc." She further stated that "there is no common meeting ground and hospital services have become almost totally unregulated. Consequently, the conditions in our capital city are chaotic. The poor and the needy flock towards the larger, better known hospitals in the hope of better treatment and care, only to find that they have to wait for days to be examined, much less to find a place to stay. Patients wander from hospital to hospital. Besides facing considerable inconvenience, their efforts to seek relief cause duplication of work and expenditure. It is thus necessary that every big city must have an apex body, perhaps called the hospital board, to establish referral hospitals for every zone."

How can we get out of this chaos? How to design a system of patient care? The answer is introduction of Regionalisation. Regionalisation connotes the development of graded patient care within a defined geographical or functional area from lower to higher levels adapting the health services to the characteristics and needs of the area and, thus, ensure the optimum utilisation of resources. The essential characteristics of regionalisation are:

(a) Two-way flow at patients
(b) Two-way flow of records
(c) Two-way flow of services
(d) Two-way flow of personnel
(e) Mobile units
(f) Centralised administration and decentralised execution
(g) Coordinating education programme for the region
(h) Communication and transport between components
(i) Coordination with other community health services.

Thus, regionalisation would ensure the best utilisation of time of that specialists and provision of comprehensive health care to the patients nearer their homes with all the benefits of specialities. The regional area should neither be too large nor too small but should be such as to ensure adequate span of attention. It would also automatically develop referral system scientifically. The referral system presents the following five aspects:

(a) It has to be built into the organisational structure of the medical services of a country. The role should be that only when one unit cannot provide what a patient needs should of the patient be referred to the next higher unit in the chain.

(b) The problem has to be organised both internally and externally. 'Internally' means that patients in the hospital have to be referred from the in-patients to the out-patients department just as soon as their health situation permits. The 'externally' referred system exists among the several institutions on different levels of the hierarchy.

(c) The referral system must be established for the purpose of diagnosis and treatment and used for both in-patients and out-patients.

(d) It is a two-way system. Patients should be referred to higher level institutions for diagnosis and treatment when necessary, but they should also be referred back to the referring institution as soon as possible.

(e) The referral system concerns not only patients and diagnostic facilities but also the personnel of the medical services. This is also a two-way system, so that human knowledge and skills are utilised fully and are continually developed through consultations and the interchange of ideas and experience.

The specialists from the regional hospital must come to District hospital and the specialist from that District hospital to health centre on a regular basis as consultants, to hold specialist and give guidance; the medical and para-medical personnel should institution regularly for in-services training.

FEATURES OF REFERRAL SYSTEM

I. Referral Network and Zoning

To identify the various referral levels, the whole district is divided into several zones and the referral levels are indicated for each zone. To facilitate and for convenience of patients, certain number of Primary Health Centres are grouped and linked to community health centre (C.H.C.)/Tehsil Hospital Area Hospitals/District Hospitals depending upon the distance, availability of services, facilities of transportation, etc. But adopting a grouping system, uniform referral pattern has been developed. In this system the patient will know the course of further treatment, in case one is referred for some special procedure at appropriate level of care. Similarly, a good rapport and faith in the referral system will be developed. This is called zoning.

It helps in evolving a chain for the health units beginning at the primary level moving up through the middle tier and finally reaching the tertiary hospitals. Let us explain it with the help of Kiratpur Sahib. (see Chart 1)

After dividing the district into zones, the same is to be depicted on the map. The map should reflect all the health institutions, roads, river, bridges, Bus Stand, Railway route, Railway station, Police station, Post offices, etc.

These maps will have to be displayed at the reception counter in each of the health institutions.

2. Transportation Facilities

To build up an effective Referral System, a dependable transportation arrangement has been provided where the health personnel shall be able to send the patients to the next appropriate level of care at the earliest, as the flow of patients is expected to be from primary health centres to the tertiary level.

3. Referral-cum-Feed-back Card

Referral system is a two way process. The colour coding has been done. The patient referred from CHC shall get blue cards. The patients referred from Tehsil hospital/Area hospital shall get green card. The patients referred from District hospital shall get white card. The patient referred from P.H.C. or Subsidiary Health Centres shall have pink card.

The referral card contains—General information about the patients such as name, age, gender, address, Chief complaints, clinical findings, vital signs, Investigations done, Treatment given, procedure done where referred, and purpose of referral, i.e. for admission, Investigation or expert opinion.

At the referred hospital, patients could report directly to the unit or department to which he or she has been referred through a special counter for referred patients.

4. Referral Procedure

In the referral procedure, there are two types of referral: (i) Emergency, (ii) Routine referral. In routine referral the patient will have to make his own transportation arrangement, however proper counselling needs to be done. The patient shall be given referral card. The regular hospital hours 8.00 a.m. to 2.00 p.m. in summer and 9.00 a.m. to 3.00 p.m. in winter with half an hour break 1.30 p.m. to 2.00 p.m. For investigations, the best suitable time 9.00 A.M. to 11.30 A.M. However, emergency patients who are to be attended round the clock.

5. Receiving of Referred Patients

Referral units should receive the patients directly at a place identified in each hospital without waiting in general outdoor patient department (OPD).

The receiving hospital must ensure that a referred patient enjoys the following privileges:

(i) *Queue Jump*: The referred patient will not stand in queue for general out-patients. He/She directly goes to the doctor referred on priority through a special counter of referred patients on routine.

(ii) *No need of new OPD ticket*: The referral card itself to be used as OPD ticket. The entry is to be made in the referral registers at the reception counter.

(iii) No purchase fee for referred patient with referral card.

(iv) Feed-back-After dealing with patient and at the time of discharge in case of admission, the doctor should fill up referral-*cum*-feed-back card. This will help the referring donor to know whether the patient that he had referred, had got the relief. The specialist may send the feed-back on slip (from slip pad) through S.M.O. I/C of the health institution.

(v) *Provision of low cost transportation*: In emergency patients, it is clear that the actual fuel charges are to be paid by the patient. In poor patients (unknown, yellow card holders, natural Caldmities, Disaster), this can be exempted.

(vi) From jail Hospitals, the patients are referred through the Police guard.

6. Norms of Service

Norms of Services have been worked out for institutions at various levels in terms of facilities, staffing, equipment, services, etc.

7. Maintenance of Registers

Two registers both by referring institutions and referred institutions are to be maintained to keep a proper records. Besides, there are large number of details which have been drawn to make the system functional. However, the systems has not taken roots and is still in its infancy.

For making referral system successful, Punjab Health System Corporation has taken the following steps:

1. Intensive Training to all personnel from top to bottom to make them aware of the potentialities and limitations of referral systems.
2. Equipping the health institutions with the prescribed norms of services.
3. Making the people aware through maps of zoning and also through a video casettee "Know your Hospital."

4. Arranging transport facilities.
5. Delegation and decentralisation of administrative and financial powers.
6. Overseeing the implementation.
7. Conducting research to diagnose the problems which stand in the way of efficient functioning of referral system.

By now, referral system has been introduced in all districts of Punjab. It is hoped that this would bring a revolution in health services in Punjab.

THE REFERRAL SYSTEM IN PUNJAB

The Punjab Health Systems Corporation has initiated to strengthen the functioning of the hospitals for referral system through the following measures:

- Renovating and "grading hospital buildings to provide appropriate space for services.
- Upgrading and updating clinical skills of medical officers and staff nurses through an effective training programme.
- Providing ambulances for transporting critical patients.
- Installing phone, fax and paging systems in hospitals.
- Financial powers to Senior Medical Officers in charge of the hospitals to accord necessary single sanction up to Rs. 5,000 (Rs. Five thousand only) and Deputy Medical Commissioners, Civil Surgeon, Medical Superintendent up to Rs. 10,000 (Rs. Ten thousand only) to meet the emergency.
- The user's charges are to be retained at the site of collection. These are to be used by the Senior Medical Officer Incharge of the hospital. Norms of services have been designed for each level of faculty.

The Referral Manual for health systems in the State of Punjab has been compiled to issue administrative guidelines and referral protocols. The contents have been taken from Staff Appraisal Report, State Health Systems Development Project II, document of the World Bank—Feb. 20, 1996. The norms of services at Community Health Centre, Sub-Divisional Hospitals and District Hospitals, Equipment Norms, Norm of Staff has been collected from Project Proposals for the development of Secondary Level Health Care Systems in Punjab, September 1995. Referral Registers have been designed with the help of APVVP, Hyderabad. The Referral-cum-Feedback cards in different "colours have been printed." For Primary Health Centres Pink Colour, Blue Colour for Community Health Centre and; Area Hospital, Green colour for Sub-Divisional Hospitals, White colour for District Hospital. Reporting formats for CHC/SDH/DH have been designed.

Demographic Profile of District Ropar (See Health Map I)

Ropar district came into being on the eve of reorganisation of Punjab on 01-11.1966 and is spread over an area of about 2055 sq. miles. The district has semi-hilly and far flung areas. District Ropar is bound by Chandigarh, on East; District Nawanshahr, on the West; on the North Himachal Pradesh (e.g. District Una and Bilaspur) and on the South by District Fatehgarh Sahib, and Patiala. The health services are being provided through the Primary Health Centres, Civil Hospital, Rural Hospitals, Subsidiary Health Centres and through a network of sub-centres. Seven secondary level institutions, namely, Civil Hospital, Mohali, Civil Hospital, Kharar, R.H. Kurali, Civil Hospital, Ropar, PHC Chamkaur Sahib, Civil Hospital, Anandpur Sahib and R.H., Nurpur Bedi have been taken over by the Punjab Health System Corporation for strengthening the services including development of referral system. We are taking up Nurpur Bedi and Chamkaur Sahib to depict referral design. (For zoning see R.H., Nurpur Bedi and Chamkaur Sahib and Boothgarh Plan). (See Maps 2 and Map 3)

REFERRAL SYSTEM IN ROPAR DISTRICT (PUNJAB)

Punjab is one of the vital states of Indian Union consisting of 17 districts. Punjab has a vast network of public health care facilities comprising of 217 hospitals excluding three tertiary level hospitals, 104 community health centres, 484 primary health centres and 1462 subsidiary health centres, dispensaries. The teritary care facilities in Punjab consists of three Government Medical Colleges, two private medical colleges and a prestigious Post-Graduate Institute of Medical Education and Research (PGIMER), Chandigarh under the Ministry of Health and Family Welfare, Government of India.

Punjab Health Systems Corporation established under the World Bank project aims to develop secondary health care. It has taken up 151 health institutions including all district hospitals, 42 Sub-divisional hospitals and 87 Community Health Centre, 6 Area hospitals. Under the World Bank project, Punjab Health Systems Corporation is responsible for:

1. Renovation of hospital buildings to provide appropriate space for services.
2. Upgrading and updating of clinical skills of Medical Officer and staff nurses through an effective training programme.
3. Provision of ambulances for transporting critical patients.
4. Installations of phone, fax in hospitals.
5. Strengthening of Secondary level health care shall support the primary health care and thus there is need to formulate and implement an ideal and effective referral system. This is the right time and situation for Referral System to work and is the rationale for this system to develop.

Map I

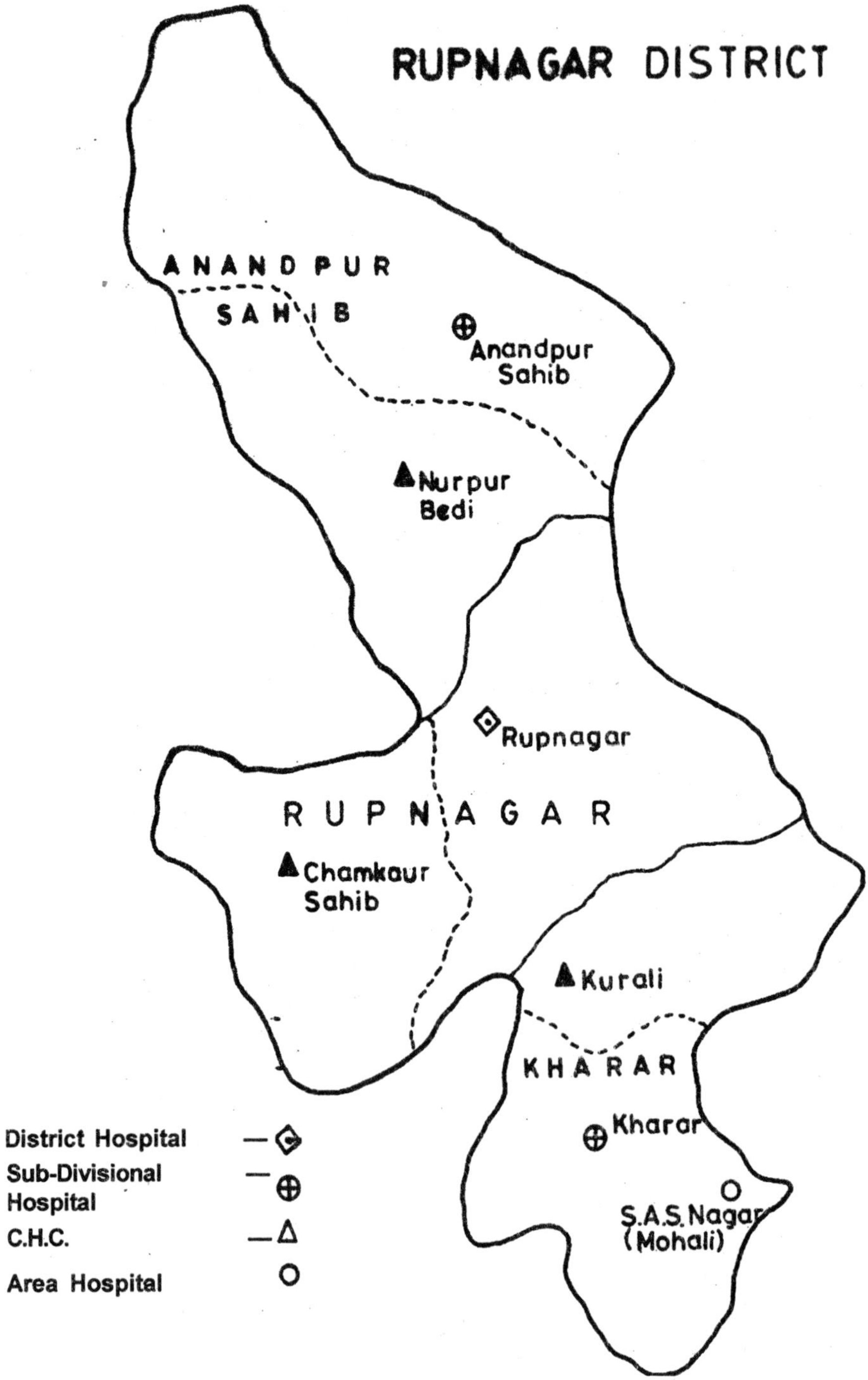
RUPNAGAR DISTRICT
ANANDPUR SAHIB
Anandpur Sahib
Nurpur Bedi
Rupnagar
RUPNAGAR
Chamkaur Sahib
Kurali
KHARAR
Kharar
S.A.S. Nagar (Mohali)
District Hospital
Sub-Divisional Hospital
C.H.C.
Area Hospital

MAP 2

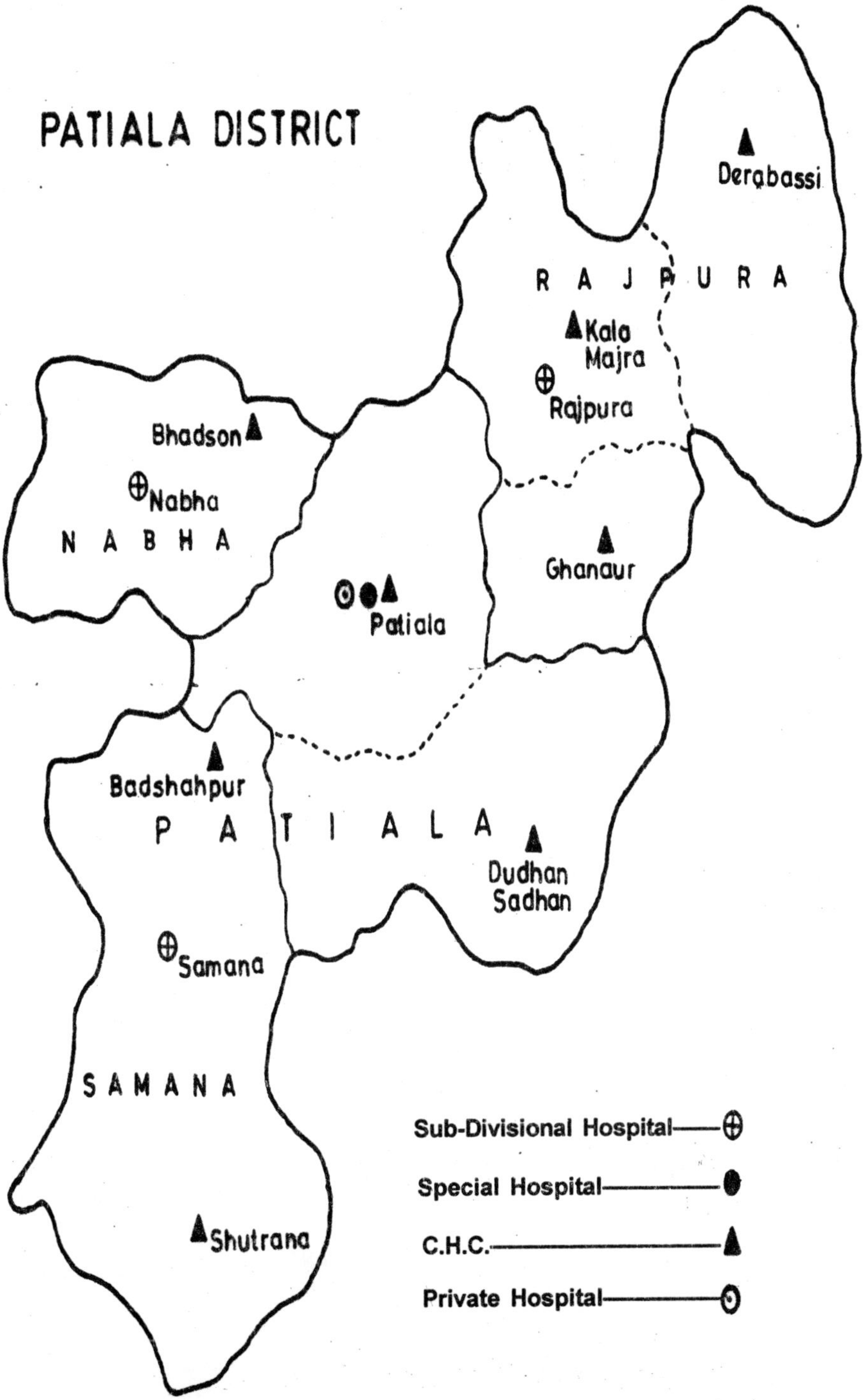
PATIALA DISTRICT
Derabassi
RAJPURA
Kala Majra
Rajpura
Bhadson
Nabha
NABHA
Ghanaur
Patiala
Badshahpur
PATIALA
Dudhan Sadhan
Samana
SAMANA
Shutrana
Sub-Divisional Hospital
Special Hospital
C.H.C.
Private Hospital

MAP 3

PUNJAB

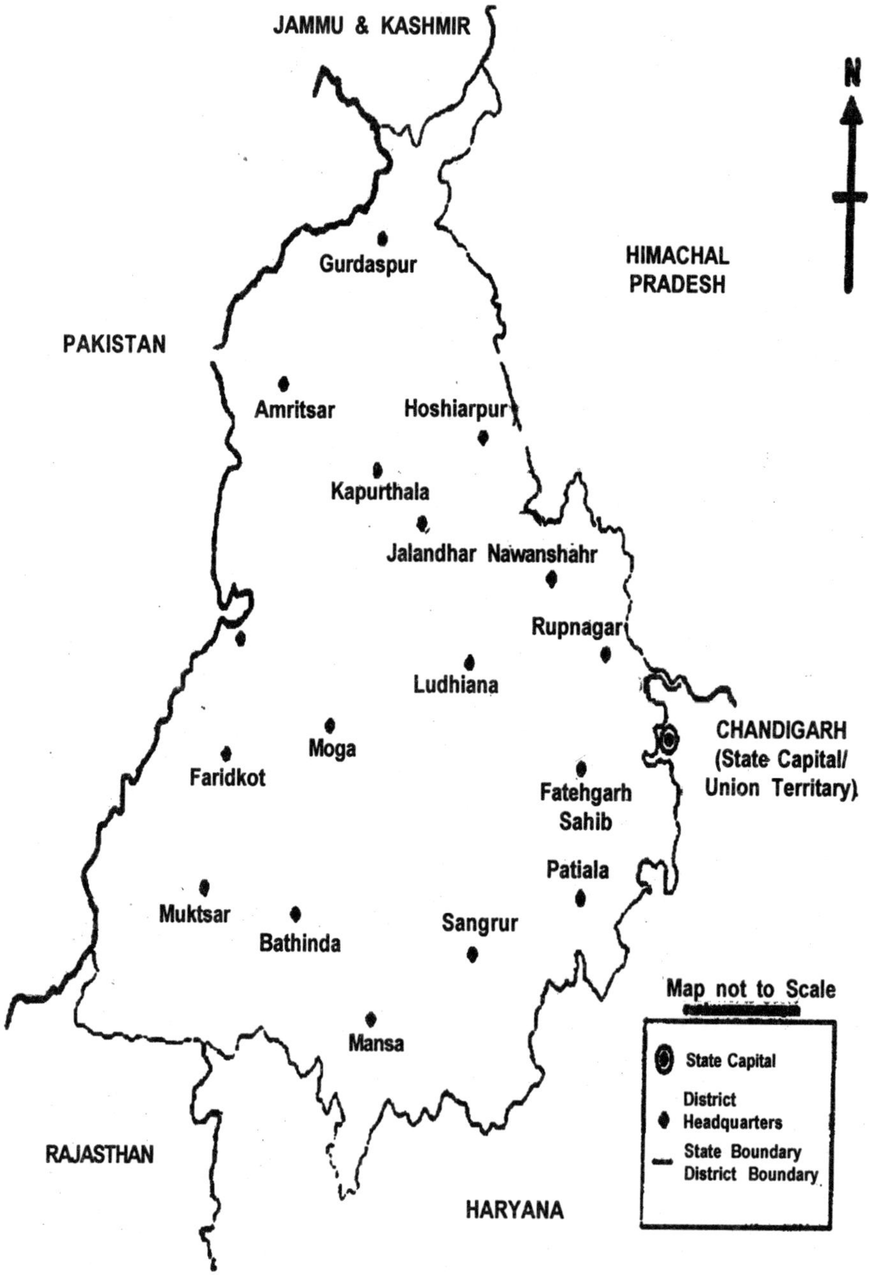

JAMMU & KASHMIR
N
HIMACHAL PRADESH
PAKISTAN
Gurdaspur
Amritsar
Hoshiarpur
Kapurthala
Jalandhar
Nawanshahr
Rupnagar
Ludhiana
CHANDIGARH (State Capital/ Union Territary)
Moga
Faridkot
Fatehgarh Sahib
Patiala
Muktsar
Bathinda
Sangrur
Map not to Scale
Mansa
State Capital
District Headquarters
State Boundary
District Boundary
RAJASTHAN
HARYANA

CRITICAL APPRAISAL

Author's personal visit to Ropar district, discussions with the health staff in various institutions and the staff of Punjab Health System Corporation revealed the following deficiencies which need immediate attention to ensure the success of referral system. It should be extended to other Districts after correcting the problems already known.

1. Half-hearted Approach in Introducing Referral System: Need of Providing Full Facilities at Each Level

Most of the doctors indicated that they do not have the full facilities as worked out by the working group. How can you expect a good referral system from hospitals which are not well equipped? Even some of the equipments supplied are not functional creating additional problems of its use. Along with it, there are no technical experts to handle the equipments supplied. It is suggested that before further embarking upon new areas, we should ensure the facilities in functional state.

2. Lack of In-depth Training to Personnel: Need of Intensive Training

At present, the training has been imparted into the mechanics of referral system but not its rationale, philosophy and utilities. It must be ingrained into the minds of the professionals that referred system is the only answer to provide graded quality health care in new millennium.

3. Professionals Leave the Working Place Daily to Nearby Metropolitan Cities: Need of Making Stay Compulsory

The first and foremost requirement of referral system is the availability of personnel otherwise patients would approach private nursing comes. They would either not entertain the referred complicated case or would try to shift to higher level. The government should make the stay of doctors in the Vicinity of hospitals mandatory with full facilities to them to make stay attractive.

4. Professionals Discourage Referral System because of their Collision with Private Practitioners: Need of Strict Control over Professionals

Professionals are cheating the Government. They are getting non-practicing allowance on the one hand while on the other hand, they work in off duty hours with private practitioners. In such a situation they would send the referral patients to private practitioners to get some money and discourage referral system. Referred patients often travel long distances only to be kept waiting in the out-patient department for hours or even days. The out-patient department must be organised to give them priority over other patients. Government should adopt strict measures to check this menace which is against medical ethics.

5. Lack of Proper Publicity: Need of Publishing in Daily Newspapers Intermittently

People being illiterate and ignorant do not understand the meaning and procedure of referral systems. They are treated in the same way as other patients resulting into agony and pain. There is a need to educate the people through press, T.V., radio, and posters.

6. No Feed-back: Need of Reporting to the Previous Level

It has been found that patients referred to higher level do not come back and report as to what was wrong and how it has been treated. Thus, one of the purposes of referral system, i.e. providing higher knowledge to lower functionary is missed. There should be some arrangements for meetings among experts at different levels to exchange notes about the referred case to keep upto date.

7. Lack of Library Facilities: Need of Allocating Sufficient Honey for Books

The professionals once appointed rarely read the latest developments in their field of specialisation and general health management. How can they learn new techniques? It is not possible always to send them for training. It is suggested that books and journals may be made available to keep them upto date, different districts can subscribe to different journals which may be exchanged after some time.

8. Van either remain out of Order or POL is not Available for Transportation: Need of Ensuring the Vans in Working Conditions

Critical patients are to be shifted immediately but delays occur due to non-availability of either vehicle or POL, or Driver. Referral systems requires good transport management.

9. Lack of Effective Communication: Need of Providing Mobile Phone Facilities

It becomes difficult to contact expert as there are no facilities. What is the consequence? Patients reach but the doctors are not available, creating critical conditions. There is a need to provide good communication system among the components of referral systems.

10. Lack of Seriousness and Interest among Top Level Functionaries: Need of Creating Interest in them

It has been seen that the top officials do not take pains to find out the loopholes during their field visit in the referral system. This lukewarm attitude spreads among functionaries at lower levels. The result is the mushroom growth of nursing homes which are fleecing the illiterate and ignorant people. Today, medical professionals are mainly interested in making money and not on excellence. There is a need to change this culture otherwise the whole of Government Medical and Health System would collapse. Under the circumstances there is no need to subsidize health services because of its inefficiency and little use to the people.

11. Insensitive to the Needs of Patients: Need of Developing Coordinal Relationships

Doctors care very less for the patients. Dr. Iqbal S. Ahuja in his article, "Self-Introspection, 1st January, 2000 *(The Indian Express,* New Horizons! New Hopes) rightly says that there seems to be decline in human relationships. Money has started playing a bigger role in the maintenance of relationship. The soul and body relationship, purity of heart, thought and action have all deteriorated. Time has come for introspection into thyself. Where are the days when the patient treated the doctor like a second God? Why have we deteriorated in thought and action? Why self has come before the service? We all need introspection in our hearts." The teachings of Swami Vivekananda can help the professionals in rejuvenating the system. To quote him: "Let us all work hard, my brethren; this is not time for sleep. On our work depends the coming of the India of the future. She is there ready waiting. She is only sleeping. Arise and awake and see her seated here, on her eternal throne, rejuvenated, more glorious than she ever was—This motherland of ours."

12. Lack of Quality Assurance and Quality of Medical Care: Need of Medical Audit

Quality assurance means delivery of efficient and effective medical care which is a *sine qua non* for referral system. The health institutions need to develop standards of quality in a comprehensive and scientific manner. They should not concentrate merely on technical competence but also ensure effective communication with patients, and develop work culture. Professional quality care can be ascertained by medical audit which can ascertain the advantage of referral systems.

Medical Audit is defined on the evaluation of medical care in retrospect through analysis of medical records of referred patients. Dr. C. Prakash, as eminent health and medical expert suggests the need of developing referral index.

The discharge reports and summaries evaluation of referred patients can provide useful indications of quality of health care. How well the hospital has passed on the information to the agencies who referred the cases? Similarly, what details the referring agencies have provided to the referral hospital, are these adequate or inadequate, appropriate or inappropriate, etc. Thus, two-way referrals should be functioning. The quality of referrals should be ascertained both-ways to find the gaps for corrective actions. The simple indicators suggested for referral functions are:

1. No. of patients referred to hospital per annum.
2. Nature of referrals made.
3. Agency referring the cases.

4. Feedback system for referrals, i.e. number of referrals for whom the referring agency was informed.
5. Higher level hospital and referrals to district or sub-division hospital for future care or follow up? and reports of such follow up if any from the periphery.
6. Similarly, referrals from one unit to another unit of the referral hospital, time lag between the admission and referral, exchange of information between the units and outcome of such referrals can be appropriate indicators for assessment of quality of referrals.[5]

World Bank deserves appreciation for providing both expertise and finances to introduce referral system in health care system in some of the states of the Indian Union. State governments should take the maximum advantage of this generous aid to improve their health system in the new millennium. World Bank can only provide facilities but cannot take the place of hundreds of health functionaries on whose shoulders the success of installation, implementation and utilisation of referral system depend.

In a report submitted to the Governing Council, Paul G. Hoffman, an ex-administrator of UN Development Programme, said: "External assistance ha.c; a limited but a vital role to play. It will help break the vicious cycle due to the fact that poverty breeds poverty and poverty of opportunity perpetuates it. Poor nations, like poor people, are caught up in the day-to-day fight for survival. Forced to live a hand-to-mouth existence, they cannot put enough to invest adequately in their own futures, poor because they cannot develop their own resources and unable to develop their resources because they are poor.[6]

Colonel Hla Han, Burma's Minister for Health, while addressing the 24th session of the WHO Regional Committee for South-East Asia held in Rangoon, stated:

> "The destinies of our nations are now once again in our hands, but as developing nations, the limitations which exist in our economic and social sectors have greatly impeded our endeavors."

Notes and References

1. Karnataka Health System Development Corporation Project, Deptt. of Health and Family Welfare, Government of Karnataka, Bangalore, January 1996, p. 109.
2. NIHFW, Management Training Modules for Health Assistants, New Delhi, 1987, p. 129.
3. Karnataka Health System Development Project, *op. cit.*, p. 103.
4. *Ibid.*
5. C.Parkash, Quality Health Care, In *Hospital Administration and Management*, Vol. III, (Editors S.L. Goel and R. Kumar) New Delhi, Deep & Deep, p. 294.
6. 12th Session of UNDP Governing Council, 7-23, January 1971, pp. 112-14. (UNDP–E/5043-Rev. 1).

CHART 12.1

Zoning Kiratpur Sahib

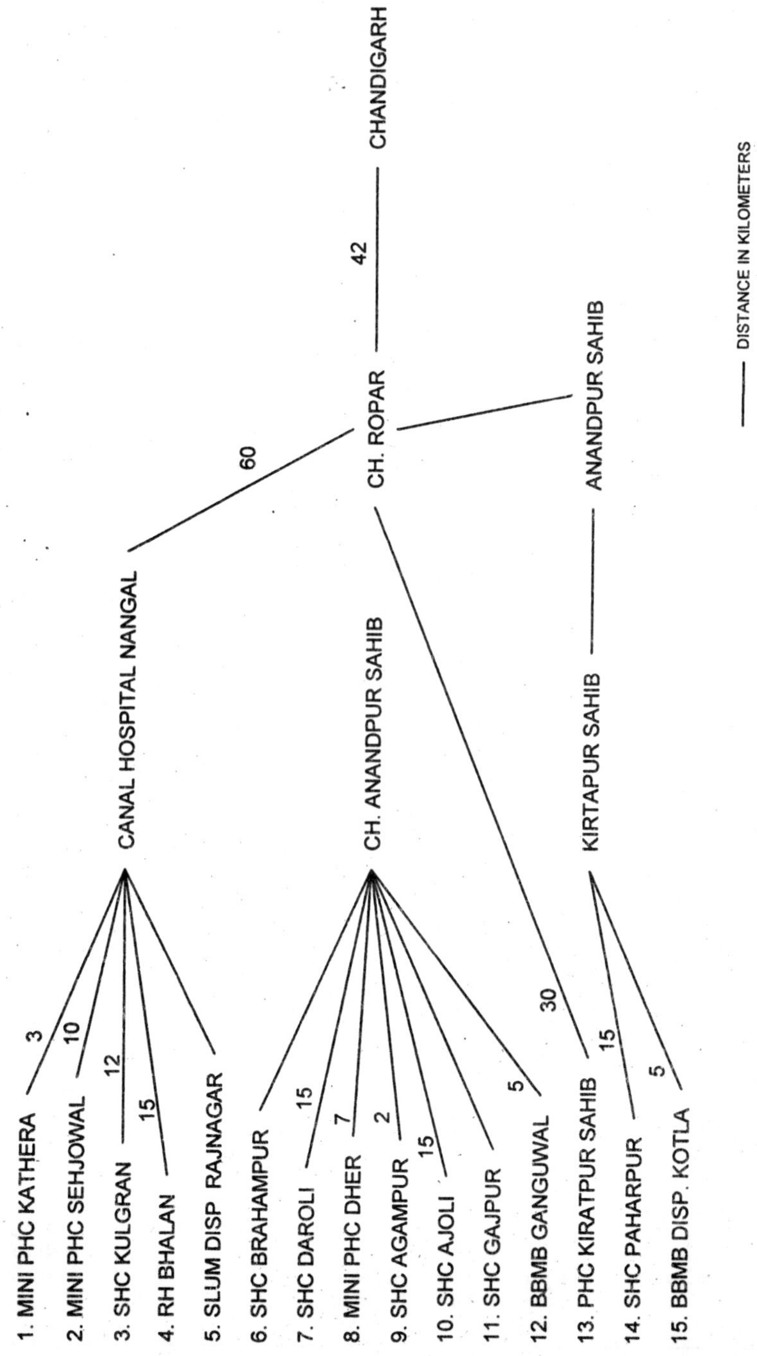

Appendix 12.1

Norms of Services

Normative Range of Services at Different Levels

Medical and Pediatric Probems

Disease of Central Nervous System

Diseases	*CHCs*	*Sub-Div. Hospitals*	*District Hospitals*
(a) Coma/ Cerebro vascular Accident	❑ To maintain vital signs and airway (Ambubag, Oxygen) ❑ To exclude Diabetes and Renal failure ❑ To provide facility of tracheostomy and Laryngoscope for intubation. ❑ To exclude head injury by doing x-ray skull. ❑ To start medical decompression treatment. Antibiotic and to treat case of poisoning if any. If coma does not improve case to be referred to district level hospital.	Same as CHC	Carry on treatment and surgical decompression if required to investigate and confirm diagnosis of CV accident. Brain tumor be referred to teritary level institution if indicated.
(b) Meningitis	To initiate symptomatic treatment and refer to district hospital for further investigation.	To do CSF examination, start treatment, if no improvement after 47 hours refer to Tertiary level hospital.	To do culture and sensitivity test, diagnose and treat.
(c) Epilepsy	Initiate medical treatment and first aid treatment, refer to district level hospital for further investigation.	Same as CHC.	Manage, investigate, do EEG, refer to tertiary level institution for surgery if required.
(d) Polio and other Acute flaccid Paralysis	Initiate medical treatment, maintain vital signs, remove discomfort, refer to district level hospital for CSF examination and stool culture.	Same as CHC.	To treat and investigate Stool culture C.S.F. exam.

Source: Punjab Health System Corporation, Referral Manual, for Health System in Punjab State, IIIrd Edition, by H.V. Jindal, pp. 14-93.

Appendix 12.2

Referral Card—Punjab Health Systems Corporation

(to be filled at the referred health institute)

1. Date and Time of receiving the Patient	Registration No.	Referring health institutions
2. Doctor/Deptt. from where referred	Date	
	Referring Doctor	Referred for
	Where referred	Admission/Invesgitation/Opinion

Signature of Receptionist

(To be filled by the attending doctor of referred institution at the time of discharge)

1. Condition of Pátient on discharge	Institution/Unit	
	1. Name of Patient	
	2. Father's/Husband's Name	
2. Investigation done	3. Age	Sex: M/F
	4. Address: H. No.	
	Village	
3. Treatment advised	Tehsil	
	District	
	5. Diagnosis	
4. Date of review if necessary		
5. Date		

Signature
(Name of Doctor)
Stamp of Hospital

APPENDIX 12.3

Respiratory Diseases

Diseases	*CHCs*	*Sub-Divisional Hospitals*	*District Level Hospitals*
Bronchial Asthma	To initiate medical treatment, if no relife send to district level for further investigation.	Same as CHC.	To investigate and Treat
Upper Respiratory and Lower Respiratory Infection	Initiate medical treatment and symptomatic treatment observe for 48 hours, if no relief refer to district hospital.	Same as CHC.	To investigate and Treat
Tuberculosis	To investigate by sputum examination and x-ray chest, initiate anti-tuberculosis treatment. Review after 15 days, if no relief refer to district hospital.	Same as CHC.	To investigate and Treat
Lung Cancer	To initiate symptomatic treatment and other supportive theraphy, refer to tertiary level health institution.	Same as CHC.	Same as CHC and refer to teritary level institute
Pleural Effusion	Initiate symptomatic treatment, do x-ray chest and diagnostic tap. Start treatment and refer to district hospital, to confirm diagnosis.	Same as CHC.	To confirm the diagnosis start treatment, if malignant refer to tertiary level hospital.
Poisonous Gases Inhalation	Start first-aid treatment, give respiratory support.	Same as CHC.	Same as CHC
Foreign Body Inhalation	Give first-aid, refer to Tertiary level hospital where facility of Bronchoscopy is available.	Same as CHC.	Same as CHC

Source: Ibid.

Appendix 12.4

Cardio Vascular Diseases

Diseases	*CHCs*	*Sub-Divisional Hospitals*	*District Level Hospitals*
Hypertension	To initiate medical treatment, of mild and moderate hypertension, refer to sub-divisional level hospital for treatment of accelerated hypertension.	Investigate and treat	Investigate and Treat
Coronary Artery Diseases	Initiate medical treatment on clinical suspicion of disease, refer to district hospital for TMT and other tests.	Same as CHC	Investigate and maintain theraphy. Refer to tertiary level hospital for active intervention, if required (Coronary, angiography, Angioplasty and Bypass surgery)
Myo-Cardial Infarction	To initiate treatment by sedation Vaso-dilator, Thromolytic theraphy (Streptokinase). If within 24 hours there is no improvement or there is complication refer to subdividional level hospital.	To manage Myo-Cardial Infarction, if evidence of heart block refer to district hospital for pace maker	To investigate and Treat
Congestive Heart Failure	Initiate treatment and observe, if decompensation persist refer to district hospital	Same as CHC	To investigate and Treat
Acute Pulmonary Oedema/ Cardiac Asthama	Initiate treatment with Bronchodilator, Diuretics, Oxygen, if no improvement refer to district hospital	Same as CHC	To investigate and Treat
Rheumatic Fever and Rheumatic Heart Disease	Start initial medical treatment, refer to district level for confirmation of diagnosis	Same as CHC	To investigate and Treat
Arrythemia	Maintain vital signs and refer to sub-divisional hospital for Defibrilator	Medical treatment and Defibrilation	Medical treatment and Defibrilation
Shock	Initiate treatment, maintain vital signs and functions. IV fluids, Oxygen and observe, if no improvement within reasnoable time refer to district hospital.	Same as CHC	To investigate and Treat

Source: Ibid.

APPENDIX 12.5

Referred Register to be maintained by the Hospital/Specialists Referring the Patients

Sl. No.	*OPD/RR Number*	*Name of patient*	*Age*	*Sex*	*Date and Time of receiving the patient for the first time*	*Name of Institute where referred*	*Diagnosis*	*Condition at the time of sending referral Date/Time*	*Sent by whom*	*Action taken*	*Feed-back received Yes/No*

Source: Ibid.

APPENDIX 12.6

Referred Register to be maintained by the Institution/Specialists who are receiving the Patients

Sl. No.	*OPD/RR Number*	*Name of patient*	*Age*	*Sex*	*Date and Time of receiving the patient for the first time*	*Name of Institute where referred*	*Diagnosis*	*Condition at the time of sending referral Date/Time*	*Sent by whom*	*Action taken*	*Feed-back received Yes/No*

Source: *Ibid.*

Appendix 12.7

Gastro Intestinal Diseases

Diseases	*CHCs*	*Sub-Divisional Hospitals*	*District Level Hospitals*
Gastro Intenstinal Bleeding	Start medical treatment and supportive theraphy, if no improvement within reasonable time refer to district level hospital for Endoscopic investigation	Same as CHC	Investigate and Treat
Jaundice/Hepatitis	Clinically diagnose and initiate medical treatment, refer to district for investigation especially if patient is in Coma	Same as CHC	Investigate and Treat
Gastroenteritis/ Dehydration	Start oral Re-hydration theraphy. Systemic antibiotics. if indicated Manage Gr 1 and Gr 2 dehydration. If condition does not improve refer to District Hospital (if there is suspicion of Cholera or other epidemic case, it be immediately referred to District hospital)	Same as CHC	Investigate and Treat
Amoebic Infection	Intestinal Infection to be investigated and treated, if suspicious of liver involvement refer to Sub-Divisional Hospital for Ultra Sound.	Same as CHC	Investigate and Treat

Renal Disorders

Diseases	*CHCs*	*Sub-Divisional Hospitals*	*District Level Hospitals*
Urinary Tract Infection	Initiate symptomatic treatment, send to District Hospital for further investigation	Same as CHC	Investigate and Treat
Haematuria	Symptomatic treatment, alkaliser, pain reliever and investigate, if cause is not identified refer to District Hospital	Same as CHC	Investigate and Treat
Acute Renal Failure and Chronic Renal Failure	Maintain vital signs and refer to Dialysis unit at Tertiary level	Investigate and Treat. For dialysis refer to Tertiary level.	Same as SDH

Musculo-skeletal

Arthritis	Start Palliative theraphy, refer to District Hospital for investigation and physiotheraphy	Same as CHC	Investigate and Treat Physiotherapy

Haematology

Diseases	*CHCs*	*Sub-Divisional Hospitals*	*District Level Hospitals*
Anemia/Infestation	Treat Nutritional Anaemia, treat worms, if no response refer to District Hospital for investigation	Same as CHC + Diagnose	Investigate and Treat
Leukaemia and Re-system Disorder	Give symptomatic treatment and refer to district Hospital for investigation	Same as CHC + Diagnose	Investigate and Treat and refer to tertiary level if needed
Bleeding Disorder	Treat Anaemia, give Haemostatic agents refer to District hospital for investigation	Same as CHC	Investigate and Treat

Infections

Diseases	*CHCs*	*Sub-Divisional Hospitals*	*District Level Hospitals*
Malaria	Diagnose and treat Malaria. In case complication develop or fever does not repond or 6-G-PD deficiency is suspected refer to District Hospital for investigation	Same as CHC	Investigate and Treat
STD	Give treatment for the symptoms, if no response refer to District Hospital WHO Regimen	Same as CHC	Investigate and Treat
Leprosy	Give treatment for the symptoms, if no response, refer to District Hospital for investigation and treatment	Same as CHC	Investigate and Treat
HIV/AIDS	All patients suspected of HIV infection should be referred for diagnosis or nearby HIV Surveillance centre	Same as CHC	Investigate and diagnose. Manage as per NACO guidelines.

Other Conditions

Diseases	*CHCs*	*Sub-Divisional Hospitals*	*District Level Hospitals*
Pleural Aspiration	Do	Same as CHC	Do
Pericardial Tap	No	Same as CHC	Do
Foreign body removal	Do Simple Cases	Same as CHC	Do
Lumbar puncture	Do	Same as CHC	Do
Malignancy	Symptomatic treatment and refer	Same as CHC	Refer to Teritary Level Hospital
Pemphigus	Initiate treatment and refer	Same as CHC	Treat
Collagen Diseases	Refer	Same as CHC	Investigate and Treat
Skin Allergy	Treat	Same as CHC	Investigate cause and treat, Refer
Sarcoidosis	Refer	Same as CHC	Investigate and Treat
Neoplasm	Refer	Same as CHC	Investiate, treat and refer to Tertiary Level hospital
Blood Safety for STD and HIV	Refer	Ensure	Ensure
Cholecystitis	Symptomatic treatment and refer	Same as CHC	Investigate and Treat including Laproscopic Cholecystectomy
Pancreatitis	Symptomatic treatment and refer	Same as CHC	Investigate and manage (for therapeutic endoscopy or surgery, refer to tertiary level)
Cirrhosis	Symptomatic treatment and refer	Same as CHC	Investigate and manage. Refer if complication
Abdominal Tapping	Yes	Yes	Yes
Congential heart diseases	Symptomatic treatment and refer	Same as CHC	Symptomatic treatment and refer to tertiary level
Head Injuries	Initial treatment, observe and refer if necessary to Tertiary level	Same as CHC	Investigate and manage
CV Accidents	Initial treatment, observe and refer if necessary	Same as CHC	Investigate and manage

Psychiatric Alements

Diseases	*CHCs*	*Sub-Divisional Hospitals*	*District Level Hospitals*
(i) Psychotic patients	To start crisis management and refer to psychiatrist at district level hospital	Same as CHC	Treat
(ii) Depression and Allied disorders	Sedation treatment and refer to psychiatrist and follow up action on psychiatrist's advise	Same as CHC	Regular psychiatric treatment
(iii) Dedication	Sedation if the patient is on withdrawal symptoms then refer to district hospitals	Same as CHC	To provide regular treatment
(iv) Mental retardation	Symptomatic treatment and counselling refer to psychiatrist/Neuro physician.	Same as CHC	Provide regular treatment

Pediatrics

Diseases	*CHCs*	*Sub-Divisional Hospitals*	*District Level Hospitals*
ARI	Treat and refer if no improvement	Same as CHC	Investigate and manage
LRI	Mild Symptomatic treatment, refer if no improvement	Same as CHC	Investigate and manage
Childhood Asthma and Allergic Bronchitis	Without respiratory distress manage	Same as CHC	Without respiratory distress Manage
Tuberculosis	Suspected cases to be investigated by sputum exam and radiography, Manage	Same as CHC	Investigate and Treat

Neonatal Services

System and Diseases	*CHCs*	*Sub-Divisional Hospitals*	*District Level Hospitals*
Resuscitation of new Born Babies			
(i) Apgarscore more than 4	Resuscitation to be done and managed.	Same	Same
(ii) Apgarscore less than 4	Resuscitation to be done. It vitals maintained—manage, otherwise refer to district level.	Same	Manage in Special Care Nursery (SCN)
Uncomplicated			
LBW babies			
(i) More than 1.8 Kg.	Manage with rooming in service and observe	Same	Same
(ii) Less than 1.8 Kg.	Resuscitation, Maintain Vitals, Refer to district level.	Same	SCN
Premature babies			
(i) Gestation less than 34 weeks	Resuscitate, maintain vitals and refer to district level	Same	Care in SCN
(ii) Gestation more than 34 weeks	Manage and keep under observation, if any problem refer to district level	Same	Same
Complicated LBW and Premature babies			
	Manage and observe. Refer if problem is unmanageable	Same	Care in SCN

Source: Ibid.

APPENDIX 12.8

Neonatal Jaundice

System and Diseases	*CHCs*	*Sub-Divisional Hospitals*	*District Level Hospitals*
(i) With 7 days and serum Bilirubin less than 10 mg (clinically)	Treat with Photo therapy	Same	Same
(ii) Early deep jaundice	Photo therapy review—refer to sub-div.-hospital	Phototherapy and monitoring of serum Bilirubin. If increase in serum Bilirubin more than 5 mg per hour requiring exchange transfusion. Refer to district hospital.	Manage in Special Care Nursery (SCN)
Septicaemia	Clinically assess, start theraphy, if no response or condition deteriorates after 24 hours. Refer to district level hospital.	Same	Manage in SCN
Septicaemia associated with serious problem like Meningitis, etc.	Initiate preliminary treatment, manage vitals and refer to SCN at district level.	Same	Manage in SCN

Congenital Defects

(i) Not life threatening	Manage and advice	Same	Manage and refer to Tertiary Level
(ii) Life threatening congenital defects like cardiacpulmonary problems	Try to maintain vitals especially take care of hypothermia and then refer to SCN at district level.	Same	Manage and refer to Tertiary Level

Source: Ibid.

APPENDIX 12.9

Proposed Facilities for Radiological Investigations at Different Levels

CHC

At CHC there should be facility for general radiography which can be interpreted by the doctors treating the patients.

Sub-Divisional Hospitals

Proposed facilities under the strengthening of referral system in Punjab are:

- ❑ General Radiography
- ❑ Contrast Studies
- ❑ Ultra Sonography for Obstetrical and Gynecological work and general abdominal work

District Hospitals

Proposed facilities are general radiography and contrast studies.

Ultra sound examination for general, abdominal, obstetric and gynae, intracavitary and cardiac work.

Laboratory Investigations to be Carried out at various Secondary Level Health Institutions

Community Health Centre	Routine Haematology
	Routine Urine and Stool
	Semen Examination
	Urine for Pregnancy
	Sputum examination
	Biochemical Tests: Sugar, Urea, Creatinine, Cholesterol and Bilirubin
Sub-Divisional Hospital	All the above tests
	Comp serology—ASO, CRP, VDRL, BH Ag. RA Factor, Widal, etc.
	Biochem-Calcium, Phosphorus, Uric Acid
	Haemogram Complete
District Hospital	All the above tests
	Seriously—Toxoplasma, Coomb's test, etc.
	Coagulation studies
	Biochemistry—Lipid profile, Liver function test, CPK, CPK—MB, Electrolytes, etc.
	Culture and Sensitivity
	Histopathology including FNAC
	Cytology, e.g. PAP Smear

Types of Services

Problem Area	*Community Health Centre*	*Sub-Divisional Hospitals*	*District Hospitals*
Surgery	Basic techniques		
	Incise and drain	Incise and	Yes
	Wound debridement	drain	Yes
	Biopsy of skin and subcu-	Yes	Yes
	taneous lesions	Yes	
Trauma and Life	Resusctiation and stabi-		Yes
Support	lisation	Yes	
	Security airway		Yes
	Circulatory support	Yes	Yes
		Yes	Yes
		Reduction and	
		stabilisation	
		of fractures	Exploratory Lap
			Yes
Trauma and Life	Tracheostomy	Yes	Yes
Support	Stabilisation of pneumo-	Yes	
	thorax and refer		Yes
	Breast abscess	Yes	Yes
		Thoracocentesis	Yes
		Management	
		of Hemo-	Yes
		thorax	
		Acute Emp-	Yes
		yema	
		Management	Stabilise medias-
		of Rib fracture	tinal injuiries
			and refer

Source: Ibid.

Appendix 12.10

Surgery

	Community Health Centre	*Sub-Divisional Hospital*	*District Hospital*
Appendectomy	Yes	Yes	Yes
Inguinal Hernia	Yes	Yes	Yes
Umblical Hernia	Yes	Yes	Yes
Rectal Prolapse	Refer to Tertiary level	Refer to Tertiary level	Refer to Tertiary level
Proctoscopy	Yes	Yes	Yes
Perianal Abscess	Yes	Yes	Yes
Anal Fissure	Yes	Yes	Yes
Cholecystectomy	—	Yes	Yes
Chest Tube	Yes	Yes	Yes
Exploratory Lap	—	Yes	Yes
Acute Bowel Rupture	—	Yes	Yes
Drainage of Abdominal Abscesses	—	Yes	Yes
Acute Intestinal Obstruction	—	Yes	Yes
Intussuception	—	Yes	Yes
Volvulous	—	Yes	Yes
Vagotomy	—	Yes	Yes

Urogenital

	Community Health Centre	*Sub-Divisional Hospitals*	*District Hospital*
Management of Acute Urinary Retention	Yes	Yes	Yes
Cystostomy	Yes	Yes	Yes
Varicocele	Yes	Yes	Yes
Vasectomy	Yes	Yes	Yes
Circumcision	Yes	Yes	Yes
Management of Rupture Urethera	—	Yes	Yes
Nephrectomy	—	Yes	Yes

Surgical Conditions

Conditions/Procedures	*Secondary Level Hospitals*			
	CHC	*Sub-Div. Hospital*		*District Hospital*
	30 Beds	*50 Beds*	*100 Beds*	*100 Beds and Above*
Abscess including breast and perianal	Incision and Drainage	Incision and Drainage	Incision and Drainage	Incision and Drainage
Wound debridment	Simple wounds	Simple wounds	Major and compund wound	Major and compund wound
Trauma and Life support	Resuscitate Stabilize and refer	Resuscitate Stabilize and refer	Investigate and managé, if needed refer	Investigate and manage, if needed refer
Musculo Skeletal	Simple Manage Complicated refer	Simple Manage Complicated refer	Manage, refer if necessary	Manage, refer if necessary
Abdominal Injuries	Stabilise and refer	Stabilise and refer	Manage	Manage
Abdominal surgeries (planned)	Refer	Yes, if Anaesthetist available	Yes	Yes
Haemorrhoids	Refer	Optional, if Anaesthetist available	Manage	Manage
Anal Fissure	Manage	Manage	Manage	Manage
Acute Retention of Urine	Catheterise and refer	Catheterise, Manage and refer	Manage	Manage
Circumcision	Yes	Yes	Yes	Yes
Hydrocele	Yes	Yes	Yes	Yes
Hemeorrhaphy	Yes	Yes	Yes	Yes
Urethral Dilation	Refer	Refer/Yes	Yes	Yes
Rupture of bladder and Urethra	Refer	Refer	Refer	Refer
Major Urological procedures	Refer	Refer	Refer	Manage, if necessary
Fracture Spine	Stabilise and refer	Stabilise and refer	Refer if necessary	Manage
Opthalmology				
Eye Problems	Removal of foreign bodies	Removal of foreign bodies Manage, Corneal Abrasions, Ulcer	Management Corneal Abrasions, Ulcer and Cataract	Management Corneal Abrasions, Ulcer and Cataract

Conditions/Procedures	Secondary Level Hospitals			
	CHC	Sub-Div. Hospital		District Hospital
Gastro Enterology	30 Beds	50 Beds	100 Beds	100 Beds and above
Endoscopy	Refer	Refer	Sigmiodoscopy	Oesophago-gastroscopy Colonoscopy
Anaesthesiology	Care of airway equipment. Management of general and regional Anaesthesia if possible	Management of general and regional Anaesthesia Pain Clinic	Management of general and regional Anaesthesia Pain Clinic	Management of general and regional Anaesthesia and blocks for Pain Clinic
Thoracic				
Simple fracture ribs	Manage	Manage	Manage	Manage
Intercostal under-water seal drainage	Yes*	Yes*	Yes*	Yes*
Flail Chest	Resuscitate and refer	Resuscitate and refer	Resuscitate and refer	Manage with ventiliatory support
Mediastinal Injury	Resuscitate and refer	Resuscitate and refer	Resuscitate and refer	Manage, refer if thoracotomy needed
Acute Empyaema	Manage by ICD	Manage by ICD	Manage by ICD	Manage by ICD
Chronic Empyaema	Refer	Refer	Refer	Rib resection and drainage Refer if decortication and resection
Thoracotomy	Yes, only in emergency	Yes, only in emergency	Both emergency and elective	Both emergency and elective
Thoracotom and Procedures**	Refer	Refer	Refer	Manage, refer if necessary
Foreign bodies in the Oesophagus and Tracheo Bonchial Tree***	Refer	Refer	Refer	Manage, refer if necessary
E.N.T.				
Foreign bodies in nose and ears	Nose remove Ear remove, refer	Nose and Ear remove	Manage	Manage
Epistaxis	Manage	Manage	Manage	Manage
Peritonsilar abscess	Refer	Manage	Manage	Manage
Tonscillectomy	Refer	Refer	Manage	Manage
Mastoid abscess	Refer	Refer	Manage, if ENT specialist available	Manage
Head Injury***	Initiate and refer	Manage stabilise, refer for advanced Management	Manage stabilise, refer for advanced Management	Manage, stabilise, refer for advanced management

* If trained in Thoracic surgery for one or two months.

** Refer all Major thoracic procedures to tertiary level

*** Refer to tertiary level

**** Refer to tertiary level for advanced Mgmt.

Conditions/Procedures	Secondary Level Hospitals			
	CHC	Sub-Div. Hospital		District Hospital
Obs. and Gynaec	*30 Beds*	*50 Beds*	*100 Beds*	*100 Beds and above*
High risk pregnancies include APH, PPH, Eclampsia	Early diagnosis and refer	Refer if necessary	Investigate and manage if possible	Manage
General Obstetric procedures Episiotomies	Repair	Repair	Repair	Repair
Craniotomy (Dead Foetus, Hydro-cephalus)	No	No	Yes	Yes
Outlet Forceps Delivery	Yes	Yes	Yes	Yes
Vaccum Extraction	Yes	Yes	Yes	Yes
Breach Deliveries	Refer	Refer if complicated	Manage	Manage
Manual Removal of Placenta	Refer	Manage if Anaesthetist is available	Manage	Manage
Inversion of Unterus	Refer	Refer	Refer if complicated	Manage
Rupture of Uterus	Refer	Refer	Yes	Yes
Threatened or Incomplete Abortion	Conservative D and C	Conservative D and C	Conservative D and C	Conservative D and C
Ruptured Ectopic Pregnancy	Stabilise and Refer	Stabilise and Refer	Laparotomy	Laparotomy
Female Sterilisation, IUD	Yes Arrange special programmes	Yes Arrange special programmes	Yes Arrange special programmes	Yes Arrange special programmes
Vasectomy, Laproscopic Sterilisation	Yes Arrange special programmes	Yes Arrange special programmes	Yes Arrange special programmes	Yes Arrange special programmes
Menstrual, Irregularities	Refer if no gynaecologist	Refer if no gynaecologist	Diagnosis and Management	Diagnosis and Management
Infertility	Refer	Refer	Diagnosis and Management	Diagnosis and Management
Planned Surgery for Prolapsed UT, DUB, etc.	Refer	Refer	Manage (Treat)	Manage (Treat)
Cervical Erosion	Refer	Refer	PAP smear, Biopsy and Manage	PAP smear, Biopsy and Manage
Malignancies, Refer to Tertiary Level for Surgery and Radio Therapy	Refer	Refer	Diagnose and Refer	Diagnose, Manage and Refer
Colposcopy and Hystoscopy	Refer	Refer	Refer	Refer
Reconstructive Surgery	Refer	Refer	Refer	Manage, if possible

Gynaecology and Obstetric Group

Problem	*Community Health Centre*	*Sub-Divisional Hospitals*	*District Hospital*
Complicated Deliveries (obstructed labour, pre-eclampsia, severe maternal foetal distress, etc.	Normal deliveries Forceps delivery Vaccum extraction	Forceps deliveries Induced labour LSCS, Extraction of retained placenta and complicated cases to be referred	Forceps Vaccum Extraction, C. Section, Induced Labour, Evacuation of retained placenta, Eclampsia with complication, Rh incompatability, Uncontrolled Diabetes, Severe Hepatitis tec. to be refered
Threatened or Incomplete Abortion	Conservative management or D and C	Yes	Yes
Family Planning	IUD Tubectomy Laproscopic tubectomy	Yes	Yes
Ectopic Pregnancy	Refer	Laparotomy	Laparotomy
Vaginal, External Genitalia	Abscess drainage	Yes Excision of Cysts Suture of Vaginal vaults EUA	Yes
High Risk and Complicated Pregnancy	Refer	Medical management and delivery Therapeutic abortion	Yes and LSCS
PID	Diagnosis and drug therapy	Yes	Yes
Mens. Irregularities including problems connected with reproduction	D and C Endometrial Biopsy Drug treatment	Yes	Yes Myomectomy Hysterectomy
Primary and secondary Infertility	Counselling Drug treatment Refer complicated cases	Yes	Yes Proper treatment and diagnosis
Cx Erosion	Cautery Biopsy	Yes Refer for further diagnosis	Yes Refer for treatment of Cx Ca treatment

Anaesthetic Facilities to be Provided at Various Secondary Level Hospitals

Anaesthetic Facilities	*Secondary Health Care*			
	PHC	*CHC*	*Sub-Div. Hospital*	*District Hospital*
Maintenance of airway	Yes	Yes	Yes	Yes
Local Anaesthesia	Yes	Yes	Yes	Yes
Use of drugs causing				
(a) I/M	Yes	Yes	Yes	Yes
(b) I/V	Yes	Yes	Yes	Yes
Block Anaesthesia	—	Yes	Yes	Yes
Endotracheal Intubation	—	Yes	Yes	Yes
Regional Anaesthesia				
(a) Sinal	—	Yes	Yes	Yes
(b) Epidural	—	Yes	Yes	Yes
General Anaesthesia				
(a) I/M	—	—	Yes	Yes
(b) I/V	—	—	Yes	Yes
Inhalational Anaesthesia	—	—	Yes	Yes
Open Ether Anaesthesia	—	—	Yes	Yes
Pain Clinics	—	—	—	—

PROBLEMS AREA—ORAL AND DENTAL HEALTH TYPES OF SERVICES AT CHC

Conservative dentistry, Tooth extractions and Tooth restorations with conventional filling materials, Dental Prophylaxis, Oral health education.

Sub-Divisional Hospital Dental Clinics

Conservative dentistry, tooth extraction, all types of fillings, extractions of embedded roots, decayed teeth, RCT of anterior teeth, Apicoectomy, Gingivectomy, Currettage of deep Peridontal pockets, Frenectomy, Simple Fractures of Jaws without displacement, Partial and Full Dentures, Oral health education.

District Hospital Dental Clinic

Removal of impacted and embedded teeth, treatment of fracture of Jaws, removal of Dental Cysts and benign tumours of Jaws, Dislocation of TM joint, restoration of teeth with composite material, crown and bridge work fixed dentures, flap operations, gingivoplastry, Alveoloplasty, treatment of Malocclusion, root canal treatment of posterior teeth, treatment of Trigeminal Neuralgia.

Source: Ibid.

APPENDIX 12.11

Equipments Norms

In the process of restructuring the facilities of the secondary health care where services to be given for each tier are well-defined, it became naturally imperative that an equipment norm need to be adopted in accordance with the norms of the services. Hence community health centre, Sub-divisional hospitals and district Hospitals will be separately equipped with a set of surgical, electro-medical and other instruments for delivering better services to the Community and satisfaction to the health providers. The equipments are inclusive of imaging, electro-medical, pneumatic, hydraulic sterilisation, laboratory and hospital utility, refrigeration, air conditioning, and support.

The Radiographer, X-Ray Technicians, Medical Laboratory technicians have been trained in preventive maintenance of equipment at C.E.D.T. (Centre for Electronics Design Technology), Mohali, Government of India, undertaking. The new equipment purchased are on annual maintenance contract. The old equipment is repaired are also made on annual maintenance contract (AMC). This is done so that the equipment remains in order throughout the year and the service are provided to the health-seekers without interruption.

Installation of such sophisticated surgical and investigative instruments will help in streamlining of the referral chain whereby patients need not travel to the tertiary hospitals for services, which now they can a vail within their own districts. Availability of proper equipment will go a long way in the proper utilisation of the secondary level health institutions as well as spare the community from unnecessary expenses hassles and time.

The Peak Quality Committee under the Dy. Medical Commissioner will monitor the functioning as well as repair and maintenance of the equipments at each level. A co-ordinated effort by all concerned can make the instrument to be provided, to be utilized optimally and to the maximum benefit to the community.

Maintenance of Equipment

A ledger should be maintained for all equipment giving details of the name of equipment, date of purchase, cost of equipment, source of supplies, life of equipment, maintenance schedule (including Calibration, if required) break downs and cost of repairs, etc. All equipment costing more than Rs. 10,000 a separate history sheet should be maintained for each of the equipment giving all the above details and the inventory of additional spare should also be maintained. The equipment may be recommended for condemnation if it breaks down repeatedly incurring heavy expenditure and becomes beyond economical repair or obsolete model. Efforts should be made to keep good Liaison with the team of Bio-medical Engineers for maintenance as and when required.

PHSC: Equipment Norms

D. Equipment

Since the secondary health systems are being restructured under the proposed project. New Equipment norms separately for each level of facility are adopted.

The following aspects are addressed to arrive at the norms:

(a) Equipment norms for each facility.
(b) Volume of existing equipment.
(c) Volume of additional equipment needed.
(d) Equipment maintenance procedures.

The equipment should ensure the improved quality of diagnosis, treatment and care delivered. These estimates should be realistic and can be affordable and attainable at each level at the end of the project.

To arrive at the norms, the equipment has been broadly classified under the following heads:

1. Imaging
2. Electro-medical
3. Pneumatic-hydraulic and sterilisation.
4. Laboratory
5. Air conditioning and refrigeration.
6. Hospital Utility support systems
7. Office
8. Transport

Separate norms have been worked out by Corporation—under these heads—for different levels of institutions depending on the normative range of clinical services offered by each level.

Similarly, norms have been worked out for minor equipment, packs, equipment for training, laboratory equipment for dispensaries and consumable.

Major Equipment

	Community Health Centre	SDH	District Hospitals 100 Beds
	1	2	3
Imaging Equipment			
500 mA X-Ray	0	0	1
300 mA X-Ray	0	1	0
100 mA X~Ray	1	0	1
60 mA X-Ray (Mobile)	0	1	1
Dental X-Ray	1	1	1
Ultra Sound Scanner (Linear)	0	a	1
Ultra Sound Scanner (Linear Sector)	0	1	0
US Scanner (Linear Sector with upgradability	0	0	1
Electro Medical Equipment			
ECG (Computerised)	1	2	3
Cardiac Monitors	0	1	2
Holter Monitor	0	1	1
Defibrillators	0	1	2
Audiometers	0	0	1
Baby Incubators	0	2	4
Photo therapy Unit	0	1	2
Endoscopes (Fibre Optic)	0	0	1
Endoscope with laprocator and accessories			1
Hysteroscopy, insuffiator, calposcope			1
Operating Microscopes	0	0	2
Cryo Surgery (Delux)	0	1	1
Foetal Monitor/Topometer	1	2	3
Short Wave Diathermy (Pliysio therapy)	0	1	1
Menlays Ventilators	0	0	2
Boyles Apparatus with circle absorber	0	1	2
Boyles Apparatus without Flutac	1	1	2
Opthalmoscopes	0	1	3
Slit Lamp	0	1	1
Retinoscope	0	1	1
Perimeter	0	1	1
Emergency Resuscitation Kit	1	2	3
Dosimeter			1
Sigmoidoscopes	0	1	1
Headlights	0	1	1
Pulse Air Tonometer	0	1	1
AMC Equipment	0	0	1
Radiant Heater (4 KV)	0	1	1
Cryo Surgery	0	0	1
Pulse Oxymeter		1	
Blood Gas Analyser			1

Pneumatic, Hydraulic and Sterilization Equipment			
Dental Unit	1	1	1
Dental Chair	1	1	1
Air Rotor	0	1	1
Ultrasonic Scalar	0	1	1
Operation Table (Ordinary)	1	2	3
Operation Table (Hydraulic)	1	2	3
Autoclave HP (Horizontal)	0	2	3
Autoclave HP (Vertical)	1	1	2
Autoclave with Burners (2 bin)	1	1	0
Shadowless Lamp (Mobile)	2	3	4
OT Lights (Shadowless)	1	2	3
Focussing Lights (mobile)	1	2	2
Suction Apparatus (High vacuum MTPL)	1	2	4
Suction Apparatus (Flectrical)	2	4	15
Foot Suction Apparatus	1	1	2
Vacuum Extractors	1	1	2
Instrument Sterilizer	3	10	25
Diathermy Machine	0	1	2
Gynae Electric Cautery	1	2	2
Automist	1	2	3
Dental Lab (Bath, Motor, Lathe)	0	0	1
Laboratory Equipment			
Microscopes (Molecular)	1	3	5
Chemical Balances	0	1	1
Simple Balance	1	1	1
Photo Electric Calorimeter	1	1	2
Flame Photometer	0	1	1
Spectro Photometer	0	0	1
Micro Pipettes	0	1	1
Electrophoresis	0	0	0
Water Bath	1	1	2
Hot Air Oven	1	1	1
Incubators	0	1	1
Distilled Water Stills	1	1	1
Centrifuges	1	2	3
Centrifuge (Haematocrit)	0	1	2
Hot Plates	0	1	1
Rotor Shaker	0	1	1
Counting Chamber	1	2	3
pH Meter	0	1	1
Glucometer	1	1	2
Hemoglobin Meter	1	2	3
Microtom	0	1	1
Oven (Wax Embedding)	0	0	1
Tissue Processor	0	0	1
Timer Stop Watch	1	1	2
Alarm Clock	1	1	2
Semi-auto Analyser	0	1	1

Refrigerator and A/C			
Refrigerator (165 Liters)	2	5	8
Refrigerator (300 Liters)	0	1	2
A/C Machines with Stabilizer	1	2	8
Water Cooler	4	5	3
Two Body Mortuary (Cold Storage)	1	2	3
Hospital Plants			
Generator 5 KVA	0	0	0
Generator 15 KVA	1	0	0
Generator 50 KVA	0	1	0
Generator 62.5 KVA	0	0	1
Hot Water Systems (Solar Unit)	1	1	3
Vacuum Cleaner on a trolley	0	1	2
Floor Scrubber	0	1	1
LPG with Burner	1	2	4
Administration			
Typewriters	1	3	4
Photocopier	0	0	1
Rhoneo Machine	0	0	1
Intercoms (15 Lines)	0	1	0
Intercoms (40 Lines)	0	0	1
Fax Machine	0	0	1
Telephone (External Lines)	2	6	12
Library	0	0	1
Minor Equip. and Furnishings			
X-Ray Viewing Box	2	6	10
Developing Tanks (X-Ray)	1	2	3
Safelight (X-Ray Dark Room)	1	2	3
Cassettes (X-Ray)	4	12	32
Intensifying Screen (Various)	4	12	32
Lead Aprons	1	2	4
Lead Protection Screen	1	1	2
Chest Stands (X-Ray)	1	1	2
BP Apparatus	6	12	24
Weighing Machine (Adult)	2	4	12
Weighing Machine (Infant)	1	2	4
lufra-red Lamps	2	4	6
Oxygen Cylinders	10	20	40
Nitrogen Cylinders	5	10	20
Regulator and Flowmeter	4	8	16
Ambo Bags	4	8	16
Angle Poise Lamp	0	2	4
Hot Place (Domestic)	1	2	6
Emergency Lamp	4	8	16
Sewing Machine	0	0	2
Fire Extinguishers	2	4	6
Laryngoscopes	2	2	4
Otoscope	0	1	2
Universal Bone Drill	0	1	2

Furnishing and Other Equipment			
Examination Table	5	15	30
Labour Table	2	4	6
Foot Steps	5	15	30
Bed Side Screen	10	20	40
Revolving stool	6	20	40
Arm Board (Child and Adult)	20	40	60
Saline Stand	10	25	50
Wheel Chair	2	4	12
Emergency Recovery Trolley	1	2	4
Stretcher on Trolley	2	4	12
Oxygen Cylinder Trolley	3	8	16
Height Measuring Stand	1	2	4
Fowler bed	0	2	4
Iron Cot	30	100	250
Cardiac bed			4
Baby Cot	4	6	12
Bedside Locker	30	100	250
Dressing Trolley	2	4	12
Mayo's Trolley	1	2	4
Instrument Cabinet	2	4	8
Instrument Trolley	2	4	8
Linen Trolley	2	4	8
Kick Bucket	4	8	16
Attendant Stool	30	100	250
Traction System	1	4	8
Computerised Traction System	0	1	2
Postmortem Table	1	1	1
Wash Basin	10	20	40
Instrument Tray	4	12	24
Chairs	12	24	50
Wooden Tables	10	20	40
Steel Cupboard	4	12	36
Swab Rack (OT)	1	2	4
Fracture Table	0	1	2
Blood Donor Table (Wooden)	1	2	4
Mattress	30	100	250
Pillows	30	100	250
Wooden Benches	10	40	100
Cheatle Forceps Jar	4	10	20
Patella hammer	2	4	8
Tongue Depressor	6	12	20
Oxygen Mask	2	4	8
Torch Ught	2	8	12
Medicine Cabinet	1	4	10
Side Rails	2	4	10
Bucket Gaiva	4	8	20
Bed Pans and Urinals	4	8	20
Bowls	24	48	100
Kidney Tray	8	20	40
Racks	6	24	48

Patient Attendant Cots	0	20	50
Wooden Tables	0	20	50
Wooden Chairs	0	20	50
Surgical Instruments Packs			
OD and C	3	6	6
MTC Cervical	1	2	4
Biopsy	1	2	4
Evacuation	2	4	8
Delivery	4	6	10
PN Sterilization	10	12	24
Episiotomy	3	6	10
Venisection	3	6	12
Copper T	2	4	6
Caesarean Section	2	4	8
Incision and Drainage	2	4	6
Vaginal Hysterectomy	1	2	4
Abdominal Hysterectomy	1	3	6
Vogotomy	0	1	1
Appendicectomy	1	2	2
Hydrocele	1	2	2
GJ Harmorrhoidectomy	1	2	2
Suture Removal	1	1	1
Suturing Tray	3	6	12
LP Tray	2	4	6
Cholecystectomy	1	2	2
Thyroid	0	1	2
Catheriterization Tray	0	1	1
IM Nailing	3	6	6
SP Nailing	0	0	2
Dynamic Compression Plating	0	0	2
AM Prosthesis	0	0	1
Dynamic Hip	0	0	1
Screw Fixation	0	0	1
Fixation of Radius and Ulna	0	0	1
Cataract Operation	0	4	8
Needling and Cataract Evaluation	0	1	2
Iridectomy	0	1	4
Iridenclisis	0	1	2
Extra Capsular Operation	0	0	2
Chalazion	0	5	10
Tarsorraphy	0	2	4
Enucleation	0	2	4
Probing of Lacrymal Passages	0	2	4
DCR	0	0	2
Lacrymal Sac Excision	0	2	4
Trabulectomy	0	2	4
Pterygium Excision	0	2	4
Entropion Correction	0	2	4
Foreign Body Cornea	0	4	8
Foreign Body in AC	0	1	2
Conjunctival Cyst Excision	0	2	4

Ear Examination	0	1	2
Mastoidectomy	0	0	2
Micro Ear Set Myringo, Tympano Stepedo Plasty	0	0	1
Nasal Set SMR, Septoplasty Polypectomy	0	0	1
DNS	0	0	1
Rhinoplasty	0	0	1
Aden-Tonsillectomy	0	2	4
Tracheostony	5	10	20
Endo Laryngeal Micro Surgery	0	0	1
ENT General	0	4	8
General Anaesthesia Kit	2	4	6
General Orthopaedic Kit	0	1	1
Dental Kit	1	1	2

Addition to Equipment Norms

	CHC		*Sub-Divisional*	*District*
	30 Bed	*50 Bed*	*100 Bed*	*Hospital*
Physiotherapy				
Shortwave Diathermy		1	1	2
Infra red and Ultraviolet ray lamps		1	2	2
Ultrasound Therapy		0	1	2
Muscle Simulator		0	1	2
Electrical Cervical and Lumbar Traction		0	1	2
Hydrotherapy Equipment		0	1	1
Interferrential Therapy		—	—	1
Suspension Pulley Electronic			0	2
Electronic Exercise Equipment		—	0	2
EMG Equipment				1
Apparatus Low Frequency		—	—	1
Electronic Electra Therapy Diagnosis				
Gathri's Men Paraplegic Apparatus		—	—	1
Ergo Meter Cycle (Adult)		—	1	2
Laser Therapy		—	0	2
Wax Therapy		0	1	1
Bio Feedback Equipment		—	—	1
Equipment for Mortuary				
Oscillating Saw		1	2	2
Hammers		1	2	2
Chisels		1	2	2
Rib Shears		1	2	2
Enterotomes		4	8	8
Measuring Jars		3	6	12
Weighing Scales		1	2	2
Measuring Tapes		3	6	6
Magnifying Glass		1	2	2
Emergency Light		1	1	2
Refrigerator			1	1
Instrument Kits		2	4	4

Norms of Furniture and Hardware for District Training Centre + HQ

Description	*No. Required per Centre*
Chairs with arms for writing	30
Table and Chair	1
Library Book shelf	3
Magazine Racks	2
Filling Cabinets	2
Colour TV with VCP	1
Audio Aids	1
Overhead Projector and Screen	1
Slide Projector	1

Source: Ibid.

APPENDIX 12.12

Norms of Staff

Sl. No.	*Category*	*District Hospital*	*Sub-Divisional Hospitals*	*Community Health Centre*
1.	Incharge CMO/SMO	1	1	1
2.	SMO/MO	7*	5*	1
3.	Casualty MO	3	—	—
4.	Dental Surgeon	1	1	1
5.	Social Scientist	1	—	—
6.	House Surgeon	5	—	—
7.	Matron	1	—	—
8.	Asstt. Matron	—	—	—
9.	Statistical Assistant	1	1	
10.	Computer	1	1	1
11.	Sr. Lab Technician	1	1	
12.	Steno	—	—	1
13.	FPFW	1	4	4
14.	Nursing Sister	3*	1	1
15.	Staff Nurse	25*	11*	7
16.	LHV	1	2	2
17.	ANM	1	9	9
18.	O.T. Attendant	1	1	
19.	Pharmacist	5	3	3
20.	Lab Tech. Gr. I and II	2	1	1
21.	Steno Typist	1	1	
22.	Lab Attendant	1		
23.	Radiographer	1	1	1
24.	Physiotherapist			
25.	Operation Room Attendant	2	—	—
26.	Cashier	1	—	—
27.	Head Clerk	1	—	—
28.	Dental Mechanic	—	—	—
29.	Dietician	—	—	—
30.	AaO/Accountant	2	1	1
31.	Clerk	3*	1	1
32.	Typist-*cum*-Clerk	—	—	—
33.	Head Cook	—	—	—
34.	Electrician	1	—	—
35.	Carpenter	1	—	—
36.	Plumber	1	—	—
37.	Driver	3*	4*	2
38.	Cook	2	2	1
39.	Helpers to Cook	2	—	—
40.	Caretaker	—	—	—
41.	Dhobi	2	2	—

* including PP Unit and Truma Ward.

42. Class IV	54*	25*	14
43. Mali	1	1	1
44. Chokidar	3	—	—
45. Storekeeper	2	1	—
46. FP Ext. Educator	—	1	1
47. Peon	—	1	1
48. Storekeeper-*cum*-clerk	—	1	1
49. Ayah	—	2	2
50. Safal Sewak	—	2	2
51. Ward boy	—	2	2
SPECIALIST POSTS			
1. General Medicine	1	1	1
2. General Surgery	1	1	1
3. Obstetrics and Gynaecology	2*	1	1
4. Psychiatry	1**	—	—
5. Pediatrics	2*	1	1
6. Pathology/Bio-Chemistry/Microbiology	1	1	—
7. Tuberculosis	—	—	—
8. Anesthetist	1	1	—
9. Radiology	1	—	—
10. Skin and VD	1**	—	—
11. Blood Transfusion Officer	1	—	—
12. Orthopaedics	1	1	—
13. Ophthalmology	1	1	—

* Includlng PP Unit and Truma Ward.

** Desirable.

Source: Ibid.

13

CHAPTER

Nursing Services and Administration in Secondary and Tertiary Hospitals

A. NATURE AND CLASSIFICATION OF NURSING PERSONNEL

Significance

The institution of nursing is the backbone of the organisation that provides health services to the community at large. Nursing is a vocation, implying dedication to the service of suffering mankind and a missionary service to be rendered at any hour of the day and night as the need arises. It is a demanding and exacting profession. The ideal relations of a doctor, patient, nurse and the medicine are the four pillars upon which a cure must rest.

Definition of Nursing

A study carried out by the International Council of Nurses defined nursing as:

> The nurse is a person who has completed a programme of basic nursing education and is qualified and authorised in her country to supply the most responsible service of a nursing nature for the promotion of health, the prevention of illness and the care of the sick.[1]

Nursing in its broadest sense, may be defined as the provision of nursing care to individuals, families or communities in connection with the restoration or preservation of health, and comprising the nursing component of the organised health care and preventive services. Such care may be provided by personnel ranging from the nursing aide to the professional nurse and nurse-midwife. The National League for Nursing has adopted the following principles of nursing care:

CHART 13.1

Nursing Organisation of Post-Graduate Institute of Medical Education and Reserach, Chandigarh

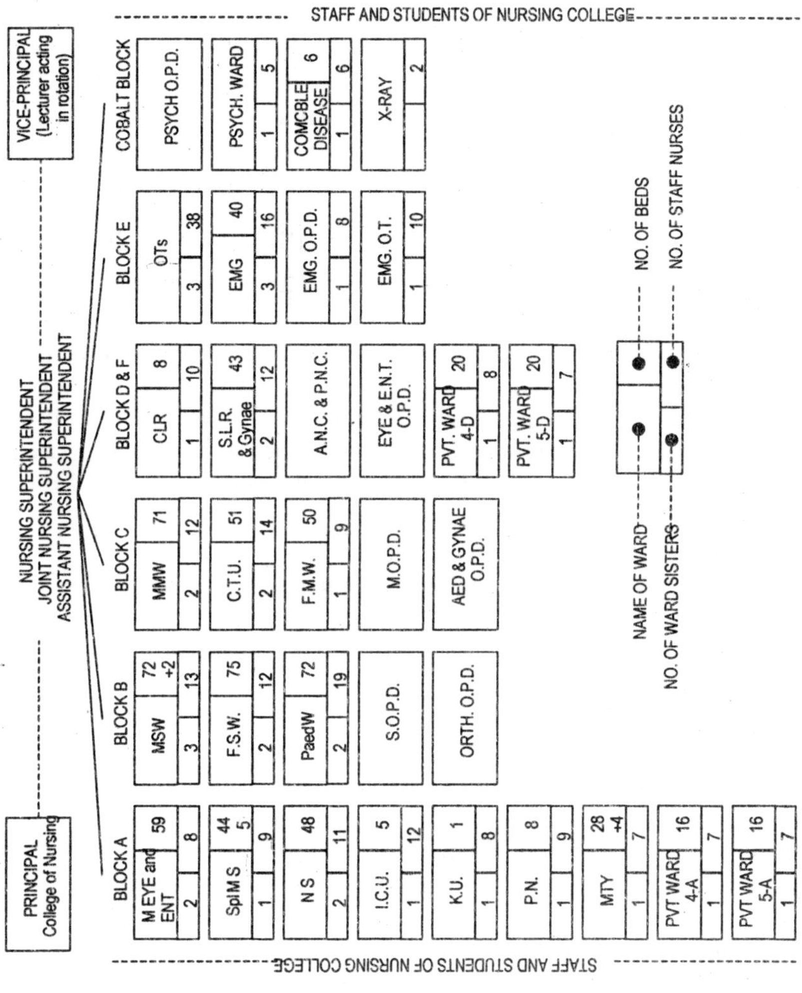

Nursing care encompasses health promotion, the care and prevention of disability, and rehabilitation, and involves teaching, counselling and emotional support, as well as the care of illness. Nursing care is an integral part of total health care and is planned and administered in combination with related medical education and welfare services. Nursing personnel respect the individuality, dignity and rights of every person regardless of race, colour, creed, national origin, social or economic status.[2]

The following is a statement taken from the Code of Ethics as Applied to Nursing published by the International Council of Nurses:

> Nurses minister to the sick, assume responsibility for creating a physical, social and spiritual environment which will be conducive to recovery and stress the prevention of illness and promotion of health by teaching and example. They render health service to the individual, the family and the community and coordinate their services with members of other health professions.

The words and expectations appeared vary a great deal, and, as with many other professional groups, the nurses role is a shifting one. A unique function of the nurse has been identified as "to assist the individual, sick or well, in the performance of those activities contributing to health or its recovery or to peaceful death that he would perform unaided if he had the necessary strength, will or knowledge, and to do this in such a way as to help him gain independence as rapidly as possible."[3]

From these definitions, we infer that nursing is-to nurse the patients or to serve the patients. It is the duty of the nurse to ensure the healing touch of sympathy for the patients. In view of these, Florence Nightingale felt a nurse should be chaste, sober, honest, truthful, trustworthy, punctual, quiet, cheerful and kind.

Categories of Nurses and their Education

There are a large number of categories of nursing personnel depending upon the duration and purpose of training and the level of general education. Let us discuss these categories briefly:

1. Auxiliary Nurse-Midwives

This category of nurses are trained to function as multi-purpose workers in rural areas. Their functions are: care of the sick, home visits, treatment of minor ailments, maternal and child health care, family planning follow-up, nutritional education, etc. The entrance qualification for training to such category is Middle Standard and the age between 18-30 years. The duration of the training is two years and includes shorter and simpler courses in nursing and midwifery. Students are provided stipends and free accommodation.

2. Lady Health Visitors' Course

This is of 1/2 year's duration. This is a modified Auxiliary Nurse-Midwives Course with more emphasis on maternal and child health. The minimum entrance qualification is matriculation.

3. General Nursing and Midwifery

Minimum education is matriculation with 45 per cent aggregate marks, having science subjects. Duration is 3 years. They are trained to function efficiently both in hospitals and in the community. It is also called Grade Nursing Course.

4. B.Sc. Nursing Degree Course

This is a University Programme, in General Nursing and Midwifery of 4 years' duration. Educational requirements are higher secondary or intermediate with science subjects. Degree programmes are conducted in colleges of nursing in our country at Delhi, Bombay, Bangalore and Chandigarh.

5. Post-Certificate B.Sc. Degree Course

This course is conducted for diploma-holders in seven colleges of nursing in India. Duration of this course is two years.

6. Masters in Nursing

This is of 2 years' duration and is conducted at Delhi, Vellore, Chandigarh and Bombay.

7. Specialised Courses

A large number of specialised courses are conducted for diploma-holders. They are:

(a) Ward Sister's Course for efficient management in the wards.
(b) Public Health Nursing is for better community health services.
(c) Tutor's Course.
(d) Administration in Nursing.
(e) Operation Theatre Training.
(f) Paediatric Nursing.
(g) Psychiatric Nursing.
(h) Orthopaedic Nursing.

These are essential for efficient functioning of specialized departments

8. Nurse Technician

This category includes Senior Dressers, Assistant Nurses and Community Nurses. More than one but fewer than three years of nursing education and training is required with a minimum of nine years of general education.

9. *Nursing Aides*

This category at present includes servants, messengers or other personnel actually performing certain nursing functions. Although aids must be literate, formal training is not generally required, since they are trained on the job to assist in patient care. On examining critically, we find that it is illogical to classify all the personnel engaged in the assistance of health care as 'Nursing Personnel'.

We must restrict the classification of nursing personnel to the nurses formally trained to do the job. We may give different names to the personnel helping the nurses. This would enhance the status of nursing personnel and would focus our attention on a definite category of personnel. The numerous categories of nurses diffuse functions and responsibilities. Dr. Gunaratne, the former Regional Director of the South-East Asia Regional Office of WHO observed that Sri Lanka had experienced some difficulties because of the numerous categories of nursing personnel, including staff nurses (who underwent three years' training), emergency nurses (with three to six months' training), assistant nurses, nursing aides and ward attendants. The Government intended to have only two categories of personnel-staff nurse (a fully qualified nurse) and ward labourer (who would have nothing to do with patient care). The same is the problem in many countries. There is a need of rational classification of nursing personnel so that their duties may be clearly demarcated.[4]

In order to provide incentive and motivation to nursing personnel, five per cent of the seats in the proposed short-duration course of medical education may be reserved for the nursing personnel who fulfil the minimum qualifications and have set good standards of service. This would also attract good candidates to this profession.

Changing Concept to Meet Present Needs

There has been a change today in the concept of nursing care. In the words of the WHO Expert Committee on nursing, "Minor modifications of existing nursing systems will be inadequate to meet new situations and demands in a rapidly changing society . . . nursing must break with some of its traditions as well as alter existing stereo-types."[5]

The current trend is to involve the nurse in the planning, implementation and evaluation of health programmes rather than simply expecting from her a subservient role in patient care. This requires a great change in the contents and methodology of nursing education. The present nursing education does not encourage research. The nursing journals contain articles of descriptive nature. There is a need to encourage research among the post-graduate nursing students and the faculty members to prepare them for senior positions in the health care delivery system. In a report of an international seminar on Research in Nursing, Brotherston has summarised the position thus:

"Whereas the ability and opportunity to carry out research must be limited to a minority in any profession, an urgent and understanding sense of the need for research should be part of the mental equipment of every member of any profession worthy of the name."

He further adds that there is a need for the profession to cultivate research-mindedness which he defines as, "readiness to look analytically at the events or working methods, a willingness to encourage scientific study or experimentation and an ability to accept the proven conclusions and act accordingly.[6]

Research is a fundamental function of a profession which is necessary to ensure its growth and progress. The professional competence of nursing personnel also greatly depends on the availability of research reports based on basic as well as applied researches. A recent book on Essentials of Nursing Research by Notter says that "Research is serious business. It should not be entered into lightly, but neither should it be feared." Nursing research in India still remains neglected.

In order to keep the nursing service up-to-date it is necessary to organise programmes of in-service education and training for all nursing personnel as a means of improving the quality of patient care. The contents of these programmes may be carefully scrutinised. At present, wherever such programmes are being carried out, they are few and lack in seriousness and purpose.

The literature available for the study and research in nursing services and administration is in the context of the developed world and is written by the writers and their professional associations from the developed world. This situation needs to be improved by rejuvenating the nursing professional associations to inculcate professional standards among their members and produce stimulating literature in the context of the needs of their countries. Dr. Chitt (Thailand) while speaking in the Regional Committee meeting of the WHO suggested that steps should be taken to stimulate the establishment and development of professional nursing associations. The essential part to be played by them in the overall growth of the profession has not been fully appreciated even by the nurses themselves.[7] Besides, the nursing associations can help in building professional standards for the professional growth of their members. According to Gardner:

"Standards are contagious. They spread throughout an organisation, a group, or a society. If an organisation or group cherishes high standards, the behaviour of the individual who enters it is inevitably influenced."[8]

The future of the nursing profession is in the hands of its members who must strive for creativity, academic excellence and the pursuit of a lofty standard in their professional activities.

Critical Appraisal of Nursing Education

The quality of nursing education needs immediate change so that qualitative nursing care can be assured. The following facts and suggestions can be taken into consideration to improve the situation.

1. There should be two categories of nursing personnel-Graduate Nurse and an Auxiliary Nurse/Midwife. The nursing aides may not be included while classifying or defining nursing services.
2. The entrance qualifications should be higher secondary with science. At present, there is no admission policy, i.e. a fixed criteria for admission to nursing schools. It was learnt from direct interviews of some nurses that "merit is no criteria to get admission in a nursing school. Those who have political and other pressures get admitted leaving the best available candidates." It is suggested that nursing schools and colleges should declare their admission policy to ensure fairness, impartiality and proper selection. This would go a long way in improving the nursing profession.
3. All nursing education should be continuous and not terminal. Besides, the in-service training programmes may be arranged to keep them abreast of the latest development. The nursing leaders do not appreciate the need for higher education among nurses as they think that nurses are to carry out only routine and mechanical duties which, as already mentioned in the earlier part of this chapter, is quite short-sighted and wrong. A nursing superintendent of a big hospital informed the present author that the nurses did not need higher education as they were responsible only for elementary activities like bed-making, sponge-bath, noting the temperature, pulse-rate, respiration, etc. The same view is held by the doctors in a hospital about the status of nurses. Mrs Narinder Nagpal, Secretary, Trained Nurses Association of India, in her article, 'Noble Profession in Neglect' in *The Tribune* (Nov. 15, 1979) rightly mentioned, "The nursing profession is treated as an auxiliary to the medical profession. We have been telling the medical men that they should leave the nursing profession to the nurses. But, so far we have not met with success." This is the reason why most of the nursing superintendents and hospital authorities are not in favour of deputing their nursing personnel for higher education. Some nurses even seem to feel that they are not allowed to improve their qualifications so that they may not become more qualified than the existing nursing leaders thereby posing a professional threat. It is strange to find that most of the nurses have improved their general qualifications through correspondence courses or by appearing in examinations in a private capacity. Many of them have completed the university degree courses while some of them have passed M.A. examinations from first rate universities. It is suggested that correspondence courses in B.Sc. Nursing may be instituted by some universities to ensure professional growth of nurses otherwise they would be misutilising their energy for improving general qualifications.

4. Nursing schools and colleges should be independent institutions. There may be arrangement for formal and informal coordination between the hospital and the nursing institutions. This would save the exploitation of nursing students—perhaps relieve them from excessive clinical work and thus neglects of their studies. Miss Simmone Liegeois, Secretary, International Committee of Catholic Nurses, New Delhi, has rightly mentioned that the shortage of nurses led to the use of student nurses for services much to the detriment of theoretical instructions. This problem needed to be studied in order to raise the quality of basic training."[9] Besides, nursing schools should adopt some hospitals to enlighten and develop the existing nursing personnel with the latest developments in the field of nursing education and administration. The nursing personnel in the hospital should be encouraged to study in the library so that they keep themselves aware of the latest developments.
5. The nursing teachers of right quality and calibre should be prepared. Some research degree may be instituted. This would encourage research among the nursing educators. Their conditions of service must be the same as of lecturers in a college. Besides, the time devoted by them in the nursing institutions is about 9 hours which is too much. This leaves no time for research and library reading. They must be encouraged to do independent work by reducing their duty hours.
6. Most of the nurse educators interviewed by the writer were unaware of the system of health care prevailing in the country. They were only equipped in the paper they were teaching. It is suggested that an independent paper on "Health Care Administration" may be started to inform them of all the developments in this sector from the international to the local levels.
7. Whenever a new post-graduate course in a particular medical specialty is started for doctors—a course for nurses and other workers should also be started simultaneously to prepare a team and provide effective services to the patients.
8. The school and college subjects may include 'Nursing' as one of the papers which can create interest among the students to pursue this profession.

The dearth of nurses especially really well qualified and the unsatisfactory standards of education are because of the poor status of nursing as a career. Besides, the teachers of nursing institutions are not at par with their counterparts in schools and colleges. Professor P.K. Devi has suggested that: "In order to improve the image of nursing, the profession has to consider three aspects. First, the independent way in which nursing benefits humanity, by taking crucial decisions at critical times where timely action by nurse-in-charge has led to saving of life, e.g., early diagnosis of fatal complications like pulmonary oedema, embolism, collapse, hyper-pyrexia, etc. Secondly, administrators must recognise the place of nursing in the medical team and nurses must prepare themselves to take their due place and accept this challenge.

Thirdly, economic rewards must be commensurate with the nature of their responsibilities. Employment conditions must not be laid down unilaterally, nursing personnel must have a voice in determining how best and efficiently their services can be utilised."[10]

9. There is a need of introducing principles of management and administration of health care in the curriculum of B.Sc. and M.Sc. Nursing. At present, the principles of administration are taught without making them understand their application in the provision of health care. It is suggested that an independent paper on 'Health Care administration' may be started at B.Sc. and M.Sc. levels.
10. There is a need to open more colleges/schools for imparting nursing education. The delegates at the Third All India Nursing Education Conference held at Chandigarh from 14 to 16 November 1979, strongly demanded a sizable increase in the number of seats in nursing colleges to tackle the growing need for nursing personnel in the country. The conference also urged that the nursing education curricula may be improved so that nurses are able to manage minor ailments on their own.

Role of Indian Nursing Council: We may mention here briefly the role of the Nursing Council. It is a statutory body constituted under the Indian Nursing Council Act, 1947. The Council is responsible for regulation and maintenance of a uniform standard of training for nurses, midwives, auxiliary-nurse-midwives and health visitors. The Council prescribes syllabus and regulations for various nursing courses. In every meeting, the council discusses the issues pertaining to education and training of nursing personnel. Recently, the Council organised a workshop of the Registrars of the State Nursing Councils and Secretaries of the Examining Board from 8th August to 13th August 1983, at New Delhi, to review and study the functioning of various councils. At the 36th Meeting of the Council held on 16th April 1983, many issues were discussed. Some of them are:

(a) recognition of the B.Sc. (Nursing) degree granted by P.G.I., Chandigarh, College of Nursing, Ludhiana, and College of Nursing, Trivandrum;
(b) to approve the recruitment rules for various posts of nursing personnel prepared by the Nursing Education Committee at its meeting held on 8th and 9th February 1983; and

(c) to incorporate section 23 of the Indian Medical Council Act, 1947, regarding registration in the Indian Nursing Register.

B. PLANNING NURSING SERVICES

Meaning of Nursing Service Administration

According to Shanks and Kennedy, "Nursing Service Administration is that organisation through which nurses in a hospital or another type of health agency are able to provide the best possible nursing care for patients in the hospital or under the jurisdiction of another type of health agency.[11]

According to Finer, Nursing Service Administration is a coordinated system of activities which provides all of the facilities necessary for the rendering of nursing care to patients. Nursing Service Administration is the system of activities directed towards the nursing care of patients and includes the establishment of overall goals and policies. Administration is the selection, provision and employment of resources for a purpose—the fulfilment of which is desirable or compulsory.

Objectives of Planning

The objectives of planning of the Nursing Service should be:

(a) to ensure total patient care;
(b) to see that the nursing component at the operational level is properly organised;
(c) to ensure optimum utilisation of nursing services by avoiding non-nursing duties of nurses;
(d) to provide a congenial environment for the professional development of the nursing personnel;
(e) to encourage staff education and training so that they can take up positions of higher responsibilities in the future;
(f) to ensure effective participation of all nurses through team work in the planning and implementation of nursing services and the total hospital plan;
(g) to promote effective public relations through effective communication; and
(h) to evaluate the quality of the nursing service.

In order to achieve these objectives, we need nursing administrators who possess administrative capability, capacity and ability; good professional knowledge and skill; good communication skills, problem-solving ability and a scientific attitude enabling them to be involved objectively.[12]

Indices of Nursing Care

Some of the indices that have been used as measures of nursing care are discussed here. At least two indices will be needed for each kind of service studied, one for the total staff per care unit, and one for the staff pattern, or the proportion of each category of personnel, per care unit or per service.

1. Indices of Total Nursing Supply

(a) The ratio of number of nurses to total population is a crude index that is useful in comparing the supply of nurses in one country with that in another. Within a country, it is useful only if hospitals and health services are uniformly distributed throughout the country.

(b) The ratio of number of nurses to number of physicians is helpful in ensuring the realistic allocation of medical and non-medical tasks.

2. Indices of the Nursing Staff Pattern

(a) The ratio of the numbers in any category of nursing personnel to those in any other category is a useful index in analyzing the quality of nursing service.

(b) The percentage of total staff in each category is a useful way to express levels of nursing because it makes comparison possible between more than two levels.

3. Indices of Hospital Nursing

(a) The nursing time provided per patient per day is the most useful and realistic index since it takes account of occupancy rates, working hours, and days absent from work. It is also easier to interpret since it provides a picture of the amount of care each patient receives, but requires more information and is more difficult to compute. The following steps are involved in the computation:

Step 1. Find the average number of days worked per year by nurse by subtracting from 365 the total number of days taken, on the average, as annual leave, sick leave, holidays, and regular days off.

Step 2. Find the average number of hours worked per year by a nurse by multiplying the average number of days worked by the number of hours per working day.

Step 3. Multiply the hours worked per year by a nurse by the total number of nurses to obtain the total number of nursing hours per year.

Step 4. Divide the total number of nursing hours per year by 365 to obtain the number of nursing hours per day.

Step 5. Divide the total number of nursing hours per day by the average daily patient census to obtain the number of nursing hours per patient.

(b) The number of nursing hours per hospital bed per day is calculated as above except that in step the total number of nursing hours per day is divided by the total number of hospital beds.

(c) The number of hospital beds per nurse is easily computed and is a useful rough index. It is not an accurate measure of the amount of service given, because it does not reflect differences in hours worked, absence from work, number of shifts in a 24-hour period, hospital occupancy, or the condition of the patient.

(d) The average daily number of patients per nurse is an index having the same advantages and disadvantages as (c) above except that it reflects differences in hospital occupancy and is therefore a little more accurate.

(e) The number of nurses per 20 (or 50 or 100) hospital beds or patients provides a rough indication of the staff needed for planned new facilities. It may be preferable to use the number of beds or patients in an average nursing care unit rather than an arbitrary figure of 20, 50, etc.

4. Indices of Public Health Nursing

(a) The number of persons per public health nurse is a useful index where health services are well developed and distributed fairly uniformly over the country.

(b) The number of live births in the population per nurse or midwife may be a useful index when the major emphasis of a particular programme is on maternal and child health, as with the number of persons per public health nurse. It is unsuitable for use in planning when coverage of the population is limited and distribution of services uneven.

(c) The number of public health nurses per health centre of a given size is a practical index that allows plans for nursing to keep pace with the programme of a developing health centre. It is not as useful for purposes of comparison between countries or different kinds of services.

(d) The number of hours or minutes of nursing service per activity (e.g., home visit, clinic, consultation, immunization, etc.) is a useful index if the plan of action for the health plan is drawn up in terms of activities. An accurate calculation must be based on a time study.

5. Indices or Nurse-Teacher Supply

(a) The number of students per nurse-teacher is a good rough index for use in planning recruitment and training programmes for nurse-teachers.
(b) The number of nurse-teachers per education and training programme of a given type is also workable index. For a realistic school staffing plan, both this and the preceding index must be used.

Planning Nursing Services

Nursing in 1948 lacked the status of a profession in most of the countries in South-East Asia. This can be seen from the figures by the Regional office:

> For Afghanistan's 12 million population, there were 44 mid-wives and 303 nurses (1954); Ceylon (now Sri Lanka) with a population of 8.25 million had 1785 midwives and 2056 nurses (1953); for India's 375 million population, the figures were 17,000 and 22,100 (1954); Indonesia had 1035 midwives and 5548 nurses for 79.5 million (1954), and Thailand, 915 and 3874 for its estimated 19.5 million people (1954).[13]

The third session of the Regional Committee passed a resolution and requested the Regional Director, "to take active steps in collaboration with governments, to promote the expansion of training facilities, particularly through the provision of specialised international staff and essential teaching equipment."[14]

Since then the governments with the help of the WHO have been striving to prepare an adequate number of nurses with good training arrangements. The conditions are the worst in Nepal where there is yet one professional nurse per 52,755 people and one auxiliary per 22,570 people. However, the conditions are better in Sri Lanka and Thailand. The conditions in India and Burma are satisfactory. Still, the doctor/population ratio is better as compared to nurse population ratio in the developing world while in the developed countries, the nurse/population ratio is six times the doctor-population ratio.

Thus, the staffing of the services in the developing countries at a reasonable level of adequacy and efficiency obviously calls for vast expansion of nursing education and training. Besides, these countries must take energetic steps to build-up a nucleus of highly trained nursing personnel for manning positions of administrative and teaching responsibilities. This requires effective planning and should include all the steps required to develop health manpower plans. As stated in a WHO Health Paper, "Systematic planning for nursing is the orderly development of a system of nursing that will enable the most effective service possible to be provided with the resources available. Such a system will be based on an analytic study both of the nursing service currently provided and that needed in proposed health services."[15]

C. PLANNING A NURSING UNIT OF A HOSPITAL AND PUBLIC HEALTH NURSING

Need and Functions

The nursing unit is an integral part of the hospital complex. The hospital is divided into blocks and each block is divided into wards. A ward is that area of the hospital where all the amenities—physical, social and especially medical care—are made available to make the patients feel at home till they are discharged. In other words, a ward is a temporary home for the patients admitted there. Evidently, there is a need to ensure a healthy environment to help early recovery of the patients and to win their confidence. In each ward, there is a nursing unit to take care of the patients for all the 24 hours. The efficient planning of this unit would ensure maximum care of the patient. The broad categories of functions that should be discharged by the nursing unit are:

(a) Meeting personal needs of the patients.
(b) Efficient ward management.
(c) Proper maintenance of records of the patients.
(d) Provision of basic institutional services.
(e) Availability of diagnostic and treatment equipment.
(f) Arranging formal and informal health education of the patients and their relatives.

Planning a Nursing Unit

Planning is preparation for action. The proper advance planning would ensure best patient care. Dimock defines planning as "the use of rational design as contrasted with chance, the reaching of a decision before a line of action is taken instead of improving after action has started."[16]

The aspects of planning a ward include—Space Planning, location of Nursing Unit, Materials Planning, Personnel Planning, etc. The planning here must be practical and operational and not theoretical. In the words of Millet, "Planning is the process of determining the objectives of administrative effort and of devising the means calculated to achieve them."[17]

Hudson succinctly defines it as "the process of devising a basis for a course of future action."[18] In each nursing unit, planning may be done to provide the following basic facilities:

(a) Patient rooms with attached or separate toilet and bathing facilities.
(b) Nurse's duty room.

(c) Treatment area.
(d) Waiting room for the relatives.
(e) Storage of linen and other supplies and equipment.

Besides, there is a need of manpower planning, i.e. identification of actions which personnel have to take in order to perform activities, and identification of positions by which personnel requirements may be grouped to determine types, number and qualifications.

Administration of a Nursing Unit

The American Hospital Association and National League of Nursing Education (1950), Hospital Nursing Service Manual, New York, indicates the following steps to administer the ward:

(1) Assisting the patient with those physical services necessary for his well-being and comfort which he cannot do for himself or cannot do unaided, and planning such services to meet his individual needs as they are affected by his physical condition and his emotional reaction.
(2) Observing, recording, and reporting to the physician for the 24-hour period the physical, emotional and mental symptoms which may have significance in diagnosis and in the direction of therapy.
(3) Preparing the necessary equipment for and assisting the physician with diagnostic tests and therapeutic measures.
(4) Giving medication and carrying out treatment prescribed by the physician.
(5) Observing the patient for reactions which may follow treatment, and taking the necessary measures to combat them, should they occur.
(6) Assisting in providing a clean, orderly, well-ventilated environment for the patient, and protecting him from infections, accidents, and fire hazards.
(7) Helping the patient to feel secure in his new environment and to adjust himself to his condition and to any limitations he may have as a result of his illness.
(8) Teaching the patient how to maintain and improve his health and to carry out his treatment when he goes home.
(9) Establishing good rapport with the patient's family and his friends.
(10) Meeting emergency situations and unforeseen situations with promptness and good judgement.
(11) Making contacts for the patients with others concerned with, his care, such as the medical social worker, the dietician, the occupational therapist, or the clergy, or nursing agencies when he leaves the hospital.[19]

Planning Public Health Nursing

Public Health nursing is a recent development. The real foundation of health can be laid if the public health nursing is properly developed. This is meant to provide preventive and promotive health education. The objective of planning public health nursing may include:

(1) health counselling to individuals, families and community groups;
(2) provision of nursing care when necessary, and teaching and supervision of others providing nursing care;
(3) assistance during physical examination and medical, diagnostic, and preventive procedures;
(4) promotion of environmental sanitation in homes, schools and industry;
(5) case-finding related to the agency's programmes, and participation in epidemiological investigation;
(6) cooperation in community studies and other special research of the agency; and
(7) participation in educational programmes for nurses, other professionals, and members of the community.[20]

Nurses and Primary Health Care

Besides we must plan the use of nurses in the promotion of primary health care.

The International Council of Nurses (ICN) representing nurses throughout the world, supports the present WHO/UNICEF concept of Primary Health Care (PHC). In so doing, ICN affirms the commitment of nurses to effect changes in nursing education, practice and management which are conducive to the implementation of PHC. ICN recognises that to effect the necessary changes in the nursing contribution, nurses must continue to influence governments in their own countries to take the following action (ICN/78/142/E):

- review the role of nursing personnel in the context of the primary health care approach within the national health services, and the overall development of the country;
- develop a health manpower system which is relevant to the country and its need;
- review legal instruments which protect the public and health personnel;
- involve nurses in the policy-making, planning and management at national and local level;
- utilise nurses as teachers and supervisors in PHC activities; and
- utilise suitably prepared nurses in PHC research and as project planners/participants when planning, implementing and evaluating PHC programmes.

ICN declares its intent to cooperate, at international level, with government and non-governmental organisations, and at national level with its member associations, in making PHC an effective reality.

WARD ADMINISTRATION

A Case Study of the Ward Administration of a Teaching-cum-Research Hospital/P.G.I., Chandigarh

The whole hospital has been divided into blocks. Each block is further divided into wards. The overall responsibility of planning, implementation and supervision of nursing personnel vests in the Nursing Superintendent who is assisted by one Joint Nursing Superintendent and one Assistant Nursing Superintendent. Below them are 62 nursing sisters and 366 staff nurses. The main responsibility of administering a ward or nursing unit is of the ward sister. She looks after some particular ward as assigned to her. Let us take the case study of Male Surgical Ward to understand the dynamics of Ward Administration.

It is located on the 5th Floor, B-Block of the Nehru Hospital, PGI, Chandigarh. It consists of ten cubicles for the patients, class-room, intensive-care unit, a store, a room for doctors and nurses, and nurses' and doctors' duty room (see Chart 13.1). Let us mention some of the facts about the ward:

Bed strength	74
Number of units	4
Number of patients in each unit	18-19
Number of consultants	3 consultants in each unit
Number of junior doctors in each unit	10-12 in each unit
Total number of medical personnel	60

Nursing Staff:

Ward Sister	1
Staff Nurses	12
Ward Aide	1

Class IV Employees:

Ward Servants	4
Sweepers	5

Sanitary Annexes for the ward consisting of:
6 Latrines; and
3 Bathrooms.

The working of the ward has been examined on the basis of personal observation, interview and discussion with the staff in the ward and the patients and their relatives. Let us mention some of the problems which need the attention of hospital authorities for better performance and decent patient care.

1. Defective Construction of the Ward

The ward is made up of cubicles with a brick wall in each cubicle. This type of construction is not good as it is not possible for the ward sister and other nursing personnel to keep a watch on the patients from the duty room which is essential for effective medical care. It is suggested that the Hospital Engineering Department should always involve nursing personnel while planning for the hospital construction or alterations of existing structures to ensure better facilities and better use of the buildings. At present, the sanitary arrangements are not sufficient to meet the needs of the patients. It is suggested that more latrines and bathrooms should be provided in every ward to ensure that there should be at least 1 latrine for 8 patients. It means that four more latrines need to be provided in this ward.

2. Big Size of Ward

It is very difficult to control big wards having 70-80 patients by a ward sister. This creates the problem of span of control. In the words of Dimock:

The span of control is the number and range of direct, habitual communication contacts between chief executive of an enterprise and his principle fellow officers.[21]

It is very difficult for the ward sister to supervise 12 staff nurses effectively. Besides, she has to supervise and coordinate the activities of doctors and sweepers to ensure smooth functioning. This can be improved if the following facts and suggestions are taken into consideration:

(a) Smaller wards involving about 40 patients may be designed or earmarked.

(b) Male and female wards may be combined so that the consultants concentrate at one place and their number can be reduced. Too many consultants in a ward create confusion. Private wards pertaining to a particular specialty may be located nearer their general wards. This would make the inter-ward coordination easy and more manageable. This experiment has been a great success in some of the hospitals like General Hospital, Sector 16, Chandigarh. Even in this very hospital, this arrangement exists in cardio-thoracic ward.

3. Lack of Effective Inter-personnel Relationships

As we already know a ward has a large number of personnel—doctors, nurses, sweepers, etc. The efficiency of the ward depends upon the team spirit among all these persons without any distinction of status. Most of the staff members interviewed were of the view that there is absence of harmonious relationship among the personnel working in a ward as all individuals think in terms of their own interest rather than that of the group. It is suggested that the hospital authorities should see that the ward is conceived of as a team or group of people so related that the efforts of each duly contribute to the best patient care and most satisfying to all. The trend should be to encourage the growth of informal relations which would create better understanding and appreciation of each other's role. Such an atmosphere would germinate administrative vitality and ensure access to group opinion by extending and broadening the avenues of institutional planning and thought. Henry Fayol (1841-1925) recommended the principle of *esprit de corps,* i.e. in union there is strength. The organisation ought to function as a team and every team member should do his best to accomplish organisational goals.

4. Defective Materials Management

The efficiency of the ward depends to a great extent upon the proper and timely supply of equipment and goods by the Central Supply and Laundry Departments. There is lack of coordination between the wards and the supportive services. On holidays, wards either do not get the supply or get partial supply resulting in poor performance. It is suggested that the personnel of Central Supply and Laundry Departments may adjust their duties on holidays and compensation may be provided to them in lieu thereof.

5. Pilferage of Goods and Poor Maintenance of Equipment

It was told to the writer that the doctors do not use the equipment carefully resulting in great losses. Nursing personnel are considered by them as servants. It is suggested that the doctors may be taught health economics and the proper use of equipment as we cannot afford wastage. The main reason of the mounting cost of hospital expenditure is the improper utilisation of hospital resources.

Besides, the Class IV employees do not care much for the orders of the ward sisters and nurses. These employees are under the direct control of the Medical Superintendent. This vitiates the principle of 'Parity of responsibility and authority.' The ward sister has no effective control over the sweepers, etc. Herbert A. Simon has rightly said that, "Those who have the authority to issue orders should be willing to accept responsibility for the consequences."[22]

How can we expect responsibility from the ward sisters without granting them sufficient authority? There is a need to inculcate discipline among the employees which would generate obedience, application, motivation, energy and respect.

6. Low Morale among Nursing Personnel

If we examine the hospital structure, we find that the hospital authorities have not given due status to the nursing personnel—the backbone of the hospital system. Staff nurses get the chance of being promoted to nursing sisters but the avenues of promotions are blocked after that. A sound policy of promotion fosters a feeling of belonging and dedication among the personnel and leads to building up of healthy traditions and conventions. It is suggested that more posts of Assistant Nursing Superintendents, Deputy Nursing Superintendents may be created, to provide suitable avenues of promotion. Besides, the ratio of ward sister to staff nurse may be decreased to 1:6 from 1:12 at present.

This would provide better avenues of promotion to staff nurses. Moreover, the hospital authorities should encourage higher education among nurses and provide facilities for their growth. Henry Fayol has rightly said that: "a sign of good administration is the steady methodical training of all employees required at all levels."

Most of the nurses were very sore and mentioned that they are not encouraged to undergo higher education. It is suggested that the nursing personnel should be encouraged to undertake higher education and their promotion avenues may be increase increasing their status in the hospital system. Most of the nurses feel that there is hardly any job satisfaction. It was mentioned by (Mrs) Nagpal in her interview to *The Tribune* (Nov. 15, 1979), that when the patient is cured, it is the doctor who gets the credit. "The nurse who must have spent hours together by the patient's bedside is more often than not ignored."

7. Unsatisfactory Nurse/Patient Ratio

The present ratio of 1 nurse to 12 patients is against the recommended norm 1:3. Secondly, the number of staff nurses on night duty further decreases as compared to day time. It is a strange paradox as the patients feel more necessity of medical care during night hours. This need to be by appointing more nurses. It should be practised at least in Central Institutes which are to set standards for other hospitals.

8. Non-nursing Duties by Nursing Personnel

There are many duties which are clerical and can be performed by non-technical personnel. Most of the nursing personnel in the ward were having 40 per cent of their work which was non-nursing. This would result in the wastage of resources. It is suggested that the hospital should appoint a committee to demarcate the nursing duties so that they can devote more time to patient care and non-nursing duties may be transferred to other personnel:.

D. PLANNING NURSING ORGANISATION AND ADMINISTRATION

After the formulation of the plan, the organisation is designed to implement the plan. According to Mooney, "Organisation is the form of every human association for the attainment of a common purpose."[23]

And this is what Dimock and Dimock have to say of organisation.

"Organisation is the systematic bringing together of inter-dependent parts to form a unified whole through which authority, coordination and control may be exercised to achieve a given purpose. Organisation is both structure and human relations."[24]

Herbert A. Simon has concluded:

Organisation affects the people who work for it in five different ways:

(i) The organisation divides work among its members; by giving each employee a particular task, it limits and concentrates his attention on that task;
(ii) The organisation establishes standard practices by working out detailed procedures, it relieves employees of the need to determine such procedure, each time they use crossways;
(iii) The organisation transmits authoritative decisions by despatching such decisions downward, upward and cross-ways;
(iv) The organisation provides a communication system; and
(v) The organisation trains and indoctrinates its member by providing for the internalization of influence relating to knowledge, skills and loyalties; training enables employees to make decisions as the organisation would like them to be made.[25]

It would, therefore, be of utmost significance to stress that organisation is not merely a structure; in fact, it embraces a structure as well as the human beings who man and run it in order to realise the pre-conceived objective.

Organisation can be formal and informal. According to Simon, formal organisation means, "a planned system of cooperative effort in which each participant has a recognised role to play and duties and tasks to perform. The key to the whole process is effective cooperation among the persons engaged in the operation."[26]

But the actual working of any organisation is not according to the formal plan. The informal relationship of the persons working in the organisation may be different from the formal expected relationship. It is better to encourage informal relationships among nursing organisations to promote decent patient care.

Keith Davis has enumerated the following five practical benefits which can be derived from informal organisations which may be kept in mind by the Nursing Superintendent and other hospital administrators:

1. It blends with the formal organisation to make a workable system for getting the work done.
2. It lightens the workload of the formal manager and fills in some of the gaps in his abilities.

CHART 13.2

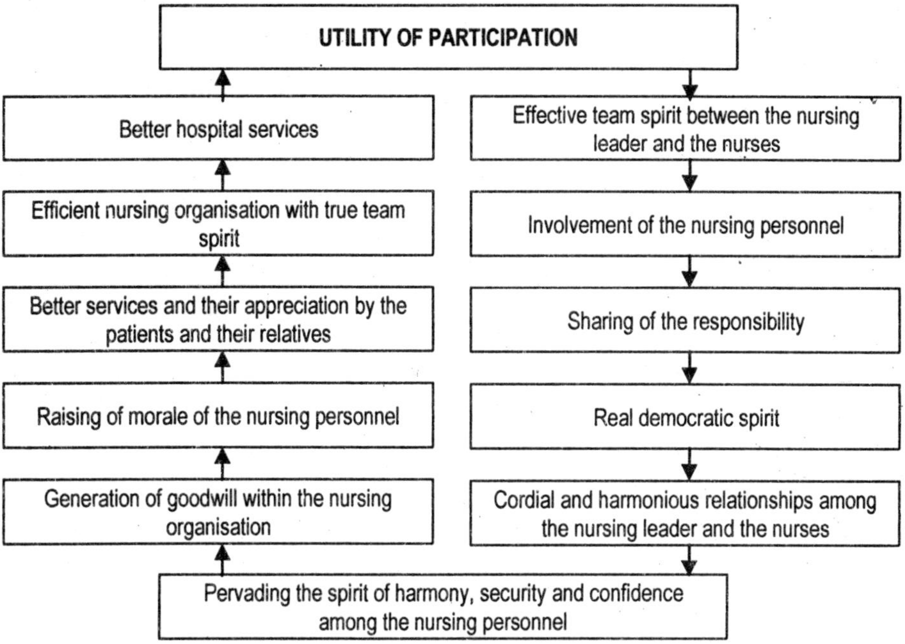

3. It gives suggestion and stability to work groups.
4. It is a very useful channel of communication in the organisation.
5. Its presence encourages the manager to plan and act more carefully than he would otherwise.[27]

Likert has called this general principle, the principle of 'supporting relationships', in which decision-making, leadership, motivation, communication and control move together. He states, "the leadership and other processes of the organisation must be such as to assume a maximum probability that in all interactions and all relationships with the organisation each member will, in the light of his background, values, and expectations, view the experience as supportive and one which builds and maintains his sense of personal worth and importance.[28]

Thus, the Nursing Superintendent and other top nursing personnel should strive as far as possible to create the atmosphere of an informal organisation which would develop the genuine feeling of goodwill and mutual trust among the nursing personnel. It should not be understood that the Nursing Superintendent should not follow the formal plan. The idea is to supplement the good elements of formal organisation with informal organisation to get the best out of the employees.

There are many aspects or problems which must be taken care of while planning an organisation. Let us discuss some of them which are important

(i) Authority and responsibility-Development of team nursing.
(ii) Delegation and decentralisation.
(iii) Public relations.
(iv) Communication.
(v) Coordination within the nursing unit and coordination with the entire hospital system.
(vi) Supervision and control.
(vii) Personnel management.

Authority and Responsibility

Authority is the right or power of a person to command other people to do things and to get work done from them. This authority in a hospital organisation relating to nursing services is exercised by the Nursing Superintendent subject to the overall control of the Medical Superintendent/ Director. It requires complete understanding of the decisions by the Nursing Superintendent and communicating them to the subordinates for implementation. Responsibility means a charge for which one is responsible or accountable. Since it would not do just to hold a person responsible for performing a task without first giving him/her the authority necessary to get the job done, responsibility should always be coupled with commensurate authority. If a Nursing Superintendent and her team is to perform efficiently, she should know what her job is and with how much authority she has to perform it. This parity is not mathematical but rather co-extensive, because both relate to the same assignments. According to Ernest Dale:

> Authority should be equal to responsibility. That is, if a man is responsible for the results of a given operation, he should be given enough authority to take the action necessary to ensure success.[29] The trend today is to make use of authority in collaboration with colleagues-developing team work. Team nursing is a plan of nursing care which makes possible utilisation of all levels of personnel to provide optimum patient care. The nurse should be a team member. This means that the nurse is to be totally integrated into the function of the team. It means involvement of all nursing personnel in the planning and implementation of patient care. It implies "expert planning and assigning of the duties to be performed by all those concerned with the care of the patient, so that nursing will be improved and the entire staff will function smoothly, efficiently and happily."[30]

The team leader must ensure effective communication to ensure effective participation. We can represent the merits of team work with the help of the diagram.

Thus, the fuller staff participation is important both as a means of tapping the practical and intellectual resources of all the nursing personnel for the benefit of the organisation and as a way of making work in the organisation more meaningful for each nurse. Such participation though theoretically available in one form or the other is practically non-existent. Most of the nurses interviewed revealed that the nursing leaders allow superficial participation which serves as an eyewash indicating the presence of distrust in the mind of the nursing leaders. The consequences of this can be represented with the help of the Schematic Chart.

The following advantages would result from the participative management:

- participation yields personal commitment and involvement of nurses toward organisational goals;
- participation produces the free flow of communications for an informal work force and atmosphere;
- control systems are primarily for self-monitoring and guidance and not needed for external control;
- it produces a high degree of mutual respect and trust among organisational members;
- through participation a nursing superintendent is likely to obtain stronger motivation towards an objective. Even those who disagree will feel compelled to loyalty by the sheer weight of the group opinion; and
- a high degree of confidence is shown in subordinates which facilitates interpersonal processes.

Therefore, we should encourage nurses' participation in the promotion of patient care, employee's participation would build his morale and ultimately his efficiency. An ILO document mentions that the individual worker "is not just a cog in the very big wheel, but that his personal effort is essential for the achievement of the overall production plan."[31]

The research theory in social organisational psychology has also suggested that participation in group decision-making enhances satisfaction among members and removes tensions. Micheal R. Cooper and Micheal T. Wood have shown that satisfaction is affected by the participation. Satisfaction was greater where participation was complete than where it was partial.[32]

There is a need to practise 'Management by objectives' to ensure fruitful participation. Management by objectives shifts the focus to goals, to the purpose of the activity rather than the activity itself. It is a process whereby the superior and subordinate personnel of an organisation jointly identify its common goals and ensure performance. The Nursing Superintendent must encourage such concepts to develop among nurses. The Nursing Superintendent/Nursing leaders should check the nursing organisation in the context of the essentials of a good organisation to ensure parity between authority and responsibility.

CHART 13.3

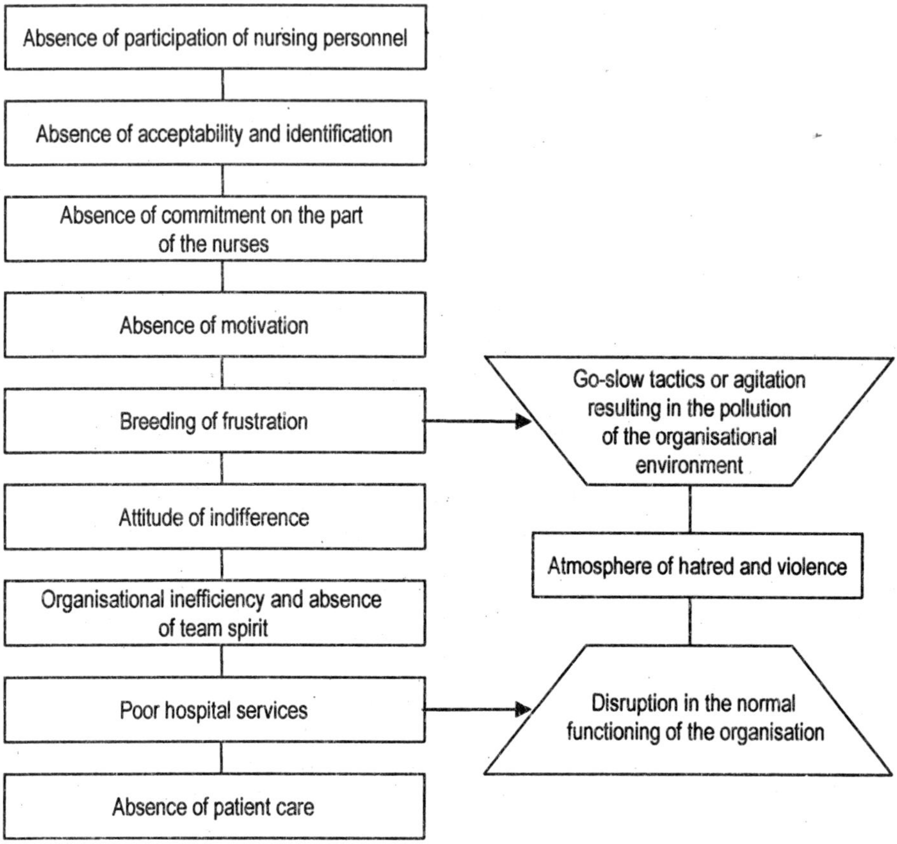

(a) Clear definition of objectives.
(b) Systematic grouping of related activities.
(c) Maximum delegation of authority.
(d) Minimum layering.
(e) Clear demarcation of line and staff functions.
(f) Unity of command.
(g) Correct span of control.
(h) Proper conditions of work.
(i) Provision for easier communication.

For a Nursing Superintendent it is one thing to have the legal right to command, and quite another to have effective direction over the nursing personnel. The former is a matter of formal power. The latter is largely a matter of appeal and influence. It requires, first of all, evidence of interest, intelligence, and energy. Unless there is single-mindedness that will enable the Nursing Superintendent to generate and sustain a general concern for the fufilment of the goals of his/her programme he/she cannot hope to assert the authority that signifies the true leadership.

These qualities-interest, intelligence, and energy—are fundamental to strength of personality. But they must also be in balance. Unless the individual's traits are so combined that they enable one to win and hold the devotion of other colleagues, one will have little chance of meeting the demands made on him or her. The nursing personnel must be able to feel that they know the Nursing Superintendent and can trust her because she is the leader of their team. More specially, an executive must have that quality about his or her personality which enables him or her, without sacrificing integrity of purpose, to lubricate human relationships. Let us understand the psychological reasons for participative management with the help of extracts from the scholars of organisational psychology. This would help the Nursing Superintendent and hospital authorities to manage their personnel efficiently. McGregor categorised the traditional motivational assumptions as Theory X, a string of self-considered notions about human nature. Firstly, the theory X assumes that the ordinary man is selfish, lazy and stimulated by only economic rewards. Secondly, the average man is not interested in work unless goaded by the superior. Thirdly, the individual and organisational goals are contradictory and tend to clash against each other. Fourthly, the average man is devoid of self-discipline and self-control. Finally, he tends to submit himself to the control and direction of others and avoids responsibility.

McGregor, however, points out that man's motivation is far too complex and varied to be explained away wholly by the aforementioned assumptions. In line with other thinkers of social psychology school, McGregor describes his alternative model of motivation as theory Y. The assumptions of theory Y may be stated as:

1. The average man is not really against doing work.
2. The ordinary man can show self-control and self-direction, depending upon the involvement in the work he is doing.
3. The average man craves self-actualisation and it is the responsibility of the management to provide genuine conditions for satisfying his creative abilities and yearnings.
4. The ordinary man, under suitable conditions, would willingly shoulder responsibility.
5. The average man is capable of making significant contributions to the solution of many administrative problems but his potentialities are not fully utilised.

McGregor's assumptions in theory Y roughly correspond to what Maslow and Argyris have stated about human motivation. The running theme of all these thinkers has been to show that adequate attention has not been paid, so far, to the actual potentialities, creativity and responsible behaviour with which the ordinary man is endowed. That way, McGregor has successfully discarded the assumptions of classical school of thoughts. Douglas McGregor has rightly given his preference for theory Y which helps in true Organisational building and development. He states:

Theory X leads naturally to an emphasis on the tactics of control to procedures and techniques for telling people what to do, for determining whether they are doing it, and for administering rewards and punishments. Since an underlying assumption is that people must be made to do what is necessary for the success of the enterprise, attention is naturally directed to the techniques of direction and control. Theory Y, on the other hand, leads to a preoccupation with the nature of relationships, with creating an environment which will encourage combinent to organisational objectives and which will provide opportunities for the maximum exercise of initiative, ingenuity, and self-direction in achieving them.[33]

Elton Mayo and his colleagues who pioneered 'the Human Relations' school also recognised and emphasised the use of techniques as given in theory Y. They outlined the following principles, which may be followed by the Nursing Superintendent and other top personnel of the hospital to develop and maintain sound organisational health:

(i) The need for recognition of the 'human' element and the well-being and motivation of the working teams.
(ii) Good supervision is exercised with proper understanding of the subordinates.
(iii) It is important to have proper communication and consultation between the managers and the workers. This creates a sense of participation and involvement among the employees. There should be means of keeping the management informed of what the employees are thinking, fearing, hoping and equally of keeping the employees informed of what the management is thinking or proposing to do.
(iv) The Hawthorne experiments showed that economic incentive is far less powerful than the personal or social incentives.
(v) The flow of work and arrangements of operations should give full play to the informal organisation of the workers.

In Argyris' view an organisation following these principles would be able to achieve efficiency as well as keep its employees satisfied. He says:

Every individual has 'psychological energy' to expand. Exerting that energy in a way that helps him fulfil his own social and egoistic needs is what motivates an individual. Therefore, provided a company is structured in such a way that an individual is able to meet these self-fulfilment needs, the psychological energy will be used in the company's interests. If the reverse is the case the psychological energy can easily be used to thwart the company's aims.[34]

This would promote dynamism. To quote Howard P. Smith: Dynamism in an organisation cannot be declared by fiat, nor can it be generated by the artificial insemination of imposed systems, procedures, and job demands. The enthusiasm people express about their jobs, about each other, and about their organisation is a priceless corollary of effective management. Without it, the whole management effort can easily become and of drudgery, never moving beyond a mechanical process with little sense of personal involvement. A spirit of dynamism in the organisation, a sense of personal involvement in the organisation's affairs, is particularly necessary as the setting for meaningful appraisal and development because of the high personal elevance of this activity. Good leadership is the real determinant of such a spirit.

Thus, we can say that the Nursing Superintendent must encourage participative management among nursing personnel to raise their morale. Such a situation will be conducive to the growth and development of nursing personnel and they, in turn, would do their best to provide decent patient care. In such a situation, the energy and initiative among the nursing personnel would be self-generating. Besides, all their latent potential energy would be changed into kinetic energy which can be utilised for the promotion of health among the persons visiting the hospitals.

Delegation and Decentralisation

The decentralisation and delegation can lighten the burden of the Nursing Superintendent and enable her to devote attention to important aspects of planning, policy-making and coordination. She should clearly make use of delegation and decentralisation through Sisters and Staff Nurses to achieve the objective of best patient care. According to Fayol, "Everything that goes to increase the importance of subordinate's role is decentralisation. Everything which goes to reduce it is centralisation."

Let us first understand the meaning of delegation and decentralisation and their utility.

Delegation is a process whereby a superior divides his total work assignment between himself and subordinates or operative personnel in order to achieve both operative and management specialisation. It is the entrustment of responsibility and authority to others and the creation of accountability for performance. It is to be clearly understood that delegation is not a process of abdication. The person who delegates does not divorce himself from the responsibility and authority which he entrusts.

There are three aspects of delegation: "the entrustment of work of responsibility to another for performance, the entrustment of powers and rights, or authority to be exercised and the creation of an obligation, or accountability, on the part of the person accepting the delegation to perform in terms of the standards established."[35]

Speedy and realistic decision-making is one of the essentials of efficient administration. In a big and complex organisation like the hospital, the number of decisions to be taken from time to time is so large and the points at which decisions are to be implemented are so many that it becomes necessary to distribute decision-making powers among a number of organs, rather than concentrate in one organ. This is expected to prevent the emergence of bottlenecks which bedevil highly centralised power structures. Thus, one of the important problems of organisation is to reconcile the administrator's desire for centralized control for the sake of uniformity and certainty of decisions and actions, with the people's view that administration should be so organised as to deal with the needs of the different segments of the society in an effective manner.[36]

Effective decision-making can be facilitated by decentralisation and delegation of powers. The word decentralisation is derived from Latin.[37] In modern times, it has been so widely and differently used that, as Norman D. Palmer says, it has become less precise.[38]

Decentralisation is a twin process of deconcentration and devolution. In deconcentration, a superior officer, in order to make his department function effectively and efficiently, delegates to his sub-ordinate field officials the power to act in his name without transferring to them the authority he enjoys.[39] Devolution, which also implies dispersal of authority, is a process wherein power is transferred from one organ of government to another by means of a piece of legislation or constitution. A certain sphere of jurisdiction, either functional or territorial, is set apart for a legally-constituted body which while administering its authority, enjoys "some power of self-determination."[40]

Besides, proper delegation of authority promotes effective control over operations, due to a clear definition of responsibility and action at each level. When decisions are no longer to be referred up the line, the delay in execution is minimised.[41]

Such delegation can prove to be of considerable value. It can lighten the burden of the Nursing Superintendent and enable her to devote her attention to more important things. The Sisters/Staff Nurses under her may feel more responsible and act more effectively if they are entrusted with responsibility and authority.

The importance of delegation was also stressed by Goddard: "Delegation of responsibility and authority is an important aspect of successful administration, to place the responsibility for decision at the lowest possible organisation level in order to attain decision as speedily as possible. No administrator can do in detail all the work he is administering, for by definition an administrator manages the work of others. Therefore, the principle of delegation of responsibility should be followed to the utmost extent consistent with efficiency and coordination of policy. The responsibility and authority of individuals should be clearly defined in writing, and the authority placed in each position must correspond to the responsibility which the position carries."[42]

Public Relations

Public relations is the establishment of a climate of understanding. It means interpreting the programme of an organisation to the public and *vice-versa*.

According to J.L McCany:

Public relations in hospitals is the composite of all the primary and secondary contacts between the hospital personnel and the patients and all the interaction of influences and attitudes established in these contacts.

According to Harwood:

Public relations may be defined as those aspects of our personal and corporate behaviour which have a social rather than private and personal significance.[43]

The purpose of public relations is not only to supply information, but also to encourage an understanding and cooperation between the patients and the hospital staff. This is very important in a hospital situation as the patients and their relatives are demoralised and psychologically insecure. It is the duty of every member of the nursing personnel to maintain public relations in the hospital at various stages of contact with the patients and the visitors.

At present, we find a great deal of alienation between the patients and nursing personnel. A large number of patients who were contacted in various hospitals were of the view that the attitude and behaviour of the nursing personnel were negative and they lacked sympathy and courtesy. Some even went on to say that their tone was biting and insulting. This has undermined the legitimacy, effectiveness and credibility of the hospital system in our country. We need to promote harmony and mutual trust among the patients and hospital authorities. The objectives of public relations should be to increase prestige and goodwill and to protect the life of the hospitals by safeguarding it against unwarranted attacks as well as to remove the genuine complaints and grievances of the people. This would be possible only if all the employees of the hospital, especially the nursing personnel, make it a point to remove the prevailing grievance in the minds of the people about the nature and scope of hospital services.

To improve understanding between the citizens and the hospital personnel, public relations need to be developed in an effective manner to create favourable community opinion towards the hospital services. This would create confidence in the minds of the people towards the competence, fairness, honesty, impartiality and sincerity of the hospital personnel.

Communication

Communication is central to the exercise of authority in an organisation. In the words of Ordway Tead,

Communication is the touching of mind by mind, of person with person whether it be one man, to a thousand. . . It can include conversation, interview, dialogue, visual technique carefully used.[44]

This is of great significance as any wrong communication or misunderstanding can be responsible for the death of the patient. There is a need to issue orders, instructions and participation implemented clearly, simply and understandably. The Nursing Superintendents should not think that their job ends after conveying the commands to the subordinates. He or she should encourage effective participation from the nursing personnel to ensure proper understanding. Most of the nurses complain that the Nursing Superintendent issues orders as these are received from hospital authorities above her. She does not take pains to understand the implications resulting in confusion. It is her duty to clearly spell out the details of the orders before passing these on for implementation. Nursing Superintendent and Sisters may keep the following facts in mind to achieve effective communication:

(a) Clarity of Thoughts

The first *sine qua non* of good communication is that the idea to be transmitted must be absolutely clear in the mind of the communicator. It must spring from a 'clear' head. It should be understood by the nursing personnel so that it may be fully appreciated and acted upon.

(b) Attach Importance to Action Rather than Words

In all communication, actions are more significant than words. Example is better than precept. A Nursing Superintendent or Sister who is not punctual cannot succeed in enforcing the time-rules on the subordinates.

(c) Participation

In this connection the essential is that both the parties (communicator and the recipient) should participate in the communication. It is the only way to make the communication effective.

(d) Transmission

In this connection the communicator must plan carefully what to communicate, to whom to communicate and how to communicate. How can the Nursing Superintendent/Sister communicate with the workers when they themselves do not know or cannot understand all the facts about the new plans? Further, delegation of authority without responsibility breaks down the spirit of communication.

(e) Keep the System always Alive

The system of communication should be kept open and alive all the year round. It is only by honest attempts that good communicative relations can be developed.

(f) Cordial Employer-Employee Relations

Effective communication requires good employer-employee relations which enables mutual appreciation of different viewpoints. According to Terry, eight factors are essential to making communication effective:

(a) Inform yourself fully.
(b) Establish a mutual trust in others.
(c) Find a common ground of experience.
(d) Use mutually known words.
(e) Have regard for context.
(f) Secure and hold the receiver's attention.
(g) Employ examples and visual aids.
(h) Practice delaying relations.

According to Millet, seven factors make communication effective viz., it should be clear, consistent with the expectation of the recipient, adequate, timely, uniform, flexible and acceptable. To quote Goddard:

Efficient communications are essential to all aspects of effective administration. Staff must be adequately and currently informed about plans, methods, schedules, problems, events and progress. It is necessary that instructions, knowledge, and information be passed on for practical application to all concerned, and that they be so clearly presented as to make misinterpretation or misunderstanding impossible. Proper and adequate communication is not just in one direction; it requires a two-way passage.

Administrators must be certain that they know and understand the problems of workers for whom they are responsible. Communications must flow from the bottom upwards, as well as from the top down."[45]

Because of the lack of proper communication and resultant misunderstandings, we observe a lot of conflict among the nursing personnel and between the nursing personnel and other staff working in the hospital. This causes a lot of inter-personal rivalries and jealousies. Such conflict may not be treated as an evil. According to Mary Parker Follett, it is possible "to conceive conflict as not necessarily a wasteful outbreak of incompatibilities, but a normal process by which socially valuable differences register themselves for the enrichment of all concerned."[46]

According to her, there are three ways of dealing with conflict. She says, "By domination only one side gets what it wants; by compromise neither side gets what it wants; by integration we find a way by which both sides may get what they want."[47]

She favours integration through uncovering the conflict and bringing the whole thing into the open. The Nursing Superintendent and hospital authorities should encourage methods to remove conflicts in a positive manner.

Coordination

In the nursing organisation, different nurses perform different duties because of the adoption of specialisation and division of work to achieve maximum results. This is possible only if all the nurses work to achieve the common purpose—welfare of the patient. This can be achieved by devising a proper system of coordination. According to I.C. Charlesworth:

"Coordination is the integration of the several parts into an orderly whole to achieve the purpose of the undertaking."[48]

It is the centripetal force in administration. It is the duty of the Nursing Superintendent to ensure this coordination among the different wards in the hospital and among the nursing personnel in the same ward through effective communication and sharing responsibility. Besides, the Nursing Superintendent has also to coordinate with the hospital authorities. This is very important as she has to plan her activities only in consonance with the total needs of the hospital. She has to liaison with the different departments, e.g. Stores, Central Steriles, Pharmacy, Dispensary, Registration, Laboratories, etc. to ensure smooth functioning.

Where the central purpose of the organisation is known, understood and considered to be worthy by workers, it binds them together as a coherent group and unifies their separate efforts into a common endeavour to realise the goal. A stimulating leadership of Nursing Superintendent/ Nursing Sisters can create enthusiasm among the nurses for the common cause and spur them to overcome difficulties. Ideally, coordination should be achieved through voluntary co-operation of the members of an enterprise. Each member should be ready and willing to adopt his work to secure unified action, Coordination can be secured by:

(a) instilling dominant objectives among the members of the group;
(b) developing generally accepted professional standards and norms making it easy for nurses to work with one another enthusiastically;
(c) promoting informal contacts to supplement formal communication;
(d) encouraging Nursing Sisters to maintain close contact with nurses working under them; and
(e) using group methods for informal exchange of ideas and views.

Supervision and Control

Planning, communication and supervision are the three main steps in the process of directions. Like every other aspect of organisation, supervision is also becoming very complicated and complex. The responsibilities of a supervisor has increased and of a good supervisor it is expected that he should have the qualities of head and heart. There is an old saying, "that which is not inspected is not done." Hence, inspection, overseeing and supervision, arise in response to needs inherent in the functioning of an organisation.

Supervision is a compound word and its two parts are 'super' and 'vision' which means overseeing. In a hierarchical organisation no one can claim to work without proper supervision. Generally, each officer is given certain powers and responsibilities and is supposed to be responsible to the officer above him for proper execution of the decisions and use of delegated powers. Moreover, for proper functioning of an organisation it is very essential that there should be proper coordination and link among different parts and organs of an organisation. It is also to be ensured that departments of an organisation do exactly the same work which is expected of them. In common parlance, by supervision we mean direction accompanied by authority. In a broad sense we mean superintendence and overseeing. Margaret Williamson has defined supervision as a process by which workers are helped by a designated staff member to learn according to their needs, to make the best use of their knowledge and skills and to improve their abilities so that they do their jobs more effectively and with increasing satisfaction to themselves and the agency.

The purpose of supervision and control is to ensure that the purpose of the organisation is being fulfiled. In nursing organisation, the supervision and control is still on the old philosophy, i.e. to find faults and award punishments. The purpose of supervision is not only to inspect and inquire but to encourage and inspire, and thus achieve team work. To quote Pfiffner:

The supervisor on the lower levels secures cooperation and production by de-emphasizing his own ego, stimulating group participation, and encouraging the maximum satisfaction of individual egos that is consistent with coordination.[49]

The supervisor should have training in human relations, public relations and human dynamics. Supervision and control should ensure higher efficiency through clarification and encouragement by the supervisors. John D. Millett rightly observes: Supervision is more than a process, it is a spirit which animates the relationship between levels of organisation and which induces maximum administrative accomplishment, or when unsuccessful, generates administrative paralysis. Effective management is concerned to realise the first and to avoid the second.[50]

According to Newman and Summer, "The aim of control is to assure that the results of operations conform as closely as possible to established goals."[51] Henry Fayol says that "Control consists in verifying whether everything occurs in conformity with the plans adopted, the instructions issued and principles established. It has for its object to point out weaknesses and errors in order to rectify them and prevent recurrence."[52]

Nigro has identified the following aspects of the supervisor's job:

(i) To satisfy the employees' desire for recognition.
(ii) To keep them informed.
(iii) To allow subordinates to make as many independent decisions as possible.
(iv) To avoid invading the specialist's bailiwick.
(v) To keep the door open for conference and consultations with subordinates.
(vi) To accept the probability of being unpopular with at least a few subordinates.

(vii) To avoid over-optimism.
(viii) To assure the proper interpretation and execution of orders.
(ix) To abolish useless regulations.
(x) To recognise that assistants will sometimes be more intelligent than oneself.
(xi) To make no promises that cannot be fulfiled.
(xii) To expect loyalty and give it too.
(xiii) To avoid discrimination even in favour of a friend.
(xiv) To resist undue pressure and fight for the interests of subordinates.

According to Chester Bernard, subordinates obey authoritarian command only when: (1) they understand what the order is and what purpose to achieve through their collective effort; (2) they feel in their cognition that the command is consistent with the organisational purpose and obeying that they are trying to be moral beings respecting a commitment; (3) they realise and understand that the command is the authority as issued and is compatible with their personal interests. If they see some gain or their personal interests are served in obeying the command, they generally accept it; (4) they know that they are qualified, competent and capable of complying with the orders. In other words, the nature of the command is such that they are mentally and physically fit to execute it.

The Nursing Superintendent and other nursing leaders must understand the implication of the true meaning of supervision and control, if properly understood, supervision and control would ensure good healthy cooperation among the nursing personnel. Such a situation would be beneficial and rewarding both to the supervisors and employees working under them. The Nursing Superintendent should see that the supervision and control should promote better understanding and cooperation rather than conflict, jealousies, heart-burning, enmity, which are detrimental to the smooth functioning of an organisation, through her role as a friend, guide and philosopher.

Personnel Management

Management of nursing personnel — training, promotion, conditions of service, etc.—is an area which holds the key to the success of health care administration especially the hospital services. Bacon, philosopher and administrator, has rightly said: It is vain for princes to take counsel concerning matters if they take no counsel likewise concerning persons; for all matters are as dead images; and the life of the execution of the affairs lies in the good choice of person.

Therefore, the first and foremost task is to pay attention to the administration of personnel in nursing organisations if we expect the effective performance of such organisations. Several steps, however, need to be taken if the health systems are to succeed in their avowed attempt to attract, retain and utilise the best talents available in the country. This includes healthy internal environment, competitive wage structure, potentialities of rapid growth and advancement and opportunities to create change/challenge and work for the promotion of decent health care.

In spite of the inherent merits of attending to personnel management, nursing manpower planning has not received due attention in the hospital management in spite of the expansion and diversification of hospital services. The image of the hospital services depends to a great extent upon the requisite skills, aptitudes, integrity and organizing capacity of the personnel working in the hospitals. In order to optimize the performance of the nursing personnel as a component of health care administration, we have to harness, coordinate and channelise their capacities and energies in meaningful and fruitful ways. It is very difficult to deal with all aspects of nursing personnel management as it is a subject by itself. We may mention here briefly one of the serious challenges facing the performance of nursing organisations, i.e. unsatisfactory terms of employment. The importance of payor compensation is very great for every employee. The standard of living and the social prestige of an employee depends to a great extent on the pay he draws. A man chooses his career on the basis of pay which he expects to receive. Rightly does Mason Haire remark, 'Pay in one form or another is certainly one of the mainsprings of motivation in our society.[53]

The tempo of challenging and arduous tasks to be undertaken by the nursing personnel can only be accelerated in case they have the right number of employees, with the right level of talent and skills, in the right job, at the right time, performing the right activities and to achieve the right objectives. But the health care systems cannot attract such talented and motivated nursing personnel unless they are able to provide good conditions of service and good status.

Because of the poor conditions of service, it is very difficult to attract better qualified people to take up the nursing profession. Besides, their avenues of promotion are very limited. A staff nurse can be promoted to a Ward Sister and it is very difficult to be promoted beyond that as the positions are very limited. The status of Nursing Superintendent in a hospital is very low which affects the morale of the nursing personnel. In many hospitals, it is the Superintendents who are all in all. The Nursing Superintendents are mere decorative pieces. They have no authority. Even the Nurses' duty rosters are made by the Medical Superintendents. This leads to a deterioration in the quality of Nursing care. It is suggested that the status of Nursing Superintendent should be raised to the level of Medical Superintendent and more avenues of promotion may be made available to Nursing Sisters. It has been the feeling of most of the nursing personnel interviewed by the writer that, "inadequate salary structure, poor service conditions, want of scope for career development, long duty hours, are the general features of employment causing frustration and low morale."

Thus an adequate and sound salary structure together with healthy working conditions is the *sine qua non* for the organisational efficiency and effectiveness. Otherwise, as the Administrative Reforms Commission aptly observes, the lack of those conditions has been: "one of the major factors for strikes, agitations, inter-service tensions and rivalries, indifferent attitude to work, poor performance, frustration and low morale of the employees."[54]

In other words, the aim of health care systems should be to create and maintain such conditions whereby an employee feels like giving his best, gets satisfaction out of his job and is suitably rewarded. Besides, the conditions of service, the personnel management may look after the following aspects of nursing personnel:

(a) to treat the nursing personnel as partners along with the other members of health and medical team;
(b) to help the nursing personnel reach self-actualisation and thereby help release their creative energy for the promotion of health;
(c) to create facilities for continuous growth, development and training of nursing personnel to make them fit for higher jobs;
(d) to ensure adequate working arrangements and maximum participation in management and decision-making of the health system by nursing personnel;
(e) to provide institutional safeguards for redress of grievance by nursing personnel;
(f) setting good professional standards by senior nursing personnel; and
(g) development of unity, energy, initiative and loyalty among nursing personnel.

Notes and References

1. International Council of Nurses (1965), Special and Committee reports presented to the IGN Board of Directors and Grand Council meetings in Frankfurt, June 1965, p. 6.
2. National League for Nursing, What People can Expect of Modern Nursing Service? New York, 1959.
3. Henderson, Virginia (1969), Basic Principles of Nursing Care, Gen. International Council of Nurses, p. 4.
4. WHO, SEA/RC/19/2, p. 96.
5. WHO, Technical Report Series, 1966, No. 347, p. 7.
6. Brotherston, J.H., Research Mindedness and the Health Profession, quoted in International Council of Nurses, Learning to Investigate Nursing Problems, London, 1960, p. 24.
7. WHO, SEA/RC/21/2, p. 111.
8. Gardner, John W., Excel/Enc., New York, 1961, Harper and Brothers, p. 74.
9. WHO, SEA/RC/21/2, p. 111.
10. The First All-India Nursing Education Conference, Chandigarh, April 19-24, 1971, Proceedings of the Conference, p. 26 (Address of Prof. P.K. Devi, P.G.I., Chandigarh).

11. Mary, Shanks D. and Dorothy, Kennedy A., The Theory and Practice of Nursing Administration, London, McGraw-Hill, 1965, p. 3.
12. Herman Finer, Administration and the Nursing Service, New York, 1952, The Macmillan & Co., p. 19.
13. SEARO, Summary of Vital and Epidemiological Statistics, 1956, New Delhi, p. 28.
14. WHO, SEA/RC/3/RS, September 1950.
15. WHO, Public Health Papers, 44, p. 18.
16. Dimock and Dimock, Public Administration, Rinehart, New York, 1956, p. 83.
17. Millet, Government and Public Administration, the Quest for Responsible Performance, New York, McGraw-Hill, 1959.
18. Seckler Hudson, Organisation and Management: Theory and Practice, The American University Press, Washington DC, 1957, p. 102.
19. American Hospital Association and National League of Nursing Education (1950), Hospital Nursing Source Manual, New York.
20. Goddard, H.A., Principles of Administration applied to Nursing Service, World Health Organisation, Geneva, 1958, pp. 35-36.
21. Dimock and Dimock, *op. cit.*, p. 110.
22. Herbert, Simen A., Administrative Behaviour, 2nd Ed., New York, the Macmillan Co., 1958.
23. Mooney, J.D., Principles of Organisation, p. 1.
24. Dimock and Dimock, Public Administration, p. 104.
25. Simon, H.S., Administrative Behaviour: Study of the decision-making process in administrative organisation (2nd Ed.), New York, Macmillan, 1960.
26. Simon H., Public Administration, p. 5.
27. Keith Davis, Human Behaviour at Work, 4th Edition, New York, McGraw-Hill, 1972, pp. 257-59.
28. Rensis Likert, The Human Organisation, New York, McGraw-Hill Book Co., 1967, p. 103.
29. Ernest Dale, Management—Theory and Practice, 1973, Tokyo, McGraw-Hill, p. 149.
30. Elizabeth Jones and Joan Grube Ellsworth, U., "An Experiment in team assignment", *The American Journal of Nursing*, 49, 146 (March), p. 34.
31. ILO, International Labour Conference, 3rd Session, Provisional Records, p. 34.
32. Micheal, Cooper R., and Micheal, Wood T., "Member participation and commitment in group decision-making on influence satisfaction and decision riskness", *Journal of Applied Psychology*, Vol. 59, No. 2, April 1974.
33. Douglas McGregor, *op. cit.*, p 132.
34. Fayol, Henri, General and International Management, London, Pitman, 1956, p. 26.
35. Lyndall Urwick, The Element of Administration, New York, 1953, pp. 41-42.
36. James, Charlesworth C., Government Administration, New York, 1951, p. 207.
37. Arthur, Macmohan W., Delegation and Autonomy, New Delhi, 1961, p. 15.
38. Norman, Palmer D., "Experiments in Democratic Decentralization in South Asia", *The Indian Political Scientist Review*, Delhi University, Vol. 1, Oct. 16-March 1967, Nos. 1 and 2, p. 49.
39. White, L.D. (Ed.), Encyclopedia of the Social Science, The Macmillan Company, 1951, Vol. 5, p. 43.
40. *Ibid.*, p. 18.
41. *Ibid.*, p. 16.
42. Goddard, H.A., Principles of Administration Applied to Nursing Service, World Health Organisation, Geneva, 1958, p. 85.

43. Harwood, Childs L., An Introduction to Public Opinions, *op. cit.*, p. 2.
44. Ordway Tead, The Art of Administration, New York, McGraw-Hill, 1951, p. 45.
45. Goddard, H.A., Principles of Administration Applied to Nursing Service, World Health Organisation, Geneva, 1958, p. 85.
46. Mary Parker Follet, Creative Experience, New York, Longman's, 1924, pp. 101-2
47. *Ibid.*, p. 300.
48. J.C. Charlesworth, Government Administration, N.Y., Harper and Brothers, 1951,
49. Pfiffner John M., The Supervision of Personnel, Human Relations in the Management of Men, N.Y., Prentice-Hall, 1951, p. 215.
50. Millett John D., *op. cit.*, p. 122.
51. Newman and Summer, The Process of Management, p. 561.
52. Henri Fayol, General and Industrial Management, p. 107.
53. Mason Haire *et. al.*, "Psychological Research in Pay: An overview" in *Personnel Administration*, Paul Pigos and Charles A. Myers, New York, 1969, p. 491.
54. ARC, Report of the Study Team on Promotion Policies, Conduct Rules, Discipline and Morale, Vols. I and II, Delhi, 1967, p. 72.

14

CHAPTER

Quality Control in Health Care in a Hospital

Meaning

> Proper performance (according to standards) of interventions that are known to be safe, that are affordable to the society in question, and that have the ability to produce an impact on mortality, morbidity, disability, and malnutrition.
>
> —*Roemer, M.I. and C. Montoya Aguilar, WHO, 1988*

> The quality of technical care consists in the application of medical science and technology in a way that maximizes its benefits to health without correspondingly increases its risks. The degree of quality is, therefore, the extent to which the care provided is expected to achieve the most favourable balance of risks and benefits.
>
> —*Dr. Avedis Donabedian, 1980*

Quality is of great significance to both the providers of health care and the receivers of health care and in the process builds a solid foundation of health care institutions. Press Reports, personal discussions and observation reveal the poor functioning of health services as there is no emphasis on quality health care. Such situations create unnecessary sufferings to people and even become cause of death in many cases. This situation can be improved by injecting quality in health care system rigorously and meticulously. Talveen Singh in an Article, "What is wrong with Indian Hospitals" in *the Daily Tribune*, May 6, 2000, rightly observes, in India I notice that we are very far from world standards even when it comes to basic things like cleanliness. My room is cleanish but there are visible layers of dust encrusted on the venetian blind and the window panes and the bathroom is less clean than those you find these days. A friend's mother had been taken to the intensive care unit of a smaller

CHART 14.1

Quality Control

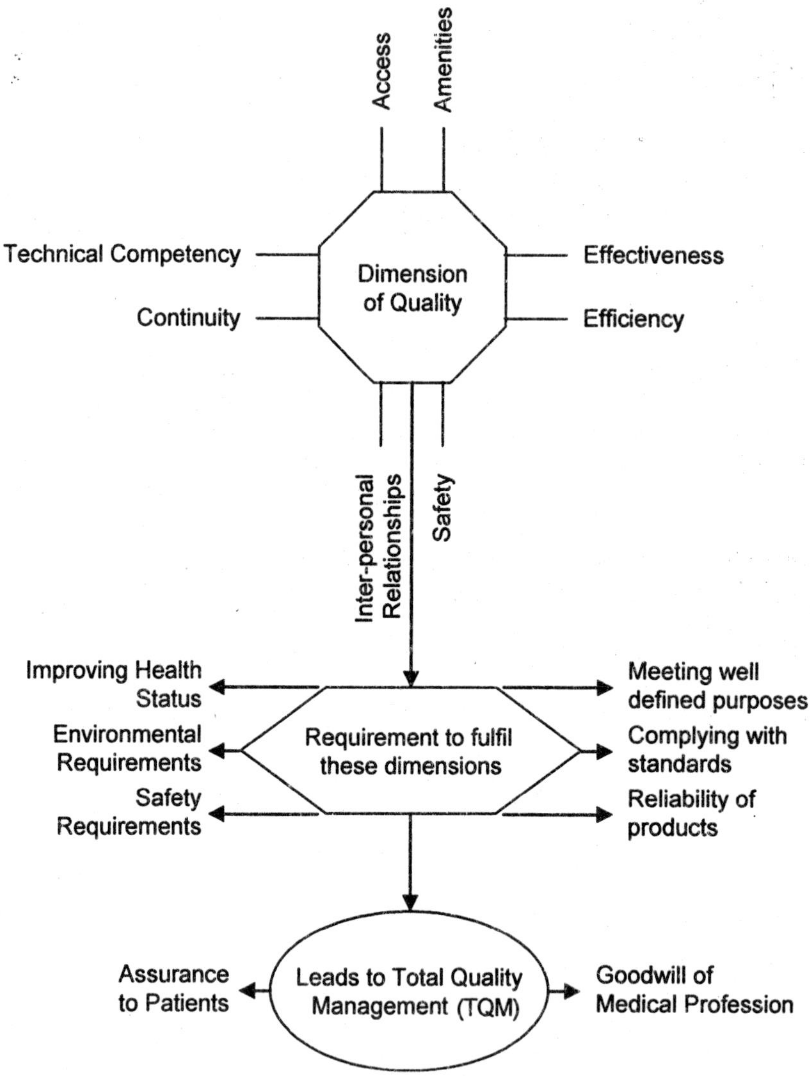

Mumbai hospital and I had gone to see her only to find myself in a place of dark, dirty corridors and wards that looked more like prison cells than places of healing. Garbage lay uncollected amid piles of old furniture in forgotten corners. It is also true that you put your life at risk when you go into an Indian hospital for treatment. In Delhi I know personally at least two women who went into hospital for minor gynaecological problems and came out with hepatitis C. I know of a young boy who went into hospital with a broken arm and ended up nearly dying of septeicemia. I know of

CHART 14.2

The Cost of Poor Quality

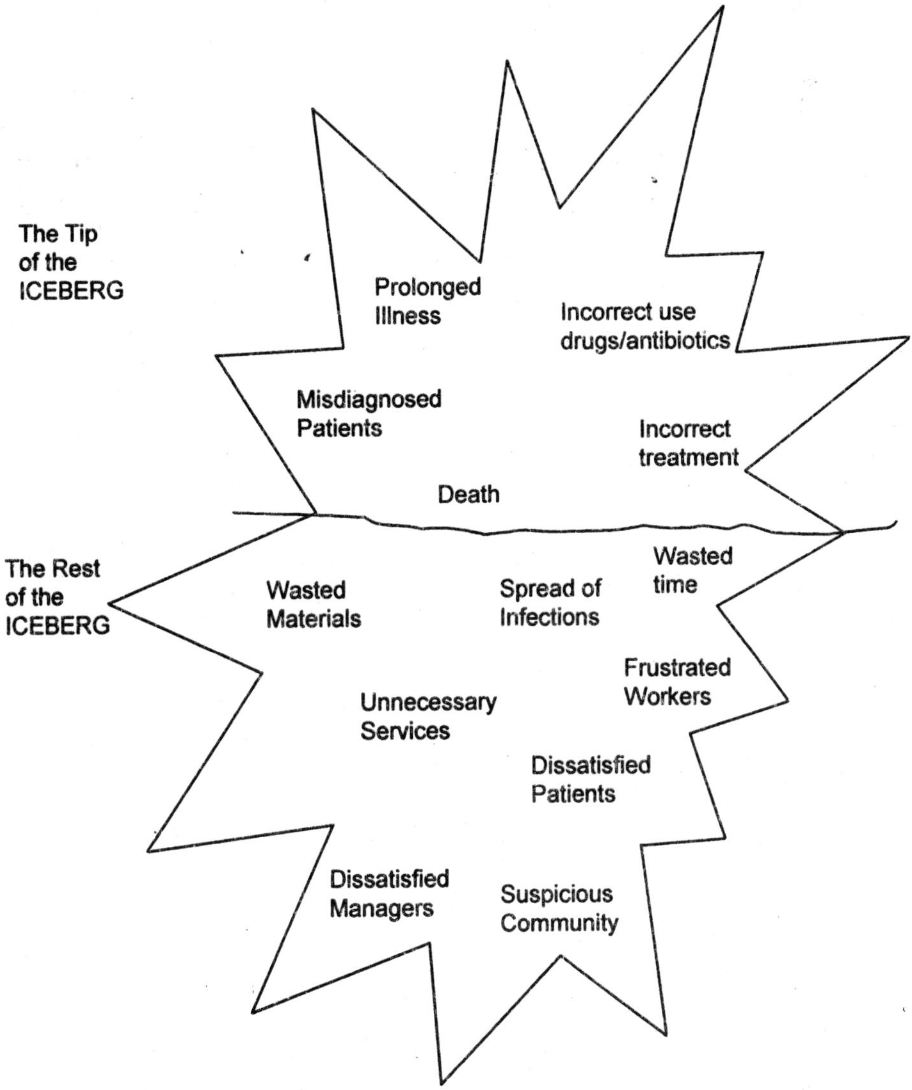

heart patients at the best hospitals in India who worry not about whether the surgeon will be able to perform their bypass properly but about whether they will survive the aftercare." ORA, AI-Assaf, WHO consultant, defines the concept of quality health care as:[1]

Quality is doing the right thing right the first time and doing it better the next, and that quality is simply the process of incremental improvements. Quality in health care should also be client focused and should emphasize meeting the clients' needs and expectations in the most effective and efficient manner. Quality, however, does not have to be luxurious or expensive. It should also be the responsibility of everyone involved and should be based on a learning environment rather than a disciplinary environment. Quality is simply a process of continuous improvement of the *status quo*.

Quality is described as having eight dimensions: effectiveness, efficiency, interpersonal relationships, safety, technical competency, access, continuity, and amenities. Each of these dimensions should be met at least minimally to meet the definition of quality. The concept of quality has been defined as "The totality of features and characteristics of a product or service that bear on the ability to satisfy stated or implied needs." The features or characteristics may be: (1) Meeting well defined purposes; (2) Satisfying patients and job satisfaction to health personnel; (3) Complying with applicable standards; (4) Reliability of products/ services; (5) Excellence; (6) Complying with safety requirements; (7) Complying with Environment requirements, and (8) Improving health status. Quality is not obtained by chance. Efforts must be made by everybody at every level and at various phases of health care delivery system. In this context, the concept of total quality management (TQM) which is being adopted by almost all excellent institutions throughout the world appears to be the only hope for establishing quality standards.[2]

TQM may be thought of as a way of organising and involving the whole health institution—every department, every activity and every single person at every level towards achieving excellence, high quality health care and research, growth of institution, patient satisfaction, and finally, moulding doctors of highest calibre. TQM can work well where culture and environment in the institution reflects academic quality as a way of life for all its employees.

Sri R. Venkatraman, former President of India, delivered the Convocation Address at the sixteenth convocation of Gandhigram Rural Institute, Gandhigram. He said: "A quality conscious system has been described as one which produces people who have the attributes of mental ability, efficacy and reliability and, above all, the capability to take initiative and innovative measures to meet situations."

Dill (1992) grouped Deming's fourteen points management into six basic themes in providing a framework for academic quality management (Williams, 1993).[3] The imperative of continuous quality improvement if an enterprise is to hold or enhance its place in the market:

- The emphasis on obtaining consistent quality in incoming resources through careful management of suppliers,
- The active participation of all members of an organisation's productive work force in the improvement of quality,
- The importance of meeting customer needs as the fundamental basis for the improvement of goods and services,

- The need for co-operation and coordination as the basic way in which an enterprise can improve its quality, and
- Quality improvement comes not from inspection but design, that is the establishment of procedures which make it impossible for bad quality to be inducted and encourage the primary aim of continuous improvement.

Murgatroyd and Morgan (1993) defined three quality-related terms:

Quality Assurance

The determination of standards, appropriate methods and quality requirement by an expert body.

Contract Conformance Quality

Some quality standard has been specified during the negotiation of forming a contract.

Customer Driven Quality

Those who are to receive a product or service make explicit their expectations. Quality assurance means delivery of efficient and effective medical care in accordance with the professional standards. The health system need to develop standards of quality in a comprehensive and scientific manner. They should not refer only to the technical aspects of effectiveness but to other aspects as well, like compatibility of service and work environment, communication with patients and their relations, and promotion of collective responsibility for medicare and health of the community. In the context of hospital systems quality assurance has to be understood in terms of entire hospital care system. The concept of quality assurance should not be fragmented for the different aspects of medicare system in a hospital rather the totality of the medical and health care provided to the patients in a hospital should be kept in view.

In Public Administration quality control is also equated with Good Governance. Quality of health services can be achieved only by efficient administration of health services that is by optimising the use of health resources.

NEED

Quality control is essential to make the efficiency of health institutions possible through:[4]

(a) Improvement of existing obsolete processes and procedures.
(b) Improved layout of office and working environment.
(c) Economy in human effort.
(d) Suggesting the best use of money and material.
(e) Improved design of the goods or services provided by the organisation.

(f) Improved performance.
(g) Job satisfaction.
(h) Improved flow of work.
(i) Standardisation of processes and products.

In brief, it aims at optimisation of resources which are:

- Manpower: Brain, skill, morale and effort.
- Materials: Inventory, Quality, Standards.
- Equipment: Design and Operation.
- Services: Communication and Information systems.
- Space and Building: Availability, design, utilisation.

Environment of Quality Control

Quality control cannot be initiated in isolation. It depends upon a number of factors both internal as well as external to the health system. Let us analyse some of them.

1. An Urge and Desire on the Part of the Personnel in the Health Organisation to Find Better Methods of Quality Health Care through Analysis of Existing Practices

Dr. M.K. Mani, Chief Nephrologist, Appolo Hospitals, Chennai, delivered the convocation address at the third annual convocation of NTR University of Health Sciences, Vijaywada on Thursday the 4th Feb., 1999.[5] He said, "What we get by reading is the distilled wisdom of others. It is necessary, and we must do it, but there is something more important, and that is to learn from our own experience. Reason, Observation and Experience are the Holy Trinity of Science. Why do we not trust ourselves? An important reason is that we do not really know what we are doing. The patients we remember are the spectacular successes or the dismal failures, but they are always the exceptions, and do not represent the true behaviour of the disease. We cannot draw on our experience if we do not record it. Documentation is our Achilles heel. We must make sure that all our experience is recorded. That is half the task. The other half is to review the records from time to time. This has two advantages. If we make an honest appraisal, we will find deficiencies in our own performance, and can improve on it. The second is that we may make genuine contributions to the world's body of knowledge. The doctors must always examine critically the work they are performing so that they can think better ideas to promote better health care.[6]

2. Need of Requisite Skill, Attitudes, and Ability in the Persons Engaged in Quality Control

Dr. K. Kasturirangan, Chairman, Space Commission and Secretary to the Government of India, Department of Space said that:

"Medical profession is one of the noblest professions that serve the humanity. It has a rich legacy of countless men and women who, through their selfless dedication and devotion, added new chapters to the long history of medicine."

The future environment is going to be dynamic and you have plenty of scope and challenge to play your part. Our society critically depends upon your contributions—which can make its members healthier, stronger and more prosperous.

Prof. J.S. Bajaj, Member, Planning Commission, Government of India, delivered the Convocation Address at the Second Convocation of the Nizam's Institute of Medical Sciences, Hyderabad. He said:[7] "Medicine is now undergoing a paradigm shift from organ physiology and cell pathology to molecular biology and reverse genetics. The recipients of post-graduate and post-doctoral degrees today are indeed fortunate that they would be practicing medicine in the twenty-first century when contemporary fundamental research and resultant basic discoveries shall be transcribed into diagnostic tools and therapeutic modalities of everyday use."

The dawn of the age of acquarius for bio-sciences seems to be tantalizingly close. However, the concern and compassion of a physician, and his inherent capacity to develop an inner vision and in-depth perception, shall always go beyond the hitherto known frontiers of bio-sciences. Indeed, this is where the sublime art of medicine surpasses the narrow confines of the advancing horizons of the science of medicine. This is when a physician attains the divine gift of healing. Yet, how many strive for both? And how few achieve either. To quote Dr. M.K. Mani again:

The medical profession has become rapacious, viewing every sick man as a gold mine. An ancient Sanskrit verse which means,

> "Hail to thee, oh physician, brother of Yamaraja, Elder brother, for Yama takes life, but you take life and money too."

We need to earn money to live, and to support our families, but we should remember that the source of our money is a human being, and one who is in distress and suffering.

You are fortunate in that your profession enables you to do good to others in the normal course of your work. You need not go out of your way to make opportunities for social service. If there is nothing that pleases you, then make yourself useful. That action is best, which procures the greatest happiness for someone in distress. By giving happiness we will receive it multiplied many-fold.

3. Need of Vision among Medical Professionals to Inject Quality

Medical profession through Indian Council of Medical Research, Medical Council of India and other organisations should define the role of the medical profession in the new millennium in the context of social development and improvement of the quality of life of the people.

A nation without a 'Vision' perishes. It is the vision that drives the progress of the nation. More than 500 experts drawn from various fields have prepared the "Technology Vision 2020" document for the country, which was released by the Prime Minister in August 1996. This vision document consists of 17 major technology packages. It deals with agricultural infrastructure and production, food-processing, health care, electric power, water-ways, life sciences and bio-technology, inland transportation, civil aviation, engineering industries, electronics, information and communication technology, material technologies and strategic industries, etc.

The Technology Vision Report aims to develop variety of indigenous technologies to transform India into a developed nation by the year 2020. With effective use of indigenously developed technologies in the next quarter century some of the visible results by the year 2020 will be, enhanced wealth of the nation, abundant production in various areas, well-being of the people and national security.[8] ICMR should prepare a document for the new millennium to ensure quality health care which should not be second to developed countries so that our people do not rush to the health institutions of advanced countries and waste financial resources and bring discredit to the country. We should develop our own health system which should possess all quality standards.

4. *Need of Initiative and Creativity among Medical Fraternity Gained through Critical Examination*

The critical examination is the crux of the quality control as it helps us to arrive at the true basis underlying each event and to draw up a systematic list of all possible improvements for designing of the most efficient, economic and practical way in which the job could be done. As stated in the report of the Secretariat Training School, Ministry of Home Affairs, Government of India (p. 91):

> "Critical Examination is a disciplined questioning technique. The questioning technique attacks the governing considerations of a specified activity under study in a systematic, logical and objective manner." The questioning technique is the means by which the critical examination is conducted, each activity being subjected in turn to a systematic and progressive series of questions.

In short, we can say that critical examination challenges the existing purpose, the resources used, the processes employed, environmental considerations of health organisations, etc. to prove quality health care. The critical examination is an intellectual exercise and must be used cautiously. It is perhaps worth-mentioning a few points which should be borne in mind:

(a) Facts must be examined as they are, not as they appear to be, or should be, or said to be.

(b) Preconceived ideas, which often colour the interpretation of facts, must be allowed no play.
(c) All aspects of the problem must be approached with a challenging and sceptical attitude. Every detail must be examined logically and no answer accepted until it has been proved correct.
(d) Hasty judgements must be avoided.
(e) Experiment resulting from 'hunches', which should have been immediately committed to paper as they occurred, should be reserved to the appropriate place in the investigation.
(f) New methods should not even be considered until all the undesirable features of the existing method have been exposed by systematic examination.[9]
(g) Details must have persistent and close attention.

We can thus say that the critical examination for its success presupposes the existence of the following ingredients—an analytical mind, freedom from prejudice, absence of pre-conceived notions, willingness to learn, strength of mind to avoid going off a tangent in pursuit of bright ideas, and concrete evidence.

Let us cultivate the valuable resources of creativity to creatively respond to the changing situations and become the 'Masters of Change' in every field.

C = Customer satisfaction leading to customer delights,
H = Honour and dignity to all the people,
A = Accountability from every area of service,
N = New ideas and commitment to innovation,
G = Growth as a continuous discipline, and
E = Excellence expressed as yardstick for performance and evaluation.[10]

The health institutions that will survive and thrive in the future, are those that foster creativity today among their health professionals. Without creativity, health professionals would become junk after a decade or so and would be a liability for the health system and even on themselves. Creativity only can keep health professionals alive in the true sense.

5. Need of High Quality Research Both in the Area of Medical Science and Human Behaviours towards their Health

According to P.V. Young, "Social Research may be defined as a scientific undertaking which by means of logical and systematized techniques, aims to:

(1) discover new facts or verify and test old facts;
(2) analyse their sequence, inter-relationships and casual

explanations which were derived within an appropriate theoretical frame of reference; and

(3) develop new scientific tools, concepts and theories which would facilitate reliable and valid study of human behaviour.

As stated in the Encyclopaedia of the Social Science, Social Research is systematic method of exploring, analysing and conceptualising social life in order to "extend correct or verify knowledge, aids in construction of a theory or in the practice of an art." The purpose of research is to discover answers to questions through the application of scientific procedures, i.e. Research Methods. There is no guarantee that any given research undertaking actually will produce reliable, relevant and unbiased results. But scientific research procedures are more likely to do so than any other method known to man. According to Young, "A researcher's primary goal, distant or immediate—is to explore and gain an understanding of human behaviour and social life."

Quality is more important than quantity in research. What is required is an increased quantity of quality research. The institutions must realise that high quality of work is a permanent asset which builds the foundations of science. A healthy climate is necessary for quality research. Openness, enthusiasm, trust, independence and team spirit is essential for the development of a scientific culture.[11]

Prof. J.S. Bajaj, Member, Planning Commission, Government of India, delivered the convocation address at the first annual Convocation of the University of Health Sciences, Vijaywada. He said, "The major goal of the new policy would be to usher in our fellow citizens a positive change in their health status where health benefits are Maximized and health hazards minimised, if not altogether eliminated. The new health policy must provide a reliable and relevant framework for not only effecting but also measuring and monitoring the health policy direction during the first quarter of the next century."

Dr. A.P.J. Abdul Kalam, Scientific Advisor to Raksha Mantri and Secretary, Deptt. of Defence R & D, Ministry of Defence, New Delhi, delivered the convocation address at the Second Convocation of the National Institute of Mental Health and Neuro Sciences (Deemed University), Bangalore, he said, "There is an urgent need of unified approach to the planning of health care delivery in our country. Besides traditional medical education and research programmes, the emphasis must be made on poly-clinic level training programmes in clinical technologies. Indigenisation of costly diagnostic and curative equipment to make them cost-effective and establishment of a nation-wide maintenance mechanism of medical equipment using indigenous skills and spares is also equally important.[12]

Dr Myint Htwe and Dr. Stephan P. Jost, in their article, "promoting the Application of Research Findings in Health Development" rightly concludes.[13]

Public Health programmes can be conceptualised as a pyramid. Research knowledge forms the base of the pyramid. Standards, norms, methods or procedures are developed on this basis. The public health information and documentation systems serve as supporting pillars. The top layers are bound by evaluative research. Therefore, research-based practice, whether derived from fundamental or evaluative findings, is a necessity. This is especially true in today's health care climate where increasing demands for high quality and cost-effective health care prevail.

Successful application of research therefore depends upon the interest and commitment of both researchers and users. It cannot be achieved by individuals working in isolation (Bircumshaw, 1990). If the ultimate benefits must be understood and implemented by health managers at all levels of the system. This does not happen rapidly. It requires commitment and willingness to learn because this process is cyclical as well as continuous. Research utilization is an organisational responsibility. It is best accomplished if there is real commitment to apply research findings at the organisational level. Therefore, translating health research into health care practice is neither easy nor quick (Sheehan, 1986). It remains an enormous challenge.

6. *Need of Commitment and Empathy*

Quality health care needs team work and mutual understanding. Medical personnel must work in a team to achieve quality health care.

S.S. Maricodoss mentions two ingredients of team work commitment and empathy. To quote him:

> "Commitment is a deep and profound value of emotional intelligence. It means aligning oneself with the goals of a group or organisation. It is applying oneself completely for a cause. People possessing this competence readily make sacrifice to meet larger organisational goals. Hence more than the individual interests, the group's mission or interest takes priority. It is very deep to the extent of sacrificing oneself. It also involves taking sides or taking stance. Emotionally balanced and committed people don't yield to any pressure or threat. Instead they courageously proceed whatever may be the consequences. Emotionally balanced people are generally empathetic and not sympathetic. Sympathy perpetuates oppression and makes people dependent. Sympathy is a form of judgement. We should therefore avoid being sympathetic towards others. Empathy means understanding the issue or concern that lie behind another's feeling. It is an ability to look at things from others' point of view or to read another's emotions or to put oneself into other's shoes and think from their angle. Avoiding pretension, it enables sensing and responding to a person's unspoken concern or feelings. It can be called the foundation skill for all the social competencies. Empathetic listening is a tremendous deposit in the Emotional Bank Account. Empathy

includes understanding others, service orientation, developing others, leveraging diversity and political awareness.[14]

7. Outstanding Leadership and Strength of Character

Health services must also develop the normative linkages, i.e. they must develop professional standards which should help them in their performances. Standards are contagious. Standards depend upon the quality of Leadership.

Eminent Industrialist, Mr. Rahul Bajaj, Chairman and Managing Director, Bajaj Auto Limited and President, CII, delivered the Convocation Address at the 49th annual convocation of the SNDT Women's University, Mumbai. He said, "To realize our goals and aspirations, we need outstanding leadership in every field and at every level. Leadership means that there is no substitute for excellence, no tolerance of mediocrity and no compromise with integrity. Leadership is not just charisma, not public relations, not showmanship. Leadership is performance, consistent behaviour and trust-worthiness.[15]

Leadership depends upon strength of character. Honourable Mr. Justice A.M. Ahmadi, Chief Justice of India, delivered the Convocation Address at the thirty-ninth convocation and special convocation of Sardar Patel University. He said, "In the final analysis, what really matters is one's character and not the outward signs of achievement. It requires character to face the unending tests that life constantly puts one through; when faced with a crisis, it is only a person possessed of true character who is able to keep his head steady whilst others around are losing theirs.[16]

Samuel Smiles says in Self Help:

> Character is the noblest possession of an individual. It exercises a greater power than wealth and secure all the honour without the jealousies of fame. Men of character are not only the conscience of society but in every well-governed State they are its best motive power. The strength, the industry and civilization of nations-All depend upon individual character. Mind without heart, intelligence without conduct, cleverness without goodness, are powers in their way, but they may be powers only for mischief. We may be instructed or amused by them. But it is sometimes as difficult to admire them as it would be to admire the dexterity of a pickpocket or the horsemanship of a highway man. Even in the noble medical professions doctors are fleecing the customers to make maximum wealth rather than take pride in the profession.

CONTENTS OF QUALITY

Health Care quality encompasses many attributes. It is very difficult to enumerate all of them. Let us discuss the important ones.

1. Effectiveness and Efficiency

Effectiveness is an expression of the degree of attainment of the re-determined objectives and targets of a programme, institutions, or activity seeking to reduce a health problem or improve and satisfactory health situation. This factor depends on whether the various activities and measures undertaken work (efficacy) and the degree to which they are accepted by those for whom they are intended. Efficiency is an expression of the relationship between the results obtained from a health programme or activity and the efforts expended in terms of human, financial, and other resqurces, health processes, technology, and time. The reason for assessing efficiency is to improve implementation and gain a better idea of the progress made. Both effectiveness and efficiency came at the top of the list stressing the fact that quality can only be achieved if processes are performed appropriately and in a cost conscious environment.

Only appropriate and necessary care should be provided. Waste, duplication and re-work should be eliminated. Only most economical ways and most effective ways to provide care should be stressed. In a system of higher demands for quality care coupled with the reality of limited resources, prudent decisions regarding best possible combinations of effective and efficient care are required and expected. World Health Report, 1999 rightly states how lessons learned from past successes and failures can guide a more targeted and pragmatic approach to current and emerging health challenges. It warns of the unprecedented challenges. It warns of the unprecedented complexity of these challenges, and offers strategic directions for tackling them in the next decade. Clear conclusions emerge. Despite recent spectacular progress in disease control and extended life expectancy, more than 1 billion people today have not shared in these gains.

Consequently, health systems can no longer afford to allocate resources to interventions of low quality or low efficacy related to cost. Spontaneous, unmanaged growth in any country's health system cannot reliably ensure that the greatest health needs are met. In defining priorities and selecting interventions, decision-makers must focus their efforts on areas where the return in health gains is demonstrably greatest.

2. Equity

Equity considers the coverage of population groups and geographical areas, distribution of resources and facilities, and effectiveness of services in different areas. Equity in the distribution of health care depends on the extents to which different geographical areas and population groups, according to age, sex, or wealth, have access to essential services.

How will history judge the 20th century? Will it be seen as the era of mankind's greatest advances productivity or as the era when human development faltered and gave rise to a wave of poverty like some epidemic of medieval times? As the century draws to a close, fear that it is the latter image which future generations will hold, unless we take decisive action.

The tremendous gains made in health development in the past three decades are at risk because the increasing gaps between rich and poor pose an unprecedented challenge to the health and well-being of the people of the world. Emphasis in development has for too long been on economic advancement alone, based on a simplistic belief that an increase in national income would, of itself, result in social improvements including health. In effect the world has reverted to a latter-day trickle down theory of development, an approach that was already discredited 30 years ago. Furthermore, the promise of more money for social development, following the end of the Cold War, has not materialized. Improving the health of nations is therefore dependent on reducing inequities both between countries and between the rich and poor within a country.

The basic elements of our strategy for action need be:

- Ensuring that the poorest and most vulnerable groups of the population have access to primary health care. This means redirecting often scarce money as well as personnel to the front line of the health care system at community and district levels. It also means increasing their access to information about health.
- Protecting the poorest from risks to health which are beyond their control; protection from environmental hazards; protection from crime and violence; access to adequate food, shelter, water and sanitation; and, above all, the ability to earn an income. These are the basic minimum needs for health and development.
- Building strong commitment to health among top political leaders in all countries. This includes assuming responsibility, at the highest level, for monitoring the reduction of health inequities.[17]

There is a need to redirect our efforts to ensure social development, equity and justice in 21st century and remove the imbalance accumulated in 20th century otherwise, this would be a danger to peace and prosperity on this globe.

D.R. Gwatkin proposes two initial actions that professionals can take to begin meeting the need:

- The first is that those concerned with health inequalities and the health of the poor should look beyond the issues that divide them and focus on the much more important beliefs which they share.
- The second is that they work towards the redefinition of health goals, now expressed primarily in terms of population averages, so that the goals refer directly to improving the conditions among the poorer groups and to reducing the differences between those groups and others in society.[18]

The goal of sustainable development cannot be achieved in a society if its peoples suffer ill-health. However, healthy people can contribute to the achievement of sustainable development. Therefore, health is a part of the goal of sustainable development and, in turn, helps to achieve that goal. In this sense, especially in a crisis, health is everybody's business.[19]

The principle of equity should be widely understood as the fundamental tenet of justice, to be incorporated into health policies and programmes of every society, with the particular meaning that whereas all have a right to health care, such care should take into account differential needs, so that the care is in accord with the need. Further, extending care beyond the need is the aspirational goal of reducing disparities in health status, with particular concern for the underprivileged and the needy.

A special area of concern is that of gender equality, which calls for policies and actions that will ensure equitable health care for all, including both females and males at all stages of their lives. While much of the concern for gender equality has risen from discriminatory practices directed toward girl children and women, which must be given priority in policy and programmatic actions, it is also important to acknowledge the importance of equitable care of all people at all ages. A gender perspectives is vital to the development and implementation of equitable health policies and strategies. With increase in life expectancy, creating conditions for healthful ageing assumes a sense of urgency.[20]

3. Patients/People's Satisfaction in the Quality of Health Care

Health Administration is named by people and meant for people. People's interest and satisfaction must be ensured through quality health care. R.B. Jain in his article, "Citizen's Charter—An Instrument of Public Accountability" has nicely explained the key elements in setting of citizens' charters. These are:

(i) Standards

Setting, monitoring and publication of explicit standards for the services that individual users can reasonably expect. Publication of actual performance against these standards.

(ii) Information and Openness

Full, accurate information, readily available in plain language, about how well they perform and who is in-charge.

(iii) Choice and Consultation

The public sector should provide choice wherever practicable. There should be regular and systematic consultation with those, who use services. User's views about services and their priorities are to be taken into account for final decisions on standards.

(iv) Courtesy and Helpfulness

Courtesy and helpful service from public servants who will normally wear name budge. Service available equally to all who are entitled to them and run to suit their convenience.

(v) Putting Things Right

If things go wrong, an apology, a full explanation, and a swift and effective remedy to be offered. Well published and easy to use complaint procedures with independent reviews, wherever possible to be introduced and maintained.

(vi) Value for Money

Efficient and economical delivery of public services within the resources, the nation can afford. And, independent validation of performance against standards.[21]

For democracy to be successful at the national level, the grassroots organisations have to be strong. The local authorities have to respond to the felt needs of the people.[22] The citizens have to have faith in the efficacy of the administrative system so that the distance between people and the government is reduced. The administration, for good governance has to be accessible. In developing countries, it is the government, which initiates and implements development programmes. It must gain support of the people in the discharge of these programmes, particularly at the cutting-edge. Such support would strengthen democracy as well as a positive response of the community to development programme which should be the ultimate goal of good governance.

4. Need of Positive Role of Functionaries of Health

Health functionaries have developed negative attitudes which has damaged the reputation and prestige of health system. M.K. Gaur has rightly said: Goodness of governance emerges from positive developmental roles of functionaries, underpinned with a summation of positive values—including morality, ethics, accountability, transparency, etc. in a Weberian model of public administration operating in a democratic context. A true democracy visualises, decentralization and delegation of political power to realise true people's participation, who are the ultimate beneficiaries of all administrative activities relating to law and order, development, social welfare, etc. Assertion of this angle is clearly visible behind the demand for enforcement of people's charter. Persistence in negative tendencies, in a gradually increasing proportion over the decades, has caused serious and widespread damage not only to the capability of Indian administration to be an effective vehicle of good governance but also its very credibility to discharge even the minimal functions of regulatory nature, let alone the demanding development ones. The situation is desperate and any piece-meal or patch-work approach will not work. Hence recasting Indian administration in a new mould is the crying need of the hour.[23]

Advances in the patterns of health development cannot proceed unless the human resources that lead, plan, staff, monitor and evaluate health-related services and programmes are enlightened and enabled to define and respond to societal needs. Given the evolving understandings of health problems and the changing dynamics of health system development, there must be a close and continuous interaction between educational, research and health system development to ensure relevance of education to need.

The commitment to equity must be imbedded in the educational process. Thus, population-based education and training will include learning the skills for assessing the needs of populations, including differential needs of vulnerable groups, and responding with care in relation to need. The relevant skills include the social sensitivities for interacting with patients and populations, for defining their individual and collective health problems, for determining the appropriate clinical and health-care response, and for leadership of or participation in health teams in providing such response.[24]

5. Need of Change of Attitudes of Health Functionaries

Time has come for a strong message to be conveyed that administration is for the people and not for the public servants themselves. There has to be a change of attitudes, and public servants should realise that efficiency will be measured not in terms of what the services purport to offer, but in terms of public satisfaction. Simultaneously, there has also to be a cleansing of the services and codification of the ethics, value systems and the interface with the politicians.

There is a need for:

1. Making administration accountable and citizen-friendly,
2. Ensuring transparency and the right to information, and
3. Taking measures to cleanse and motivate Civil Services.[25]

6. Need of Developing Positive Values for Health Functionaries and Ensure their Practice

Employees in public services should avoid wastage and extravagance, ensure effective and efficient use of public money within their control, and endeavour that the benefits of schemes for disadvantage and poor sections of society are not wasted or diverted for the benefit of others. They should avoid ostentation and set examples of austerity for others.

All employees in public services should promote and exhibit public and private conduct in keeping with the appropriate behaviour and standards of excellence and integrity. They should support the juniors in the latter's efforts to resist wrong or illegal directives and in abiding by the Code of Ethics. At the same time, they should reward good work and punish any dereliction of duty or obligations, based on objective and transparent criteria.[26]

7. Setting up of Work Improvement Teams

Another innovative measure designed to achieve higher productivity in public organisations is introduction of Work Improvement Teams (WITs). Adapted from the Japanese experience of Quality Control Circle, the WIT is essentially a small group of employees in the same work area or doing similar type of work who voluntarily meet regularly for about an hour every week to identify, analyse and resolve work-related problems. Through participation of the grassroots level, the scheme seeks to generate higher employee morale, improved productivity and reduction in cost.[27]

8. Need of Congenial Environment to Provide Decent Health Services

There are a number of factors within the health organisations which must be attended to achieve best health care. To quote WHO report, "Of course in a system that strives for quality other dimension must be fulfiled. Personnel interaction is important in providing quality health care. Health Care is provided by highly educated and sophistically skilled individuals but these individuals cannot provide a holistic care to the patient without relying on teamwork. Interpersonal relationships therefore, play a tremendous role in shaping the processes of care and ensuring a positive outcome to the patient. Just think of a scenario where a highly specialized hospital with all the gadgets and whistles of technology and technical competence of its staff but without real care teams. Each provider is working on his own without regards to others in the system. No coordination of activities and no collaboration between providers. Probably a total chaos! How would the care be delivered then? It would almost be impossible to deliver any care let alone quality care. Such an environment is not conducive of quality processes and this hospital is doomed to failure. Effective teamwork is a must for health care quality. Health Care quality is a process not a programme. A programme has a beginning and an end but a process has no end. It is continuous. Another issue in regard to quality is that care should be provided in a continuum. That is to say, care should be initiated, rendered, evaluated, improved, and continuously monitored even after the patient is cured of his present illness. Care is extended to include wellness, health promotion and disease prevention. Additionally, care that is started by one provider should be continued and followed by the other provider in cases of transfer to ensure continuity of care, fragmented care and disconnected system is not a quality system and health care quality may never be achieved in such a system.

Finally, it is always more pleasant to have a care provided in an aesthetically acceptable environment. A facility that pays attention to the minute details of its customer's comfort and well-being is certainly a quality facility. Whether it is cleanliness, decor, or service, health care quality can only be enhanced with such a valuable dimension.[28]

Good governance, however, is not a finished product. It is a dynamic concept. It encompasses fast-changing political, social and economic milieu, along with international environment and conditions of operational governance. Hence, the need for periodical rethinking on and even remodeling of the concept and institutions of governance. The search for good governance has to be a continuing exercise.

9. Need of Medical Audit

Medical Audit is defined as the evaluation of medical care in retrospect through analysis of medical records. It is a review of the professional work in the hospital or in other words the quality of medical care, i.e. we try to see how far the clinicians have conformed to the norms and standards of defined medical practice while treating the patients.

According to Sanalaro some 30 years ago any auditing usually took the form of chart review. This is now regarded as highly inefficient and unproductive use of physicians time, leading mainly to biased judgement. Today perhaps we need constant and recurrent medical audit. Even such review committees like hospital. Tissue review committees' findings and feedback to professionals had lead to dramatic reduction in rate of tonsillectomy as reported. The form of medical audit which have since evolved now uses exploit written criteria for judging whether care provided meets the standard of performance of the staff.

The Medical Audit is now well established as a formal activity in most of the hospitals in west. The assessment of quality of care depends upon the quality and reliability of medical records being maintained and the nature of criteria that are being used. The medical records are of value to patients, the physicians and the hospital and also for teaching and research. The quality of medical records reveals/reflects the quality of patient care and since the main objective is good medical care, it is inevitable that the physicians should assumes the primary responsibility for the quality of the medical records compiled on patients under his care. Therefore, a good medical record section becomes an essential pre-requisite for medical audit. It may be emphasised here that medical audit is not a one time activity. The medical staff of the hospital and administrators realise and appreciate its potential in improving the quality of patient care in hospitals. Besides it is going to be of tremendous professional value to hospital doctors. Keeping all this in mind it is necessary that the medical audit must be carried out as an on-going activity. This could be facilitated by putting the hospital data on computer and having necessary software for medical audit of various diseases.

Pre-Requisites of Medical Audit

(a) To be carried out by fair and impartial clinicians who are thoroughly conversant with the current practice of medicine.
(b) The impetus must come from the medical staff themselves realising the benefits to the patients and themselves.
(c) A good system of medical record keeping and a trained medical record librarian.
(d) Well defined disease related criteria.

The purpose of Medical Audit is to evaluate the factors impinging on patient care. All the deaths in a hospital where cause of death are not certain are investigated by the Mortality Review Committee. This improves the knowledge of the medical personnel and enhances their capability of handling such cases in future. The Health Survey and Planning Committee (1959-61) recommended the use of medical audit in all hospitals. The Delhi Hospital Review Committee headed by Dr. K.N. Rao (1968) also recommended the appointment of a Medical Audit Committee in each hospital. Such committee will ensure specific checks on the quality of work performed in the hospitals. We have found the following drawbacks in some of the hospitals where such committees are functioning:

(1) Poor recording of a case history
(2) Sketchy documentation
(3) Operation notes not properly recorded
(4) Lack of inter-departmental coordination
(5) Incomplete case-notes
(6) Not proper follow-up by the senior faculty members.

Either mortality committees have not been set-up in hospitals or function irregularly. The Public Accounts Committee also mentioned that:

> "Although the recommendations of the review committee to carry out hospital mortality review periodically was accepted by the Government in February 1970, it was only after a lapse of six years (May 1976) that the mortality review committee started functioning in Willingdon Hospital (Rammanohar Lohia Hospital).

The conditions are worse in hospitals under the control of State Governments in this regard. Thus, there is a need to set-up such committees to ensure efficient and effective medical audit.

10. Need to have Transparent and Honest Administration to have Good Quality Administration

We mention here some ingredients of quality administration which can help in providing decent health are services:

1. Openness in the sense of having wide contact with men and matters.
2. A sense of justice, fair play, impartiality in dealing with men and matters.
3. Sensitivity and responsiveness to the urges, feelings and aspirations of the common people.
4. Securing the honour and dignity of all human being, however humble he or she might be.
5. Humility and simplicity in the persons manning the government machinery and their easy accessibility.

6. Creating and sustaining an atmosphere conducive to development, growth, and social change and honesty and integrity in thought and action.

Process of Quality Control: Setting Standards

Standards of quality health care are not fixed as these would vary from organisation to organisation depending upon the quality of inputs. However, efforts should be made to reach standards which are international so that people can get the quality health care in their own country. Government and private resources are wasted in getting health care from advanced countries which can be .made available within the countries themselves through the application of quality standards in our health institutions. This is not going to be expensive but only require hard work and dedication on the part of the health experts and sincerity on the part of Governments.

Talveen Singh in an Article, "What is lorony with Indian Hospitals" has rightly said (May 6. 2000). Meanwhile, until our governments are able to provide decent standards of health care to the average Indian we should seriously onsider a ban on any politician or bureaucrat being allowed to travel broad for treatment at taxpayer's expense. When they and their families can no longer be treated free at the best hospitals in the world we can be sure that things will start to improve. We now mention the steps for quality control.

(i) Select/Identifying a Function or System/Activity

It can be a study of OPD, ward, emergency, etc. It is essential to select the activity in the context of economic, technical, human, social and psychological consideration. For example, let us select the problem. How many patients old and new can be seen by an ENT specialist in an OPD with quality in focus? Standard of quality could need be developed separately for each activity like laboratory services, X-ray, Wards, Nursing Services, etc. These would depend on many factors and hence would be flexible. Therefore, Standards should be set keeping in view the profile of the organisation.

After the selection of the problem, it is necessary to get a formal approval of the sponsoring organisation. This formal approval or terms of reference should define clearly the purpose of the assignment, time dimension for completion of the study, cost involved and the inherent technical or organisational limits. This formal approval must be distributed among all the employees of an organisation whose quality is being studied so that they can properly appreciate the significance of it. Besides, the organisation must ensure cordial atmosphere for the study team to ensure fruitful results. We must always keep in mind that the quality control is not only job of the team but a joint venture where success would largely depend on the support, ethos, attitudes and interest of key personnel of the sponsoring organisation.

(ii) Recording of Data

The next and an important step in the quality control is the recording of facts relating to the existing methods/Procedure/Practice. While collecting data by any method, scientific attitude is very important. To be sure, a scientist avoids personal and vested interests. The success of the quality control greatly depends on the accuracy with which the facts are recorded. The main aims of recording are:

(a) To obtain adequate and accurate information.
(b) To present the facts in a concise and comprehensible form for analysis.
(c) To submit proposals to management in a way which is easily understood.
(d) To provide, eventually, detailed operating instructions for the use of supervisors and operators.

(iii) Critical Examination

The examination is conducted by means of the sets of detailed question: the primary questions to indicate the facts and their underlying reasons, and the secondary questions to find the alternatives and the best methods of improvements. The questions pertain to the purpose of the operation, the place where it is carried out and the means by which it is carried out. Both primary and secondary questions are asked for each aspect before passing on to the next. In order to carry out the critical examination in a scientific way, a sheet of standard layout is used. The outline format of this sheet is reproduced below:

While examining the factors impinging upon the operational efficiency of purpose, means, sequence, place and person, there is no set sequence to be followed. However, we must initiate with the purpose as other factors would be considered only provided the study of purpose is justified.

The success of the critical examination depends upon the scientific attitude of the investigating team. The aim of all critical examination is the furtherance of the quality control philosophy—there is always a better and effective way.

(iv) Develop

The critical examination will suggest a number of alternative solutions to the various aspects of the problem in hand. Besides, the critical examination does not indicate the improvement of the total situation. Therefore, there is a need to devise a composite plan, integrating all the elements, to improve quality. All the elements should be combined through the building of 'Family Tree' of all variables. This would provide the integrated plan to produce total quality improvement rather than in a particular area which can create problems and thus produce negative results. Development may be compared to the development of a photograph

Facts	*Reasons*	*Alternations*	*Implication*	*Selection for Development*
Purpose What is being achieved?	Why is it achieved?	What else can be achieved?	What are the advantages and disadvantages of each alternatives?	What can be selected for development?
Means How is it achieved?	Why that way?	How else can it be achieved?	What are the advantages and disadvantages of each alternatives?	What can be selected for development?
Place Where is it achieved?	Why there?	Where else can it be achieved?	What are the advantages and disadvantages of each alternatives?	What can be selected for development?
Personal Who achieved it?	Why that person?	Who else can achieve it?	What are the advantages and disadvantages of each alternatives?	What can be selected for development?

from an exposed film or negative. The picture needs touching with chemicals to make prints of desired quality.

(v) Define/Set Standards

Apriori, quality cannot be considered as absolute concept but is a multi-dimensional dynamic entity. It is also not a unitary concept but a phenomenon determinable by relating with the excellent or the best in the field. Consequently, for judging quality, a yardstick or standard needs to be established which is otherwise called 'benchmark'. Through standards, an organisation defines what it expects for the inputs, processes, and outcomes of the health services it provides. They are an instrumental part of monitoring the quality of health care and identifying problems and measuring improvements in health care service delivery. Through periodic updating and modifications, they become a part of an organisation's cycle of continuous improvement.

(vi) Installing the New Standard

Words written or spoken are of no use unless put to action. The actual implementation is the responsibility of health management. The study team can only play an advisory and supportive role. The implementation can be successful if the top health management has developed faith and interest in the new plan and can motivate the personnel down the line. What has been seen mostly is that such schemes are shelved on one pretext or the other. Installation can be divided into five stages, namely:

(a) Gain acceptance of the change by the supervisors.
(b) Gain approval of the middle management.
(c) Gain acceptance of the change by the employees and their representatives.
(d) Train the employees to operate the new methods.
(e) Maintain close contact with the progress of the work until satisfied that it is being done as intended.

(vi) Maintaining the New Standard

Human behaviour is averse to change. Therefore, Management must see that once a standard has been installed it should be maintained as designed and that the workers should not be allowed consciously or unconsciously to slip back into old methods. As already mentioned, the top management must be innovative to handle any situation which may prevent the working of the new model. The top leaders must learn the art of dealing with interest groups and the pressure groups who may oppose the running of the new methods on flimsy grounds.

(viii) Reviewing the Standard

The main aim of reviewing is to discover whether there are any discrepancies between the authorized quality and current practice at the time of review. Reasons for any variations in the quality must be investigated. Any changes that have occurred valid reasons should be accepted and the operating instructions amended accordingly. Where the review reveals that there are undesirable variations in the quality, measures should be taken through supervision to ensure that the quality follows the authorized procedure.

The ultimate purpose of standard should be the aim of integrating quality into normal management process so that search for improvement becomes a matter of accepted practice in an organisation. We must also ensure that standard of quality is feasible, probable in the overall frame of administration.

Misconcpetion about Quality

- Quality means goodness, luxury, shininess or weight
- Quality is intangible and therefore not measurable
- Quality is expensive; "we cannot afford it."
- Quality problems are originated by the workers.
- Quality originates in the quality departments.

Relevance of Quality

- Quality is never luxury; it is essential to improve health services, and minimize waste when resources are scrace.

- Quality of health care can be measured.
- Quality is care can be improved with the same resources.
- The majority of problems encountered are due to inappropriate functioning of health systems, and not necessarily the result of errors of individual workers.
- Quality is everybody's job.

Benefits of Quality Assurance

- Improve the health status of the population.
- Insure the right of people to access to quality health services.
- Meet customers needs and expectations.
- Minimize waste of limited resources and reduce cost.
- Increased demand for effective and appropriate care.
- Increased demand for efficient utilization of limited resources.
- Standardize care and control variation.
- Ensure safety and minimize risk.
- Fulfil the ethical duty of health professionals.

CHALLENGES TO SETTING STANDARDS

In spite of a large resource of existing standards to adapt to specific needs and the growing interest in establishing standards by various country health organisations, there still exist certain challenges to this process:

(1) Reliance on Explicit Criteria: Physicians, nurses, and other health care professionals may resist on the basis that standards impinge upon their subjective judgement that they have developed through their practice. Some professionals contend that medicine is partly art, partly science, and that standards may require them to diagnose and treat without allowing them to use their professional judgement. Others may fear that standards will be used in a punitive manner, to identify and punish professionals who don't perform within strictly defined limits. These are legitimate concerns and require the organisation to address them in some constructive manner before developing or implementing standards.

(2) Identifying Appropriate Resources, Human, Physical and Financial. Developing or adapting standards takes time and resources. Sometimes the organisation must go outside its staff to use experts in the field. Throughout all this the organisation will incur certain costs that should evaluated before hand to determine if the effort is worth the costs.

CONCLUSION

WHO in its Report of WHO Inter-country meeting on quality assurance in health care from 16-20 Dec. 1996 at Indonesia suggested the following for improving quality health care for South-East Asian countries:

(1) Ensure that quality of health care is an integral part of health services delivery at all levels of health care covering public and private sectors;
(2) Organize advocacy/awareness workshops on quality assurance for policy-makers, administrators and the leadership of health care to get their commitment for quality assurance;
(3) Establish a coordinating mechanism for quality assurance activities at national level through the nomination of focal point(s) and constitute a multi-disciplinary task force of national experts to provide advice on technical aspects of quality assurance;
(4) Initiate quality assurance of health care in selected hospitals and in primary health care through the district health system approach, document the experiences and expand gradually to more health care facilities;
(5) Organize national strategic planning workshops with technical assistance from WHO;
(6) Formulate guidelines to set standards and select national key indicators on quality assurance to monitor compliance and measure performance;
(7) Invest on building local capacity in health care quality through the creation of a critical mass of expertise.
(8) Mobilize potential resources from within the country including support from international agencies; and
(9) Ensure that orientation on quality assurance be integrated in both basic and in-service training programmes of all health care professionals.

Implementation of TQM in health institution calls for a total change in culture in terms of customs, practices and improvement by creating increased sense of caring brought about by improved communication, involvement and training. It involves the integration of all functions, processes and personnel within an organisation in order to achieve continuous improvement in the quality of health care delivery systems.

By following TQM principles we can bring about harmony and quality working style in all the facets of the health institution and help it gain the top position and maintain it. Finally, TQM consists in doing for the institution what should be done as a matter of course. The fruits of implementation of TQM may not be available instantly, like magic tree, but it is sure to show improvements in health standards over a period of time.

Notes and References

1. *Daily Tribune*, May 6, 2000.
2. *University News*, March 11, 1996, p. 14.
3. G. William, Total Quality Management in Higher Education, Panacea or Placebo, Higher Education, 25, 1993, pp. 229-37.
4. S.L. Goel, Modern Management Technique, Deep and Deep, New Delhi, 1995, pp. 375-75.
5. *University News*, Aug. 2, 1999, p. 18.
6. *University News*, Sept. 6, 1999, pp. 21-23.
7. University News, Feb. 23, 1998, pp. 13-16.
8. *University News*, March 2, 1998, p. 12.
9. R.M. Currie, Work Study, 2nd Ed., London, Pitman, 1963, p. 92.
10. S.J. Mariadoss, Creativity-Competitive Resources and Core of Education, *University News*, No. 29, 1999, p. 13.
11. *University News*, Feb. 13, 1997, p. 18.
12. *University News*, Dec. 15, 1997, p. 10.
13. Dr. Dyint Htwe and Dr. Stephan, P. Jost, Research Development.
14. S.L. Maricodos, Emotional Intelligence, Tool of Credibility, in University News, March, 20, 2000.
15. *University News*, March 13, 2000, p. 17.
16. *University News*, Feb. 17, 1997, p. 8.
17. Hiroshi Nakajima, "Growing Equity is a Matter of A Life and Death", in *World Health*, Nov.-Dec. 1994, p. 3.
18. D.R. Gratkin, "Health Inequalities and the health of the poor : What do we know? What can be done? In *Bullettin of the WHO*, Vol. 78, No. 1, 2000.
19. Robert Kim Farley and Mark Books, "Role of the World Health Organisations in the Economic Crisis", in *Regional Health Forum*, WHO, SEARO, New Delhi, Vol. 3, No. 1, 1999, p. 1.
20. WHO : SEARO : Declaration on Health Development in the South-East Asia Regions in the 21st Centruy, New Delhi, 1977, p. 21.
21. Quoted in R.B.
22. A.P. Barnbas, Good Government at Local Level, *IJPA*, July-Sept. 1998, p. 453.
23. M.K. Gaur, Political Stability and Good Governance, in IJPA, July-Sept. 1998, pp. 410-11.
24. Declaration on Health Development, *op. cit.*, p. 45.
25. Action Plan for An Effective and Responsive Govt. Document 1.
26. *Ibid.*, Appendix IX.
27. *Ibid.*, Document 2.
28. WHO, SEARO, Quality Assurance in Health Care, New Delhi, 1916, p. 20.

APPENDIX 14.1

INTRODUCTION

The Centre has set-up regulatory bodies for monitoring the standard of medical education, promoting training research activities. This is being done with a view to sustain the production of medical and para-medical manpower to meet the requirements of health care delivery system at the Primary, Secondary and Tertiary levels in the country. This chapter discusses the status of these activities conducted by the various bodies and institutions.

MEDICAL COUNCIL OF INDIA

Structure

The Medical Council of India was established as a statutory body under the provisions of the Indian Medical Council Act, 1933 which was later replaced by the Indian Medical Council Act, 1956 (102 of 1956). The main functions of the Council are: (i) Maintenance of uniform standard of Medical education at undergraduate and postgraduate level; (2) Maintenance of Indian Medical Register; (3) Reciprocity with foreign countries in the matter of mutual recognition of medical qualifications; (4) Provisional/permanent registration of doctors with recognised medical qualifications, registration of additional qualifications, and issue of Good standing certificates for doctors going abroad; and (5) Continuing Medical Education, etc.

Functions

I. Inspections

The Medical Council of India from April 2006 to 30th November 2006 carried out 34 periodical Inspections of medical colleges for continuance of recognition, 13 inspections of medical colleges for recognition of MBBS degrees, 11 inspections for increase of MBBS seats, 41 inspection for renewal of permission in medical colleges and 21 inspections for establishment of new medical colleges under Section 10A of the IMC Act, 1956 and 66 inspections were carried out for verification of inspectors compliance submitted by the Medical Colleges. Further, the Council also carried out 201 inspections for starting of Postgraduate medical courses at various colleges/institutions and 35 inspections for increase of seats for which the request was received through Central Government under Section 10A of the IMC Act, 1956. The Council also carried out 168 inspections for recognition of postgraduate qualifications, 4 inspections for recognition of non-teaching hospitals for Housemanship and 3 inspections for recognition of non-teaching hospitals for internship.

2. Registration

The Council has registered 383 doctors with their additional qualifications under Section 26 of the Indian Medical Council Act, 1956. The Council also issued 1616 Good Standing Certificates to doctors who desired to seek Registration with Medical Councils of foreign countries. Further, the Council issued 536 Provisional and 1375 Permanent Registration Certificates under Section 25(2) and 23 of the IMC Act, 1956 respectively.

3. Continuing Medical Education

During the year 2006-07 the Council has planned to hold 150 CME programmes. Till 30th November 2006, 102 CME programmes have been approved of which 76 Continuing Medical Education programmes have already been held at various medical institutions in the country.

4. Accounts and Establishment

The following outlay has been approved by the Central Government as Grant-in-aid (Plan and Non- Plan) for the year 2006-07:

	Outlay approved (Rs.)
Plan (including CME)	100 Lakh
Non-Plan	60 Lakh

A sum of Rs. 11,52,88,260 has been received by the Council till November 2006 from other resources in addition to Grants-in-aid received from the Central Government.

5. Policy regarding Establishment of Medical College

As on 30th November, 2006 there are 262 medical colleges in the country out of which 174 medical colleges have been recognised under Section 11(2) of the IMC Act, 1956 by Medical Council of India. The remaining 88 colleges have been permitted under Section 10A of the IMC Act, 1956 for starting MBBS course. Out of the 262 medical colleges, 127 are Government Medical College, 5 are University colleges and remaining 130 are private medical colleges. The admission capacity in these colleges is approx. 29,172 students per year.

DENTAL COUNCIL OF INDIA

Structure

The Dental Council of India is a statutory body constituted by an Act of Parliament viz. Dentists Act, 1948 (XVI of 1948) with the main objective of regulating the Dental Education, Dental Profession, Dental ethics in the country and recommend to the Government of India to accord permission to start a Dental College, start higher course and to increase of seats. For this purpose the Council periodically carries out inspection to ascertain the adequacy of courses and facilities available for the teaching of Dentistry.

The Council had received 104 applications in prescribed form/ Scheme from the Central Government for (i) establish new Dental colleges, (ii) starting MDS Courses and (iii) increase of seats in BDS/MDS Courses for evaluation and recommendation in accordance with the provision of the Section 10A of the Dentists Act, 1948. During the said period, the Central Government on recommendation of the Council had permitted 35 new Dental Colleges, MDS Courses in 143 specialities at 31 Dental Colleges, 2. Dental Colleges for increase of admission capacity in BDS Course and 3 Dental Colleges for increase of seats in MDS Courses in 17 specialities. The Central Government on recommendation of the Council had allowed/ renewed its permission for 2nd/3rd/14th/5th/6th year BDS course in 64 Dental Colleges and renewed its permission for increase of seats for 2nd/ 3rd/4th/5th/6th year BDS Course at 25 Dental Colleges, 313 Inspections of the various Dental Colleges in the country had been carried out by the Council's Inspectors/Visitors during this period.

The Council had granted its permission to start Dental Mechanic Courses at 5 Dental Colleges and Dental Hygienist Course at 5 Dental Colleges. The DCI had recognised the Dental Mechanic at 2 Dental Colleges and Dental Hygienist at 2 Dental Colleges. The Government of India on the recommendation of the Council had issued 4 notifications of recognition of BDS/MDS qualifications awarded by the 3 Universities under Section 10(2) and 10(4) of the Dentists Act, 1948. A sum of Rs. 18 lakhs has been provided as grants-in-aid to the Council during the year 2006-07.

PHARMACY COUNCIL OF INDIA

The Pharmacy Council of India (PCI) is a body constituted under section 3 of the Pharmacy Act, 1948 to regulate the profession and practice of Pharmacy.

The Council is responsible for Prescribing minimum standards of education required for qualification as a pharmacist; Uniform implementation of educational standards; Approval of course of study and examination for pharmacists; Withdrawal of approval; Approval of qualifications granted outside India; and Maintenance of Central Register of pharmacists.

During the year under report approval of 213 Institutions was extended u/s 12 of the Pharmacy Act 65 new institutions were granted approval u/s 12 of the Pharmacy Act.

At present, there are 461 approved institutions imparting Diploma in Pharmacy to 27,735 students per annum and 261 approved institutions imparting Degree in Pharmacy to 14,790 students per annum. The Revised Budget Estimate of the Council for the year 2006-07 is Rs. 208.10 lakh.

Continuing Education Programmes

The Pharmacist is an important member of the Health Care Team. He must possess specific knowledge and skill in support of his role as a member of the Health Care Team. Continuing Education Programmes (CEP) play an important role in the growth of the knowledge bank of the pharmacist. The PCI from its own resources is giving a financial assistance to the State Pharmacy Councils for the conduct of CEP for pharmacists.

PCI has approached the Health Ministry for sanction of 100 crores from the Planning commission under the 11th Five Year Plan for professional activities like continuing education for teachers and working pharmacists, travel grants for exchange programmes between India and foreign countries, grants to institutions for upgradation of infrastructural facilities, etc.

Appointment of Inspectors u/s 26A of Pharmacy Act

Section 42 of the Pharmacy Act provides that no person other a registered pharmacist is eligible to compound, prepare, mix, or dispense any medicine on the prescription of a medical practitioner. To ensure implementation of section 42, State Pharmacy Councils are empowered u/s 26A of the Pharmacy Act to appoint inspectors with the previous sanction of the State Government. Since many State Pharmacy Councils have not appointed inspectors, PCI has taken up the matter regarding appointment of inspectors with the State Government and also requested Ministry of Health to take up the matter with the Health Secretary of all the State Governments/Union Territories for appointment of inspectors u/s 26 A of the Pharmacy Act to ensure strict compliance of section 42 of the Pharmacy Act in the interest of Public Health.

INDIAN NURSING COUNCIL

The Indian Nursing Council is a Statutory Body constituted under the INC Act, 1947. The Council is responsible for regulation and maintenance of a uniform standard of Training for Nurses, Midwives, Auxiliary Nurse-midwives and Health Visitors. The Council prescribes the Syllabus and Regulations for various nursing courses.

The inspection of Nursing Schools/Colleges and Examination Centers is done by Indian Nursing Council to maintain uniformity and the requisite standard of nursing education in the Country. During the year 2005-06, inspection of 11.18 institutions have been done.

During the year 2006-07 upto 28.12.2006 a total number of 888 Nursing Training Institutions were inspected. The Nursing Training Institutions recognized by Indian Nursing Council as on 31st March 2006 are as below:

Programme	*Total*
A.N.M.	271
G.N.M.	1312
B.Sc. (N)	582
P.B.B.Sc. (N)	62
M.Sc. (N)	77

According to information collected by the Indian Nursing Council, the total number of qualified nursing personnel entered in the State Register up to 31st March 2005 are as follows:

Registered Nurses, Registered

Midwives GNM and B.Sc.(N)	—	9,08,962
Auxiliary Nurse Midwife	—	5,21,593
Health Visitor	—	50,715

A sum of Rs. 10.00 lakh (Non-Plan) and 100.00 lakh (Plan) has been sanctioned by the Government of India, Ministry of Health and Family Welfare for the year 2006-07 as Grants-in-aid to Indian Nursing Council. Out of Rs. 100.00 lakh plan money in the year 2006-07, Rs. 50.00 lakh has been received and expenditure of Rs. 49,97,703.00 upto 28.12.2006 has been incurred from plan money.

DEVELOPMENT OF NURSING SERVICES

In order to improve the quality of Nursing Services, the following activities are being implemented under the scheme of Development of Nursing Services:

(i) Training of Nurses.
(ii) Strengthening of existing Schools/Colleges of Nursing.
(iii) Upgradation of Schools of Nursing attached to Medical Colleges into Colleges of Nursing by providing one time non-recurring assistance of Rs. 1.50 crores to states.
(iv) Providing recurring assistance to Schools of Nursing which were opened during IXth Plan with assistance under the scheme of Development of Nursing Services.
(v) Establishment of College of Nursing at JIPMER, Pondicherry.
(vi) Strengthening of R.A.K. College of Nursing as "Center of Excellence."
(vii) Upgradation of Schools Nursing into Colleges of Nursing attached to Dr. R.M.L. Hospital, S.J. Hospital and Lady Harding Medical College, New Delhi.
(viii) Construction of Delhi Nurses Colony.

Moshe Prywes in his article "All who serve—teach" in the *World Health*, April 1984 observes that Medical education is a socio-cultural complex of values and inter-relationships, and only partly a scientific discipline. It must not be regarded as an aim in itself, but as a mission-oriented endeavour, judged by its contribution to improving the nation's health and developing new models of medical care.

Academic medicine has only rarely tried to direct health delivery systems outside its own sphere. Medical academicians have preferred to remain in the comfortable micro-environment of their university hospital and research laboratories. If they continue to disregard the community's needs for better, cheaper and more easily accessible health care, and if they do not educate health professionals who are aware of their community role, medical education will not fulfil its fundamental social objective.

It, however, the academic medical community could find the way to mobilize the university to participate in the improvement to health delivery systems in the community, we are likely to find a balance, not only between medicine and science, but also between medicine and society. Today, the University must have a wider vision. Its three functions of teaching, research and service have to be reviewed in the light of a world blemished with gross inequalities and clamorous with need. The winds of change must blow away the cobwebs of learning for its own sake (and of course Oxford itself is changing).

In the particular field of health, teaching is vital; but it must be directed towards all categories of health workers, including those in primary health care, not merely towards the medical 'specialist'. And then research too is vital; but it should seek to resolve real problems, rather than being "pure research." And the service function of a university should surely rate top priority; in any country, whether developing or developed, there are serious gaps in the public health services which can only be filled through the efforts of talents and their hard-earned skills to serving the community.

15

CHAPTER

Medical Education

The success of health and medical care delivery system depends to a substantial extent upon the quality of medical education as the product of medical education, i.e. Doctor, Superspecialists, Nursing personnel and other para-medical staff are responsible for providing medical and health care. Medical education thus occupies a significant place in the promotion and development of health services. Medical Education in turn depends upon number of factors—

(i) Quality and Quantity of teachers engaged in medical education. In addition to their qualifications, the teachers should be dedicated, creative and innovative. C.V. Raman rightly describes the role of teacher as: "Principal function of a teacher—is to discover talent and genius in the younger generation and to provide ample opportunity for its free expansion and expression." The essence of teaching lies in creating an insatiable love for knowledge in the learners, a love that will not die when they leave the educational institutions, but will continue to influence them till the end of their lives. The purpose of medical education is to provide quality education. A quality conscious system would produce people who have the attributes of functional and social relevance, mental ability and physical dexterity, efficacy and reliability and above all the confidence and capability to communicate effectively and exercise initiative, innovative and experiment with new situation.

(ii) Relevant and creative curriculum—Curriculum must be innovative, interesting and relevant and must include all the latest developments in the field of medical education. Medical education must include the knowledge of ethics, social sciences,

CHART 15.1

Medical Education

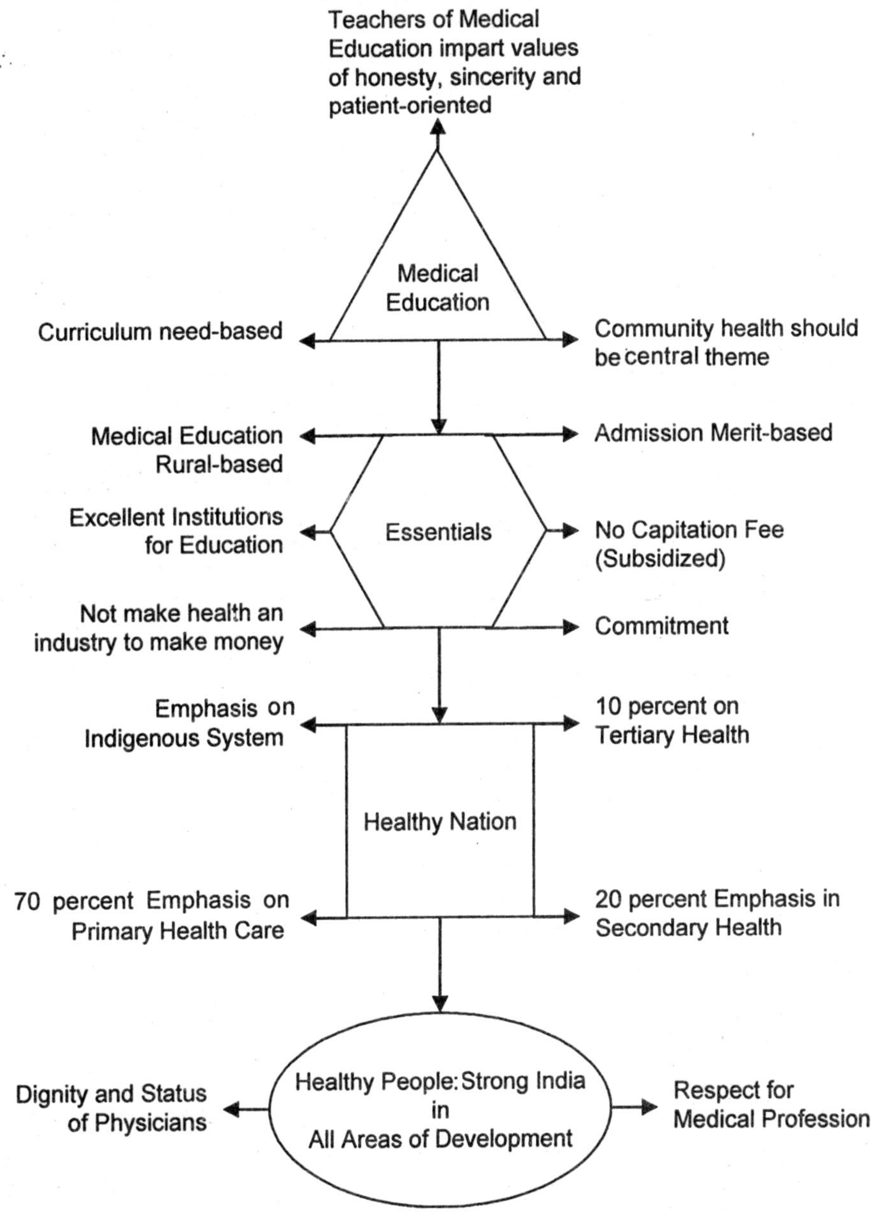

etc. as the products of medical education would have to treat human beings.

(iii) Fully equipped laboratories.

(iv) Spacious and good infrastructure with all facilities.

(v) Arrangements for indoor and outdoor games.
(vi) Hostels with full facilities.
(vii) Excellent hospitals for providing medical students rich practical experience.
(viii) Good Liaison between hospital and medical students.
(ix) Quality supervision of medical students to make them perfect in their discipline.

We may sum up that students must be provided best medical education so that they can become excellent doctors, super specialists, excellent teachers, researchers as well as can serve the ailing humanity with expertise and affection.

Medical Education is concentrating on curative aspects and for this purpose the medical institutions are providing under-graduate and post-graduate medical education. Medical Council of India, Ministry of Health and Family Welfare, All India Council for Medical Research, Tertiary and Secondary hospitals are not realizing that all the diseases are a product of malnutrition, lifestyle, alcohol consumption, lack of safe drinking water, etc. and the solution of these must be given priority in medical education. The cost of medical education is becoming very high both for those who take up these courses at under-graduate and post-graduate level as well as to the patients who are increasing in geometrical proportion. This can be visualized on surveying the market where chemists shops are increasing every day with great rush of patients purchasing medicine. Such a situation is very serious as poor people cannot afford costly treatment. So there is a need of critical examination of our medical education policy. What can be done in improving our medical education? What can be done to check increasing rate of diseases among people? What can be done to check the rising cost of medical care? An analysis would reveal that medical education should not concentrate only on diseases and their treatment but should be imparted community medicine courses intensively and seriously. Medical education should prepare doctors who play a great role in attacking the causes which create the prevalent diseases. In addition, Medical Education must include the teaching of Indigenous system of medicine like Yoga and naturopathy which are cheap and preventive. In addition, in the entire education system from primary to higher education level, students must be taught about keeping their health in perfect order and warn them the consequences of taking alcohol, smoking, environmental pollution, etc. Thus preventive health is the only answer.

Ministry of Health and Family Welfare deserves appreciation for starting Public Health M.Sc. course through a Five Year integrated courses. Ministry may also get prepared small booklets on "How to be Healthy."

Farokh Erach Udwadia in his article, "Humanity: The Core of Doctor-Patient Relationship" clearly defines that Medicine must have been surely born with the awakening of consciousness of primitive man. The trail of medicine has witnessed several twists and turns, victories and defeat, scintillating light and somber darkness. After over 5000 years of recorded history, medicine has now evolved into a powerful force, an art, a science and a profession poised to make a quantum leap into the twenty-first century. The roots of medicine lie in magic—in the magical and empirical beliefs of the shamans and priests physicians of ancient civilizations. It was however philosophy which gave the first true impetus to the evolution of medicine. The Vedas in the East and the great Greek philosophers in the West asked pertinent questions—Who was Man, what was his nature, where did he come from, where did he go, how did he relate to nature and his environment? More than any other field of human endeavor, medicine through the ages has been influenced by philosophy, religion, economics, sociology, geography, by art and culture, by war and natural calamities and by the rise and fall of mighty civilizations. Above all it has been influenced by the natural sciences so that by the late quarter of the twentieth century the science of medicine in a way seems to have overpowered its art.[1]

The need to have a competent, motivated and a sustainable health workforce in ensuring an efficient and effective health system is essential. The importance of HRH development cannot be undermined at any cost. Health workforce has a pivotal role in effective, efficient and sustainable delivery of health services.[2]

Medicine and surgery are today capable of performing feats deemed incredible a century ago. Many a life has been saved, many marvels performed, and many indeed must have reaped the benefit from the knowledge and power that a revolutionized medical science has to offer. Yet Man and Medicine stand on the threshold of the twenty-first century, sharing an uncertain future. No longer are doctors considered next to gods, as they were till the middle of the twentieth century. In fact, there is today a seething discontent against medicine and the profession—a discontent which is shared by many in the profession. I shall give you my analysis as to why this should be so.

The mechanization of medicine (as I would like to term it) has depersonalized medicine, robbed it of its very essence, its humanism. All through the ages—from Imphotep, Hippocrates, Charaka, Susruta, Hunter, Lister, Pasteur, Osler, Flemming and several others medicine meant care, compassion and a special empathy for the patient. Whatever grab medicine assumed, whatever philosophy it professed, whatever its blemishes and faults, human qualities lay deeply entrenched at its very core, central to its being and existence. The advent of machines, gadgets and sophisticated technology in medicine has lessened its humanity and adversely affected the doctor-patient relationship. Patients are made to relate more to machines than to doctors, and doctors relate more to sophisticated gadgetry than to patients. The machine has thus unfortunately become the interface between the doctor and the patient.

An inevitable accompaniment of the mechanization of medicine is super-specialization. A super-specialist is of unquestionable importance in certain well-defined situations and is an invaluable asset to modern medicine. But over-emphasis on super specialization can be self-defeating as it negates the holistic aspect of medicine. We must remember that disease is no specialist. "Patients do not consult us because certain organs are affected, but because they feel ill. They come with symptoms and the earlier and therefore more curable their malady is, the more vague will those symptoms be, the more difficult the elucidation of their cause, the greater the need in the first place of general investigation by one whose daily practice covers the whole of disease."[3]

It is also necessary to appreciate that the effective delivery of health care services would depend very largely on the nature of education, training and appropriate orientation towards community health of all categories of medical and health personnel and their capacity to function as an integrated team, each of its members performing given tasks within a coordinated action programme. It is, therefore, of crucial importance that the entire basis and approach towards medical and health education, at all levels, is reviewed in terms of national needs and priorities and the curricular programmes restructured to produce personnel of various grades of skill and competence, who are professionally equipped and socially motivated to effectively deal with day-to-day problems, within the existing constraints. Towards this end, it is necessary to formulate, separately, a National Medical and Health Education Policy which (i) sets out the changes required to be brought about in the curricular contents and training programme of medical and health personnel, at various levels of functioning; (ii) takes into account the need for establishing the extremely essential inter-relations between functionaries, of various grades; (iii) provides guidelines for the production of health personnel on the basis of realistically assessed manpower requirements; (iv) seeks to resolve the existing sharp regional imbalances in their availability; and (v) ensures that personnel at all levels are socially motivated towards the rendering of community health services.[4]

Education of Health Care Professionals

Medical and Dental Colleges are not evenly spread across various parts of the country. Apart from the uneven geographical distribution of medical institutions, the quality of education is highly uneven and in several instances even sub-standard. It is a common perception that the syllabus is excessively theoretical, making it difficult for the fresh graduate to effectively meet even the primary health care needs of the population. There is a general reluctance on the part of graduate doctors to serve in areas distant from their native place. NHP-2002 will suggest policy initiatives to rectify the resultant disparities.

Certain medical disciplines, such as molecular biology and gene manipulation, have become relevant in the period after the formulation of the previous National Health Policy. The components of medical research in recent years have changed radically. In the foreseeable future such research will rely increasingly on the new disciplines. It is observed that the current under-graduate medical syllabus does not cover such emerging subjects. The Policy will make appropriate recommendations in respect of such deficiencies.

Also, certain speciality disciplines—Anaesthesiology, Radiology and Forensic Medicine—are currently very scarce, resulting in critical deficiencies in the package of available public health services. This Policy will recommend some measures to alleviate such critical shortages.

Need for Specialists in 'Public Health' and 'Family Medicine'

In any developing country with inadequate availability of health services, the requirement of expertise in the areas of 'public health' and 'family medicine' is markedly more than the expertise required for other clinical specialities. In India, the situation is that public health expertise is non-existent in the private health sector, and far short of requirement in the public health sector. Also, the current curriculum in the graduate/post-graduate courses is outdated and unrelated to contemporary community needs. In respect of 'family medicine', it needs to be noted that the more talented medical graduates generally seek specialization in clinical disciplines, while the remaining go into general practice. While the availability of post-graduate educational facilities is 50 percent of the total number of qualifying graduates each year, and can be considered adequate, the distribution of the disciplines in the post-graduate training facilities is overwhelmingly in favour of clinical specializations. NHP-2002 examines the possible means for ensuring adequate availability of personnel with specialization in the 'public health' and 'family medicine' disciplines, to discharge the public health responsibilities in the country.[5]

The National Health Policy affirmed that the effective delivery of health care services would depend very largely on the nature of education, training and appropriate orientation towards community health of all categories of medical and health personnel. It is, therefore, of crucial importance that the entire basis and approach towards manpower development in terms of national needs and priorities are reviewed and training programmes restructured accordingly. Besides there is an urgent need to reassess appropriate health manpower mix to deliver health services at primary, secondary and tertiary level and for the purpose of training and research. As much as approximately three-fourth of the total expenditure of health services is spent on personnel. Yet, health manpower planning, production and management, which constitute key elements for effective implementation of health programme, have not received adequate attention.[6]

A sound health manpower policy is the main requirement for the development of any functionally effective health care system. Most of the countries in the developing world have never formulated or implemented such a policy.

"The most crucial factor for the improvement of the world health situation . . . is undoubtedly the development of health manpower that is properly attuned to the health problems of the people and suitably trained to respond to health programme and service need."[7]

We must find the method to achieve greater productivity, efficiency and cost-effectiveness in health manpower utilization. No society, especially the developing, can long justify investing years of education and training in individuals who later on perform rudimentary duties that could be achieved satisfactorily by people trained in half that time. The critical decisions in health manpower planning concern the kinds of personnel required, the type and adequacy of education and training and financial resources necessary to produce them, their relationship to each other in the health team, and where and how they would practice.

The objective of a good medical education should be to produce general practitioners, specialists, teachers and research workers. The factors governing this are the curriculum, medium of instruction, duration of course, admission qualifications, the examination system, teachers-students relationship, prospects of teachers and students, etc. Besides, it may be mentioned that the medical education should fit in with the needs of the country and the conditions prevailing there. For instance 70 per cent of the population of India live in rural areas. The training given to the doctor should enable and motivate him to carry on his work among the vast masses in the villages. We have been designing out undergraduate and postgraduate medical education which can fulfil this basic aim. There has been a big gap between aims and fulfilment. J. Gallagher, Regional Officer for education and training, WHO Regional Office for Europe has expressed concern about, "inadequate communication between educational systems for health personnel and the health administrations that use the products of these systems. There is very little understanding of how the manpower training and development needs of health administrations can be met in a systematic way."[8]

The Government of India launched the Re-orientation of Medical Education Scheme in 1977 with the objective of involving the various medical colleges in the country in the direct delivery of health care services to the rural and semi-rural population. Under the scheme, each of the 106 medical colleges in the country is to accept in the first instance, the total responsibility for promotive, preventive, curative health services in three Community Development Blocks in the districts in which the institution is situated. 318 mobile clinics at the rate of 3 per college have been provided to the medical colleges to render quality services nearest to the rural population. The objectives of the scheme are:

(i) To expose the Medical faculty, residents, in terms and the students to the Rural Community;

(ii) To train the students, in terms and Residents in Community Organisation and Community Participation; and
(iii) To render comprehensive health care services to the villages in collaboration with the local Primary Health Centres.

It has been expressed in the Fifth Plan document that teaching in medical colleges still requires a radical change for its orientation towards the need for community care. Medical education over the years, has been urban biased. It is hoped that in the Sixth Draft Plan (1978-83), it would be possible "to produce medical graduates who are aware of the health problems of the community, who have a sense of compassion and motivation to serve the public and who have ability to effectively meet the urgent needs of the health care problems of the rural masses and the urban-poor."

According to the Estimates Committee:

> "The National Policy should indicate in unmistakable terms the goals to be achieved and the method of accomplishment . . . Such a policy especially in the context of health being a State subject will help in maintenance of the requisite standards of medical education throughout the country in keeping with the needs of the people."[9]

The Government of India has announced the National Medical Education Policy. There is a need to set-up a Health Care Medical Service Commission responsible for planning of medical manpower, medical education, research, training of all para-medical personnel would be a step in the right direction. This commission when appointed should use Health and Medical Educational Planning as a means of rationalizing the education of health manpower. Besides, the Commission may encourage the health administrations to provide the policy and planning backgrounds required for this purpose.

Health services require large members of well-trained qualified professionals and workers, with a variety of skills and appropriate knowledge, and attitude to improve the health of the people, and to reduce suffering due to ill-health. It is necessary to have formal and informal educational centres to train persons in adequate numbers and of the requisite quality.

The biggest challenge to the health-care education institution is not just technical, managerial or financial development, but quality human resources development, which includes:

1. formation of young health professionals and supportive staff who are responsive to social, technical, scientific and management abilities to work effectively in a comprehensive health system;

2. development of a faculty team, consisting of not just good teachers but learners-oriented facilitators in educational process, who are also good role models with social vision, commitment to ethical norms and values; and inspirers of people and community-oriented vocations through precept and example; and
3. development of a supportive team of staff who will complement the faculty in the educational institutions, laboratories, outpatients, wards and other specialized clinics, field practice areas and community health: centres with needed skills and motivation.

Need of Reforms in Medical Education and Training[10]

- Selection of students (both undergraduate and postgraduate) should not be based only on the ranking at the entrance examination. Stress should be on the aptitude of the candidate. The selection should be based on their commitment to the social objectives and technical challenges of education in the State. The output from these institutions should be need-based.
- The education should be competence and value-based. Nurture the human resources holistically in terms of knowledge, skill, values, attitude and social commitment. For this process to be effective, the focus should be on three dimensions—professional, personal and social.
- A doctor has to face moral and ethical dilemmas all the time. He/she must be prepared to face these problems, just as he/she faces clinical or health problems. Then only can the doctor take appropriate decisions. Rajiv Gandhi University of Health Sciences has taken the right step in recommending teaching of medical ethics throughout the course including internship.
- The education should be scientific and evidence-based. The approach should be humanitarian and holistic, rather than disease-oriented. Day-by-day the doctor-patient relationship gap is widening. Commercialisation has eroded the doctor's concern for the patient. The education which at present is knowledge-oriented, should focus on development of required skills, and attitude so that he/she will have the confidence and competency to face the challenges in caring for the individual, family and community. The teaching and learning programmes should be oriented taking into consideration the abilities identified by Medical Council of India and other professional councils, which are required for a graduate to practice independently. The thrust should be on student-centered learning rather than to satisfy the teacher's capability. They must be encouraged to get involved in electives or small projects.

The teacher's role should shift from a mere instructor to that of a facilitator and create a situation for the student to learn by participating in the learning process. There should be stimulus to the student to apply his/her mind and provide an opportunity for self-learning.

- Medical and health professional colleges and other health care institutions must adapt to the important health reforms in the society. The students must accept a certain degree of accountability towards society's health if they wish to continue to be forces for social progress and consequently to merit taxpayers support. It is their obligation to direct education, research and service activities towards addressing the priority health concerns of the community, region and state; they have a mandate to serve.
- At the time of admission, the student should be exposed to educational objectives, skills of learning and communications. National Health Policy, values, group dynamics, team work concept, dignity of labour, use of library and computer application. Foundation courses should be organised towards development of personality and leadership qualities. During the course, equal importance must be given towards involvement of students in cultural and sports activities. To counter the enormous stress during the course, continuous counseling of students should not be lost sight off.
- Apart from concentrating only on the merit, non-scholastic capacities like: thinking skills, speed of thinking, aptitude, group behaviour and communication skills of the candidate must be given weightage. His/her knowledge in the field of behavioural sciences also need to be tested.

The students should be actively involved in social actions and disaster management. A brief exposure to National Service Scheme (NSS) would enable them to understand the fabric of the society.[11]

Essentials for Re-orientation on Medical Education

I. Need of inculcating Multi-Sectoral Dimension of Health Development

Health professionals often lack familiarity with the methods and tools which could predict health futures, and lack the skills needed to establish linkages with other sectors. A major challenge for them is to extend their horizons and pursue health as an achievable social goal.

Since medicine alone cannot deal with ill-health caused by adverse socio-economic conditions, there is a need to involve professionals of other health-related sectors such as health economists and social scientists to provide other missing but vital inputs, necessary for health planning and health development. Such inputs would also provide health planners with the vision and understanding on the ongoing demographic, social and political changes and make them responsive to such changes.

In other words, for a clear vision of the future, it is imperative that health issues in Region are viewed holistically, that is, in the context not merely of epidemiological trends and forecasts, but also within the cultures and attitudes prevailing among administrators, professionals and health workers.[12]

Thus, good health is a synthesis of physical, mental and social well-being. As stated in the First Five Year Plan: "Health is a positive state of well-being in which harmonious development of mental and physical capacities of the individuals lead to the enjoyment of a rich and full life . . . It implies adjustment of the individuals to his total environment—physical and social.

Some people even define it as a condition under which an individual is able to mobilize all his resources—intellectual, emotional and physical—for optimum living. Thus health is not static; on the contrary, if fluctuates on a scale which ranges between optimum health as defined by WHO to complete lack of health. Dr. E. Berthet, Secretary-General of the International Union for Health Education, Paris, defines health as follows:

"We no longer ought to define health only in terms of sickness, but rather in relation to the harmonious development of every individual's personality. After all, it represents a balanced measure of a person's total potential—whether biological, psychological and social; and to the notion of individual health we should and the concepts of family and community health.

2. Medical Education is not oriented to future needs

Dynamic linkages between planning, production and utilization of health personnel are essential. Imbedded within such systems are pathways for leadership development. Too often, the training of health personnel follows a pattern of yesterday's view of health care, or even of only the clinical care, and falls seriously short of meeting today's and tomorrow's requirements for personnel who can lead or participate in effective health services responding to people's needs.

3. Commercialization of Medical Education

To the mechanization of medicine is added the sin of commercialization. This is an age of consumerism where the lure of money—which brings with it power, luxury, comfort and enjoyment of life in all its varied physical forms is paramount. Dreadful as it may sound, medicine is fast becoming a business rather than a profession, and that too, not uncommonly, a nefarious, corrupt business. What could be more nefarious than charging exorbitant fees from those who cannot afford them. What could be more corrupt than the practice of doctors who on purpose refer unsuspecting vulnerable patients from one specialist to another for no reason other than profit? What could be more corrupt than the unethical practice of commissions demanded by general practitioners from a specialist to whom a patient is referred?

Another major drawback of contemporary medicine is the crippling expense an ill-patient often incurs—an expense that is often ruinous to the family. This is partly due to the fact that the physician of today has forgotten the art of medicine and remains solely pre-occupied with its science. His rapport is with machines and not with patients; it is technology that dictates his course of action and not his clinical judgement. History-taking is a neglected art; he forgets to use his senses—his eyes, ears and hands, but remember numbers, equations and formulae. Expensive investigations and expensive modes of treatment result, when simple tests and simpler measures would have sufficed.

Institutionalised medicine has also led to malpractice. Expensive glittering machines and foyers resembling five star hotels are the landmarks of modern institutions. To meet the cost, and, hopefully, make profit, machines have to be fed, and patients become the fodder for these machines. If an audit was to be carried out on the cost-effectiveness of modern day investigations, the result would indeed be shocking.[13]

5. Devoid of Human Values

Why has there been such a decline in the ethics of contemporary medicine? It is almost certainly related to the decline in the sense of values in our present-day world. This decline is observed in all professions and in the whole of society, perhaps even to a greater extent than that observed in medicine. A burning desire for material gain and wealth dominates life today. It is indeed difficult for a profession to remain an island of virtue when surrounded by a sea of filth and corruption. The island is first eroded and then gradually swamped. But please remember that we have an ancient heritage to cherish and maintain. We must therefore combine and rise to root out the canker eating into the heart of medicine.[14]

6. Theoretical and Not Practical

In the present scenario of medical education the teaching is didactic and theory based, more of information imparting than problem solving, the students are more oriented to examinations, Teachers lack training to guide the student to impart knowledge; There is sequestration of what he has learnt in the pre-clinical year with hardly any integration with clinical subjects and *vice versa*. A pre clinical student can learn with interest the functioning of heart and lungs if the clinician makes an audiovisual presentation to them on cardio pulmonary resuscitation or vascular access.[15]

7. Not Community-oriented

The primary objective of medical education is to support the health development of the nation; it should be "Community-oriented." Unfortunately the medical education system till date has been hospital-based, specialization-oriented and dependent on sophisticated investigatory procedures. The curriculum is over-crowded with factual information and this inhibits a student from developing creative and critical thinking to solve problems. The Edinburgh Declaration (1988) states, 'the aim of medical education is to produce health professionals who will promote the health of all people. Further, it states that scientific research continues to bring rich rewards, but man needs more than science alone, and it is the health needs of the human race as a whole and of the whole person that medical education must affirm. The declaration also emphasizes in shifting the training from passive to active learning. The existing medical education system does not follow the spirit of Edinburgh declaration. Health professional education is presently centered on tertiary care units, whereas it should necessarily be based on a priority of primary, secondary and tertiary care with the largest component being primary health care. Our medical colleges are sequestrated from the community and the present system of medical education is not need-based.

Physicians worldwide are trained in the academic niche of tertiary hospitals, where day-to-day discussions revolve around the obscure mechanisms of rare diseases, state-of-the-art diagnostic tools and sophisticated, high-technology medical interventions. Despite strong indications that the requirement is more of training in primary care and more investment in the critical public health issues, precious time is spent on investigation of diseases, which afflict a tiny proportion of the humanity. Graduates from the present medical colleges feel that all this learning is wasted in a primary or secondary care hospital, which in fact is the backbone of our health care delivery system. Health Care providers are not mere professionals with technical knowledge to solve health problems but are accountable to the society. Medical education and Health Care delivery should be linked. At present these are two systems going parallel, often not complimenting each other. Medical education should be linked to all levels of health care—primary, secondary and tertiary.[16]

Moshe Prywes in his article, "All who serve—teach" in the *World Health*, April 1984 observes that Medical education is a socio-cultural complex of values and inter-relationships, and only partly a scientific discipline. It must not be regarded as an aim in itself, but as a mission-oriented endeavour, judged by its contribution to improving the nation's health and developing new models of medical care.

Academic medicine has only rarely tried to direct health delivery systems outside its own sphere. Medical academicians have preferred to remain in the comfortable micro-environment of their university hospital and research laboratories. If they continue to disregard the community's needs for better, cheaper and more easily accessible health care, and if they do not educate health professionals who are aware of their community role, medical education will not fulfil its fundamental social objective.

If however, the academic medical community could find the way to mobilize the university to participate in the improvement to health delivery systems in the community, we are likely to find a balance, not only between medicine and science, but also between medicine and society. Today, the University must have a wider vision. Its three functions of teaching, research and service have to be reviewed in the light of a world blemished with gross inequalities and clamorous with need. The winds of change must blow away the cobwebs of learning for its own sake (and of course Oxford itself is changing).

In the particular field of health, teaching is vital; but it must be directed towards all categories of health workers, including those in primary health care, not merely towards the medical 'specialist'. And then research too is vital; but it should seek to resolve real problems, rather than being "pure research." And the service function of a university should surely rate top priority; in any country, whether developing or developed, there are serious gaps in the public health services which can only be filled through the efforts of talents and their hard-earned skills to serving the community.

8. Need of Collaboration between Scholars of Medicine and School of Health Science in the following area

A variety of factors influence human development both favourably and unfavourably. Some of these factors are: environmental—natural and man-made; physical, chemical, biological and social; economic, cultural factors; education, genetic factors; prenatal health development factors and nutritional factors. Thus the promotion of health cannot be achieved by measures that derive from any single health discipline, nor can health measures be considered independently of the broader educational, social, economic and administrative factors that are crucial to human development.

Obviously, the relationship between socio-economic development and progress of health is of extreme importance. In fact, every aspect of economy has a health component which has an important bell ring on the overall socio-economic development. Thus, as stated in a WHO paper on public health: "The health component and other components of the total system necessarily interact. Health not only affects the remainder of the socio-economic complex but is also affected by it, sometimes unfavourably."

Because of this intimate relationship, it has been mentioned in the First Five-Year Plan, "If this subject is regarded in the proper light as one which is concerned with everything affecting the health of the community, it must be admitted to be the biggest and the most important problem of India."

Socio-economic development consists of various components related to the productive shares of activities. Health programmes cannot be related unilaterally to either the economic or the social spheres as they influence both and are influenced by both.

There, obviously, is a need for a unified, integrated approach to public health, i.e. to combine services for nutrition improvement, communicable disease-control, better maternal and child-health and family-welfare. Thus, conventional linear planning and the execution of separate programmes cannot meet the needs of human development. As stated by T. Adeoye Lambo in his article, 'Total Health' in *World Health.*

> "It is now apparent that a more balanced consideration of the Biological, social and cultural aspects of health is needed. Life is a process and not a substance—a living system based upon the primacy of continuity and inter-relatedness throughout the universe." If man and his family are to remain in empathy with the emerging necessities in the developing milieu, an adequate design of inter-disciplinary tools will have to be made to assist in this task of providing a total health package."

In general, the factors influencing health could be classified into three broad categories, hereditary, environmental and personal. Similarly, the various conditions which play a vital role in determining one's health status can be put under three major areas, viz., mental health, spiritual health and physical health.

9. Teaching Values

- Presuming a high standard of professional and personal values in relation to patients and their care.
- Being available and accessible to patients.
- Maintaining a high standard of clinical competence.
- An ability to communicate effectively.
- An assurance to personal, and professional, development as a doctor.
- An assurance to professional audit and peer review.
- An assurance to team working in multi-professional environment.
- An understanding of the mufti-cultural society in which medicine is practiced.
- An enthusiasm for his/her specialty.
- A personal assurance to teaching and learning.
- Impressionability and responsiveness to the educational needs of students and junior doctors.
- The capacity to promote development of the required professional attitudes and values.
- An understanding of the principles of education as applied to medicine.
- An understanding of research method.
- Poetical teaching skills.
- A willingness to develop both as a doctor and as a teacher.
- A commitment to audit and peer review of his/her teaching.
- The ability to use formative assessment for the benefit of the student/trainee.

- The ability to carry out formal appraisal of medical student progress/the performance of the trainee as a practicing doctor.[17]

Dr. H. Mahler is very critical about the inability of health workers in contemporary society to influence those social and environmental factors which truly determine public health. He states: "There persist widespread negative attitudes among health professionals towards the health care of the poorest strata in the rural and urban population in the developing countries. Most of these attitudes imply—with a repetitiveness of an old gramophones records caught in a narrow, arrogant, condescending and indifferent groove—that these poor people are too apathetic, too superstitutious, too illiterate to benefit from the health cart potentially availability to them. Health professionals and those who train them should be much more radicals in accepting a social responsibility for the health needs of the people in these poor rural urban communities so that they can act as agents for change."[18]

Thus, we can say that there is a need to train health administrators and workers in the new art of Public Health Administration so that they can take the benefits of the modern science to the common man and maintain the spirit of Geneva Declaration."[19]

Now being admitted to the profession of Medicine, I solemnly pledge to concentrate my life to the service of humanity. I will give respect and gratitude to my deserving teacher. I will practice medic with conscience and dignity. The health and life of my patients will my first consideration. I will hold in confidence all that my patients confides in me. I will maintain the honour and noble traditions of medical profession. My colleagues will be my brothers. I will not per considerations of race, religion, nationality, party politics or so standing to intervene between my duty and my patient. I will main the utmost respect of human life. Even under threat I will not use knowledge contrary to the laws of humanity. These promises I make freely and upon my honour."

The same feelings has been expressed in the Tokyo Declaration quote the preamble to the Declaration of Tokyo:

> "It is the privilege of the medical doctor to practice medicine in the service of humanity, to preserve and restore bodily and mental health without distinction as to the persons to comforts and to ease the sufferings of his or her patients."[20]

Prof. S. Neki has rightly said in this connection that "to help, to heal, to reconstruct, to comfort—and all along the line to act compassion—all these bear testimony to the moral consciousness doctor. Whatever the new strains imposed upon medical ethics, structure will survive and continue to guide doctors in their professional conduct. Legal and juridical obligations they have, of necessity to fulfil. But these are not genuine ethics. Genuine ethics has to be ingrained character and does not have to depend upon external controls:[21]

10. Medical Education not oriented to Rural Needs

A group on medical education and support manpower set-up in 1974 noted with concern that "Medical Education in India over the years has been essentially urban-oriented, relying heavily on curative method and sophisticated diagnostic aids, with little emphasis on preventive and promotional aspects of community health. Programmes of training in the field of nutrition, family welfare planning, maternal and child health have tended to develop in isolation from medical education and thus do not subserve the total needs of the community. Although the number of doctors has speedily increased over the successive plan periods, the alienation of doctors from the rural environment has deprived the rural communities of total medical care." The same feeling was voiced in the Fifth Five Year Plan. The Sixth Plan also went on to point out that, "the basic problem is to produce a doctor who will be able to provide good health care and medical service to the community and will be able to work effectively in rural areas." Thus, it is high time for the State governments to take policy decisions to reorient medical education with a view to progressively make the training of the medical students more community-based. It is suggested that the internship of medical college students may be arranged in villages. The students may be asked to execute a bond to serve in the villages atleast for a period of five years. The curriculum may be curtailed and may be oriented to the community needs.[22]

Medical Education is Urban-oriented

There is national commitment to reorient medical education profession and health services, so as to serve the needs of rural people. All the expert bodies have agreed to modify the syllabus of under-graduate medical education so as to produce a basic doctor who would have the ability to cater to the needs of the rural area. It is necessary to make the medical colleges act not as ivory temples in majestic isolation but take on the responsibility for providing total health care for specified segment of the rural population. The aim of medical education should be to promote happiness through better health of most of the deprived hundreds of millions of human beings. With the contemplated changes in the contents of the under-graduate course, the students would be in a position to appreciate the problems of rural people and would develop proper motivation to help them.

11. System focus to Medical Education

A medical institution could be considered as a system where the inputs are the students and the output is the juvenile medicos, who are the products of an institution (process includes the teaching learning activities). The role of environment in a system is quite significant. The environment in this context is the society at large. We take the students from the society and after training them leave them back to the society. Society would embrace them only if they can take care of it and its needs; hence it is very important that the training imparted to them is a need-based one.[23]

12. Mushroom Growth of Medical Institution

The growth in medical institutions for imparting education to physicians and Nurses is increasing at a fast rate in the private and has become an industry to earn money at the cost of quality. The charges of fee and other expenses are very high. How can we expect values from medical graduates coming out of such institutions and not to indulge in corruption. Besides, faculty is also not of good quality. It has become heaven for petty businessmen, shopkeepers are running such institutions and even getting the status of deemed University.

13. Preparing Frontline Health Professionals with five roles

The frontline health professionals will have five principal roles to play:

Care-givers

Besides giving individual treatment. Frontline doctors must take into account the total (physical, mental and social) needs of the patient. They must ensure that a full range of treatment—curative, preventive or rehabilitative—will be dispensed in ways that are complementary, integrated and continuous. And they must ensure that the treatment is of the highest quality.

Decision-makers

In a climate of transparency the frontline doctor will have to take decisions that can be justified in terms of efficacy and cost. From all the possible ways of treating a given health condition, the one that seems most appropriate in the given situation must be chosen. As regards expenditure, the limited resources available for health must be shared out fairly to the benefit of every individual in the community.

Communicators

Lifestyle aspects such as a balanced diet, safety measures at work, type of leisure pursuits, respect for the environment and so on all have a determining influence on health. The involvement of the individual in protecting and restoring his or her own health is therefore vital, since exposure to a health risk is largely determined by one's behaviour. The doctors of tomorrow must be excellent communicators in order to persuade individuals, families and the communities in their charge to adopt healthy lifestyles and become partners in the health effort.

Community leaders

The needs and problems of the whole community in a suburb or a district must not be forgotten. By understanding the determinants of health inherent in the physical and social environment and by appreciating the breadth of each problem or health risk, the frontline doctor will not simply be treating individuals who seek help but will also take a positive interest in community health activities which will benefit large numbers of people.

Managers

To carry out all these functions, it will be essential for the frontline doctors to acquire managerial skills. This will enable them to initiate exchanges of information in order to make better decisions, and to work within a multidisciplinary team in close association with other partners for health and social development. Both old and new methods of dispensing care will have to be integrated with the totality of health and social services, whether destined for the individual or for the community.

The ideal frontline doctor of the future might be described as "the five-star doctor" someone who is equal in excellence to a five-star hotel or restaurant, but is accessible to everyone from the richest to the poorest. The skills of the doctors of tomorrow will serve the needs of all health systems and services; these abilities will be desirable to a certain degree in health personnel at every level. Far from being a dream, these goals and skills must be seen as imperative for our doctors of tomorrow.[24]

Faculty Development

(a) Trustworthiness of Medical Professors

Medical professors are the architects and builders of students behaviour using a standard program. They are also the curricular developers and thus have a pivotal role in shaping the future medicos. Charka Samhita lays down that the teacher should be one "whose doubts have been all cleared in respect of medical scriptures-possessed of experience-clever in the practice of his profession. Conversant with nature his knowledge of medical science supplemented with a knowledge of other branches of study—without malice—of a peaceful disposition—capable of bearing privation and pain-well affected towards disciples and prone to teach them-capable of communicating his ideas, etc." (Chaudhary, 1994).

(b) Training to Faculty to keep them abreast of latest development

Selecting the "right" trainer may not be always possible but improving them by periodic training program is feasible. An "effective" teacher will be one who is "competent" (has knowledge and skill) and is a "performer" (can use knowledge and skill in a classroom) to complete "teacher goal", MCI formulated its recommendations in 1981 and declared that the recommendation were oriented towards training students to undertake the responsibilities of a physician of first contact. But while depicting the situation analysis, draft "Medical Education Policy", in 1993 laments that "Advancements in medical education both in quantity and quality have not resulted in parallel achievements in the field of health care. The steps to be taken were: (a) clear delineation of goals and objectives of education, (b) Adjustment in the course structure, (c) Updating course content, (d) Rationalizing assessment strategy, (e) Emphasis on structured and skill-oriented internship (Kacker and Adkoi, 1993), and (f) The President, MCI while concluding his foreword to the document embodying the revised curriculum adopted by the council rightly mentioned that this curriculum can only be successfully implemented through appropriately oriented and properly equipped teachers. Faculty should promote values of administering medicine and service to society among medical students.[25] They should be told not to exploit poor people. Medical profession is a service and not a business.

(c) Management of Medical Students

When a medical student becomes a member of a health care team or is in a rotation where he or she is expected to participate in the delivery of health care, the supervisor and/or most responsible physician must provide appropriate supervision. This includes:

Assessing the student's level of expertise through direct observation, and ensuring ongoing evaluation to determine the medical student's clinical competence and educational requirements; authorization that the medical student to whom they are delegating has the appropriate knowledge, skills and judgment to perform the delegated act such that the patient is not put in jeopardy interaction regularly with the medical students to discuss his or her assessment, management and documentation of patient care Guided by the principles of level responsibility, students may carry out controlled acts, under direct or remote supervision, depending on their level of competence.

Criticism and countersigning documentation by a medical student of a patient's history, physical examination and diagnosis, within a fixed time period, as well as progress notes Catchword all orders concerning investigation or treatment of a patient, written under the supervision or direction of a physician, prescriptions, telephone or other transmitted order of a physician may be transcribed by the medical student, but must be countersigned at a later date.

Medical colleges must be compensated that, in therapeutic research, the foreseeable risks will not outweigh the potential benefits to the patients. The development of treatment and furthering of knowledge should never take precedence over the patient best interest.

In non-therapeutic research, you must keep the foreseeable risks to participate as low as possible. In addition the potential benefits from the development of treatment and furthering of knowledge must far outweigh any such risks.

(d) Selection of teachers should be not only be based on academic merit and professional experience, but also on social/community perspective and aptitude. Commitment to the profession should be emphasized. He/she should be a good motivator and facilitator to the student learning. Qualities such as ability to motivate and leadership must be part of the criteria for selection. Methods to assess these qualities have to be identified.

- Soon after the appointment of a teacher, he/she should be oriented to the vision and mission of the institution. Orientation or induction courses should be organized in the field of educational science and technology (including problem-based learning and examination, and assessment methods). He/she must provide quality training to the students, which is socially relevant to the community. He/she must actively participate in research, which is relevant and beneficial to the society.
- He/she must attend continuing education programmes and conferences for individual professional enrichment. Must be encouraged to take social/community oriented activities.
- He/she should not forget the obligation towards collective development of the department and the institution.
- A system of assessment of teachers by students, peer group and the head of the department, should be developed. Needless to say one must be prepared for self-evaluation also. Such assessments should be considered for promotion, etc. The services of teachers who show initiative and innovation must be recognized.
- Private practices should not come in the way of their professional obligation to the students, department institution and the patient.[26]

The process of becoming a doctor and a member of the medical profession is a social one. Professional, socialization requires a medical curriculum, which would include training in communication skill, medical ethics, health economics, and consumer right besides clinical skills and subject knowledge (Bunyan, P.S., 2000). The Medical Education Units should pay attention to the development of this collateral curriculum. It should plan a curriculum for "Tomorrow's Doctors" where "core and options" curricula are exemplified. Communication, patient autonomy and doctor-patient relationship must underpin the whole educational process (Jolly and Rees, 1998). In one of the SEARO publication (1998) Dr. Myatu had mentioned that if doctors are to remain relevant to the changing needs of the society they have to shape their roles within the context of total human development" (Sharma, 1994). For M-E-T to gel there is a need to include an educationist and human resource development manager as a part of the team (Joglekar and Bunyan, 1998).

Proposition for Improvement of Medical Education

Pedagogues Development

Professors need to be trained in framing objectives, selecting appropriate teaching-learning methods and media, and proper evaluation methodologies. To improve the quality of teaching, staff-development programs should be incorporated.

Medical Edification

This could be in the form of investigation driven system in various aspects of medical education (Consortium of Medical Institutions, 1994).

Continuing Medical Education

Technological elevation and knowledge explosion are advancing at jet pace. To keep up with the latest, the medical methodologist must be updating their knowledge at regular intervals. The need for quality care is being sought after by the society. Gone are the days of 'quantity' care.

Policy Outgrowth

This should be a joint venture between teachers and policy-makers. It should be based on economics, infrastructure and requirement of the country.

System of Evaluation

Uniform revision in the system of assessment needs to be done correlating with the objectives laid down (Mehta *et al.*, 1996).

Communication Padlock

With other institutions both in India and abroad.

Instructional Arrangement

Medical Education Technology Unit should take up the responsibility of providing guidelines to modify curriculum and implement the changes effectively. Today, in the world of knowledge explosion, emphasis should be on the processes for retrieval of information and its appropriate use. One needs to use criterion referenced evaluation to find out whether the graduate is competent to serve the needs of society. Teachers should be taught to evaluate objectively, reliably and without loosing the insight for relevance. In conclusion, we would like to say that the technological progression and knowledge explosion in medical science and pedagogy has necessitated the need for training medical teachers. For a teacher to be conversant with the latest trends he has to keep upgrading himself at frequent intervals and continue a lifelong saga. "Men are men before they are lawyers, physicians or manufacturers, and if you make them capable and sensible men, they will make themselves capable lawyers and physicians."[27]

- The students should be socially oriented with emphasis on Primary Health Care Approach.
- The public health concept, which has lot of relevance on the health of the community, has to be revived.
- The students should have an exposure to the management aspects of health care delivery system.
- Students should have an opportunity to learn through alternate parallel tracks.

- Curriculum should be reviewed periodically depending on the changing needs.

Suggestions

Public Health Administrative capability is sine qua non for the success of any programme. It is a major and crucial factor in the success or failure of development programmes. It is the scarcest of all resources in the developing world. The general administrator is fit only for the maintenance of law and order and he is not suitably equipped to deal with the problems of development and welfare economics.

According to K.N. Rao "Unlike advanced countries there is no pool of experienced and well informed leaders of thought available as potential leaders for ministerial positions which greatly handicaps their assuming policy-making and decision-making responsibilities in the Government. This results in over-dependence on the Secretaries who are non-technical general administrators.[28]

The technical experts must be given training in public health administration to make them competent in the art of health planning and administration.

The National Education Policy in Health Sciences was unanimously endorsed by the Central Council of Health and Family Welfare in 1993. The Policy emphasizes the vital role of health Planners and managers in the achievement of national health objectives, and states:

> "For the successful implementation of health programmes, health planner and health managers are extremely vital. Over the years, the area of health planning and health management has been gradually eroded. In India, it is universally accepted that the health programmes have not succeeded to the extent desired. The main reason has been identified as poor management. It is essential that the specialty of health management is recognized and appropriate steps are taken to develop it. All tertiary care teaching hospitals should offer education and training programmes so that adequate number of health planners/managers become available in the foreseeable future. Without proper health managers the task of achieving Health for All by 2000 A.D. had not been effective.

A basic doctor, to effectively deliver health care to the country must be an astute clinician, a good communicator, and a sound administrator, so as to effectively lead an ever expanding health team for a positive health action. Work and action domain of the doctor has crossed the boundaries to drugs and dispensaries and presently extends to a large extent to the families and to the communities—hence the need for the basic doctor to be a community physicians. Thus has emerged the need for developing a well designed and structured programmer of education for basic doctors with general applicability, departing from the present MBBS curriculum, and with emphasis on the primary health needs of the country. In addition, human values and medical ethics needs to be incorporated at a part of the curriculum. In essence, the National Education Policy in Health Sciences aims at, and strives towards, the production of the basic doctors equipped with adequate knowledge, requisite skills and appropriate behavioural attributes to meet the health needs of the country.[29]

Decentralization and Community Participation

For decentralisation of health care delivery services, planning and execution from the local level is crucial. The recent 73rd and 74th Constitutional Amendments and revitalization of the Panchayati Raj Institutions provide an unique opportunity for evolving a more decentralised health structure and planning health programmes based on needs of people at grassroot level. It is suggested that the Government should only play a facilitating role of providing financial and technical inputs, framing a set of policy guidelines and programmes, allowing the Panchayati Raj structure at different levels to implement the programmes as per local needs in an integrated manner. This would help the Panchayats to take initiatives for rural development and horizontal integration of various programmes including health. By making suitable policy changes and with proper orientation and training, Panchyats would be able to supervise the quality of health and family welfare services directly along with ensuring integration of socio-economic development programmes with health promotion activities at local levels. At another level, it would also help in bridging the communication as well as functional gaps which exist between the community and the providers of health services leading to 'demystification' and 'decommercialisation' of health technology in the long run.

Medical Education and Public Health Orientation

The pattern of medical education guided by market economy has concentrated on biological causes of the diseases and curative actions based on hospital care, drugs, surgery, etc. without any recognition of the socio-economic and environmental status of the population. Health problems in a country like ours can not be solved only through marketing medical therapy and interventions with a curative bias by neglecting the preventive, promotive, environmental health and the community need orientation. The lack of a holistic and community-based approach to disease control over the years has further led to over emphasis on 'quantity', rather than 'quality' of health care resulting in erosion of trust on the quality of health care services provided by the public sector and increasing dependence of the population on the private sector. Thus, during the past five decades, despite the quantitative growth in terms of hospitals, health centres, health manpower, infrastructural support services and number of Health and Family Welfare programmes, the public health situation has remained a cause of great concern as reflected in the mortality, morbidity, health status, urban-rural differentials and health seeking behaviour patterns of the population. This calls for re-orientation and reorganisation of our medical and health education system with emphasis on "holistic" and "community based" health care as well as effective and efficient administration and management of health care delivery services. Keeping in view the national needs, priorities and goals for health for all, it is essential to upgrade the managerial, technological and professional skills of health manpower through appropriate changes in the course curriculums of medical and health education institutions at different levels with greater emphasis on epidemiology, computer and management disciplines.[30]

At the same time, without minimizing the importance of scientific progress, we have to recognize that, as far as public health in the past few decades is concerned, medical interventions (apart from vaccinations) have not been the chief contributors to the improvements in health registered in the industrialized countries. Where fault lies? The problem has been that the developments in science and technology must accompany with corresponding health education to individual, community, patients, etc. The dramatic decrease in heart disease recorded in certain developed countries has been due essentially to a change in dietary habits and lifestyles created through constant health education. Similarly. some counties have shown a marked drop in frequency of lung cancer because of a reduction in smoking due to educating the smokers about the ill-effects of smoking. On the other hand, unfortunately, the threat posed by other abuses, such as drug taking and alcoholism continues unabated.

These considerations underlie efforts all over the world to strengthen activities aimed at curbing harmful habits and encouraging healthier lifestyles through well laid out health education system. These steps must be taken in collaboration with the powerful media networks, with educators and schools, with professional and local organisations, and with trade unions.

"Most of the world's major health problems and premature deaths are preventable through changes in human behaviour, and at low cost," WHO former Director-General, Dr. Hiroshi Nakajima, declared recently. Viewed in its social and cultural dimension, health is seen to be not a gift that comes automatically, nor a consumer product that can be bought, but the result of the conscious education aimed at each human being, each family, each community.

What must be done today is to educate everyone with the will to be healthy. This involves educating peoples the true meaning of health in the lives of individuals and nations, and encouraging everyone to find in their environment the motivation and the means to sustain their wish to be healthy.

To want to be in good health, to give this capital importance in life, to be able to tell oneself resolutely "health comes first"—these are ideas that can be acquired and develop. They are of inestimable value, because they make possible a dialogue between individuals and the institutions, which must serve them, a dialogue through which both can make progress.

John Bland in his article, "Health Manpower Development—Basic Skills" in the *World Health*, July 1976 observed that Medical education is a costly and long-drawn out process, so that cost becomes a paramount factor to be considered when a comparatively poor country plans to set-up a medical school. The outlay involved in training a medical graduate can be estimated by multiplying the annual expenditure on him by the number of years four to six—that his course will last, and then taking into account investments wasted on students who "drop out" before graduating. Using this formula, a study some years ago showed that if cost Nigeria US $ 33,600 and Uganda $ 26,000 to train a medical graduate. The size of these figure may be seen even more clearly when they are compared with the per capita annual income of the two countries at that time, $ 68 and $ 83 respectively.

Medical schools in the Regions with WHO collaboration have been strengthening and reorienting the medical education system to achieve a closer quantitative balance and systemic relevance to their manpower development programmes. The trends are for greater community orientation of the curricula, introduction of innovative strategies such as problem based learning and strengthening of educational management processes. Experimenting with objectively-structured clinical and practical examinations and the introduction of enquiry-driven methods for accelerating changes in medical education are being promoted. Problem-based learning programmes have been established in some medical schools in India, Indonesia, Myanmar, Nepal and Thailand.

CONCLUSION

A sound health manpower policy is the main requirement for the development of any functionally effective health care system. Most of the countries in the developing world have never formulated or implemented such a policy.

> "The most crucial factor for the improvement of the world health situation . . . . Is undoubtedly the development of health manpower that is probably attuned to the health problems of the people and suitably trained to respond to health programme and service needs."

We must find the method to achieve greater productivity, efficiency and cost-effectiveness in health manpower utilization. No society, especially the developing, can long justify investing years of education and training in individuals who later on perform rudimentary duties that could be achieved satisfactorily by people trained in half that time. The critical decisions in health manpower planning concern the kinds of personnel required, the type and adequacy of education and training and financial resources necessary to produce them, their relationship to each other in the health team, and where and how they would practice.

A basic doctor, to effectively deliver health care to the country must be an astute clinician, a good communicator, and a sound administrator, so as to effectively lead an ever expanding health team for a positive health action. Work and action domain of the doctor has crossed the boundaries to drugs and dispensaries and presently extends to a large extent to the families and to the communities hence the need for the basic doctor to be a community physician. Thus, has emerged the need for developing a well designed and structured programme of education for basic doctors with general applicability departing from the present MBBS curriculum, and with emphasis on the primary health needs of the country. In addition, human values and medical ethics need to be incorporated as a part of the curriculum. In essence, the National Education Policy in Health Sciences aims at, and strives towards, the production of basic doctors equipped with adequate knowledge, requisite skills and appropriate behavioural "attributes to meet the health needs of the country'. All the health experts from top to bottom including auxiliary health services need be taught as to how preventive health services through health education can be developed to avoid opening of more and more hospitals; and assuring an effective and efficient health services.

We may sum up with the following suggestions:

1. Community medicine must be given top priority in the syllabi of Medical Education as an independent subject which must be taught with all seriousness.
2. Medical Education must teach the doctors to give priority to preventive health while treating the patients.
3. The curriculum should reflect emphasis on preventive health through lifestyle changes.
4. The Government should come out with some legislation on Hospitals which may check fleecing the customers. This may be taught to doctors.
5. Consumer forums must give exemplary punishments to hospitals and individuals indulging in malpractices.
6. The medical education must teach the medical students to be punctual and perform their duties sincerely. This should be followed by Government to ensure compliance.

Notes and References

1. Farokh Erach Udwadia, "Humanity: The Core of Doctor-Patient Relationship", *University News*, Vol. 42, No. 34, Aug. 23-29, 2004, p. 15.
2. WHO: SEARO: The Work of WHO, July 2006-30 June, 2007, pp. 69-70.
3. Farokh Erach Udwadia, "Humanity: The Core of Doctor-Patient Relationship", *University News*,Vol. 42, No. 34, Aug. 23-29, 2004, p. 15.
4. National Health Policy, 1983.
5. National Health Policy, 2002, Para 2.8 and 2.9.

6. Public Health in India's Five Decades, 50th Anniversary of India' Independence (Vol. I), p. 5.
7. *WHO Chronicle*, 31, 123-26 (1977), "Health Challenges For J.K. Nath (Editor), 1978-83.
8. J. Gallagher: "Educational Planning and Health", in *WHO Chronicle*, 30: 70-71, (1976).
9. Lok Sabha Secretariat: 102nd Report, Estimates Committee, (Fifth Lok Sabha), p.4
10. Karnataka Towards Equity, Quality and Integrity in Health, Final Report, Family Welfare, Government of Karnataka, April 2001, p. 247.
11. Karnataka Towards Equity, Quality and Integrity in Health, Final Report of The Task Force on Health and Family Welfare, Government of Karnataka, April 2001, p. 248.
12. WHO, Regional Office for South-East Asia, New Delhi, 1997, p. 32
13. *Ibid.*, p. 17.
14. *Ibid.*, p. 16.
15. A. Rajasekaran, "Radical Changes Required in Medical Education", *University News*, Vo. 44, No. 23, June 05, 2006, p. 15
16. *Ibid.*, p. 15.
17. Vijay Pithadia and Vandana Parmar, "Appraisal of Medical Education in India, *University News*, Vol. 44, No. 44, Oct. 30, 2006, pp. 11-12.
18. Text on Address by Dr. H. Mahler, to the Thirteenth Session of Regional Committee of South-East Asia.
19. Geneva Declaration.
20. I Swear by Apollo by Christian Videma, *World Health*, July 1979, p. 28.
21. J.S. Niki, Medical Ethics, *World Health*, July 1979.
22. S.L. Goel, Public Health Administration, Sterling Publishers Pvt. Ltd., pp. 311-12.
23. Vijay Pithadia, "Appraisal of Medical Education in India", *University News*, 44 (44), Oct. 30-Nov. 2006, p. 11.
24. Charles Boelen, "Frontline Doctors of Tomorrow", *World Health*, 47th year, No. 5, Sept.-Oct. 1994, p. 5.
25. Vijay Pithadia, "Appraisal of Medical Education in India", *University News*, 44 (44), Oct. 30-Nov. 2006, p. 11.
26. Final Report of the Task Force on Health and Family Welfare, Government of Karnataka, April 2001, p. 248.
27. Vijay Pithadia, "Appraisal of Medical Education in India", *University News*, 44 (44), Oct. 30-Nov. 2006, p. 13.
28. Merle Fainsod, "The structure of Development Administration", in Irving Swerdlow, (ed.) Development Administration: Concepts and Problems, Syracuse, N.Y. Syracuse University Press, 1963, p. 1.
29. Public Health in India's Five Decades, 50th Anniversary of India's Independence, p. 6.
30. Public Health in India Five Decades, 50th Anniversary of India's Independence, p. 26.

APPENDIX 15.1

Medical Education

The quality the quantity, distribution and availability of human resources for the health sector in India at present need to be improved substantially to deliver care-driven, rural oriented and equitable health services. Over the years, health-related education and training has become more urban oriented, doctor-centric and technology-driven. The environment of medical education needs to be both nationally sensitive and globally competitive. To realize these objectives, our medical education system needs radical reforms. The National Knowledge Commission (NKC) therefore considered it imperative to carry out a comprehensive appraisal of the system. For this purpose, Working Group was constituted which included some of the most distinguished members of the medical profession in India, chaired by Dr. Sneha Bhargava, former Director, AIIMS. Based on the inputs provided by the Working Group and further consultations with concerned stakeholder, NKC recommended the following:

1. Regulation and Accreditation

Regulation

At present medical education in India is regulated by the Medical Council of India (MCI). This system of regulation is neither adequate nor appropriate to meet the needs of the profession. Therefore, in conformity with NKC recommendations on Higher Education, a Standing Committee within the structure of the Independent Regulatory Authority for Higher Education (IRAHE) may be constituted. The primary function of the Standing Committee will be to ensure that medical practice and teaching are updated and revised regularly and minimum quality standards are maintained. The members of the Standing Committee would include faculty from recognized Universities, practising physicians, members of Civil Society, students and a director from autonomous institutions representing educators. The Chairman and the members of the Standing Committee would be accountable to IRAHE. The Standing Committee would look into manpower planning and development based on disease-profile, doctor-population ratio and skill-mix ratio.

Professional Councils

The Indian Medical Council Act should be amended such that MCI functions only as a professional association, with powers to conduct nationwide examinations, and to provide licenses for those who wish to join the profession. Similar changes are needed for all the other Councils viz. Nursing Council, Pharmacy Council, Dental Council and Rehabilitation Council.

Accreditation

IRAHE should be empowered to license suitable agencies for accreditation. Accreditation agencies could award different degrees of accreditation, such as "Full" "Provisional" or "On Probation" and have the power to de-recognize. Institutions would have to ensure transparency in their admission processes, able and responsible faculties, a multidisciplinary academic learning environment, transparency in assessment of students and close linkages with regional health care and delivery systems, in order to be accredited.

Admission

Policies of admission and fee structure of private colleges have to be related, not only to stop them from becoming sources of political and financial power but also to arrest falling Standards. There should be only one All India Common Entrance Test for all students who would like to get admission to Self-Financing Medical Colleges. Since the CBSE conducted examination for the 15% All India quota in Government Medical Colleges is taken by a very large number of students, this would appear to be the ideal examination whose ambit can be expanded. All self-financing Medical Colleges should announce their fees in their prospectus so that students can make their choice for admission. Information Technology should be used to increase transparency and efficiency in the admission, examination, administration, teaching, content delivery and other related processes.

2. Quality

Curriculum

All institutions must constitute Curriculum Committee that plan curricula and instructional methods, which are regularly updated. The structure and composition of the curriculum must describe the content, scope and sequencing of the courses, including the balance been core and optional courses. Integration of ICT in the learning process is essential. Incorporating new skills like management, disciplines like health economics and frontier areas like bioinformatics should be considered.

Standards test

An independent and standardized National Exit Examination at the end of 4½ of study, is Essential to conduct a national level assessment of skills and knowledge. The National Exit Examination could be conducted immediately after the University examination, and would also serve as a postgraduate entrance exam.

Internship Assessment

The internship year must be assessed to ensure skill development. The current practice of students continuing to study in the internship year without going to clinics needs to be addressed. There must be compulsory rotation from the teaching hospital to the community and district hospital during the internship period. Duration of the term in the district hospital should be six months, in the Community Health Centre three months and in the intern care hospital the remaining three months. Each interim should be assigned a "mentor" at the district hospital and the credits should be based on the assessment by the mentor. The entrance to postgraduate programmes should be based on a summation of the pre- and post-internship examinations.

Continuing Education

There is a need to revamp Continuing Medical Education (CME) based on distance learning. All professionals should be required to undergo a re- certification process every five years, which can be evaluated by credits earned through CME. ICT can be used extensively to provide CME at the convenience of the learner.

3. Faculty Development

Teaching

Attracting and retaining quality faculty should be accorded top priority. Measures such as opportunities to attend international conferences regularly, sabbaticals, dual appointments, rewarding research fast-track promotions, and dissociating remuneration from government pay scales should be explored. All institutions must clearly lay down exact definitions of what constitutes conflict of interest for faculty members in public medical colleges, who have a private practice in addition to their official duties, and receive a full time teacher's salary. Those who flout these regulations should be penalized.

Research

With a view to encouraging research in medicine, a Mentored Medical Student Research Programme should be set-up as a catalyst to introduce medical students to a potential career in patient-oriented/ community-oriented research including interdisciplinary research. Two points of entry into PhD programmes should be considered: one after MBBS and another after MD depending on the student's interest. The government should facilitate setting up of research centres in medical colleges. Validating Indian Systems of Medicine using bio-sciences tools should form an integral component of the research effort.

Training

Five Regional Centres for teacher training/faculty Development should be set up so that teachers from the outlying regions an be sent to these centers periodically for up gradation of their teaching skills.

4. Post-graduate Education

General Physicians

The medical profession needs to be structured little a pyramid with the base made up of general physicians. At present there is link if any space for such doctors in post-graduate courses. Therefore, we suggest that adequate representation should be given to general physicians while carrying out expansion of' post-graduate seats such that 50% seats are reserved for general physicians. New streams for post-graduation should be looked at based on needs.

Admissions

Admission to post-graduate courses should be done on the basis of credits received in the National Exit Examination and pre and post-internship clinically oriented exams after internship. There is a need to reserve post-graduate seats (up to 20% of total available seats) for graduates who have worked in rural areas for at least three years.

5. Regional Balance

Location Priorities

The number of medical colleges in relation to population in some states is much higher than in other states. The Central Government should aid new colleges in these states to address this regional disparity. For instance, north-eastern states require urgent attention in this context. The Central Government can develop a list of priority sites for establishing new colleges where the impact of new clinical facilities would benefit the surrounding rural population.

Role Models

Further at least one institution should be identified in each State that can serve as a centre of excellence and role model for the other institutions of the state. These institutions should have State-of-the art infrastructural equipment such as research laboratories, teacher training facilities, and libraries as well as talented faculty of adequate strength to act as a common resource and also to serve as a benchmark of excellence.

Medical education cannot be stand alone. It requires support in the form of trained nurses, pharmacists. Paramedic workers, it must also serve the essential purpose of delivering health care to the people. Therefore, NKC also set out some recommendations on education for supporting services and public health.

6. Education for Support Services

Nursing

There is a need to create additional capacity for training nursing staff. In addition, every district hospital should have attached to it a nursing school, which offers diploma in nursing specifically to operate primary health centres as nurse practitioners. A career growth pathway should be ensured for nurses after a specific period of primary health care service. For graduate nurses in city hospitals, specialized courses for family nurse practitioners, nurse anesthetists and in areas of tertiary care are recommended.

Pharmacy

Pharmacy education should be popularized and the number of seats for pharmacy education should be increased substantially. Gradual phasing out of untrained pharmacists should be considered.

Paramedics

The role of Paramedic workers should be expanded. A Paramedical Council needs to be immediately established, which would prepare training programmes for multi-skill and specialty technicians and oversee their delivery and quality. Paramedics, such as compounders, dressers, and laboratory technicians can also perform public health functions, such as health education, providing immunization, and first aid. Such a health worker could be trained through vocational training at the higher secondary level followed by a one year diploma. Career paths should be built into their service in order to retain them because international demand is high.

7. Public Health

Education

A three tiered structure consisting of a one year diploma course, a three year B.Sc. course and three year Master's course may be introduced. These programmes can be attached to departments of Community Medicine in all medical colleges for providing hands on training. All universities, all district hospitals and the Public Health Foundation of India can run them.

ASHA

The role of Accredited Social Health Activists (AHSA) needs to be re-conceptualized within this framework, and ASHA must be viewed as an accessible and effective health worker. The training period of the ASHA needs to be lengthened from its current duration. Steps should be taken to review the system of remuneration and improve the working conditions of the ASHA workers.

16

CHAPTER

Management by Objectives in Hospitals (MBO)

"MBO (Management by Objectives) is a system wherein the superior and the subordinate managers of Hospitals jointly define its common goals, define each individuals major areas of responsibility in terms of the results expected of him and use of these measures as guides for operating the units and assessing the contribution of each of its members."

—*George Odiorne*

Belatedly, service institutions are becoming an important segment of our societal landscape today. Broadly speaking, service institutions subsume educational institutions like schools and universities, research institutes, public utilities and hospitals, etc. Just how well we manage our service institutions today will not only determine the quality of life(QOL) our country men enjoy today but it would also largely influence , the mental and physical health of our posterity. Since the advent of Industrial Revolution which brought in its train a radical shift in our work pattern the human society has made rapid strides and has undergone mega-changes and our country in particular since it liberated itself from the foreign yoke and started its "Tryst with destiny" under the able leadership of Jawaharlal Nehru has again renewed its promise to embark on modernisation quality for the 21st Century when poverty, unemployment, illiteracy, squalar and diseases will be considerably reduced if not completely eliminated.

Management-by-objectives (MBO) is fast becoming one of the most influential yardsticks of contemporary management. The hospital administrators and professionals are becoming increasingly concerned with the quality of services their organisations are rendering. Today, there is a greater awareness and desire to achieve their missions effectively and this

CHART 16.1

MBO

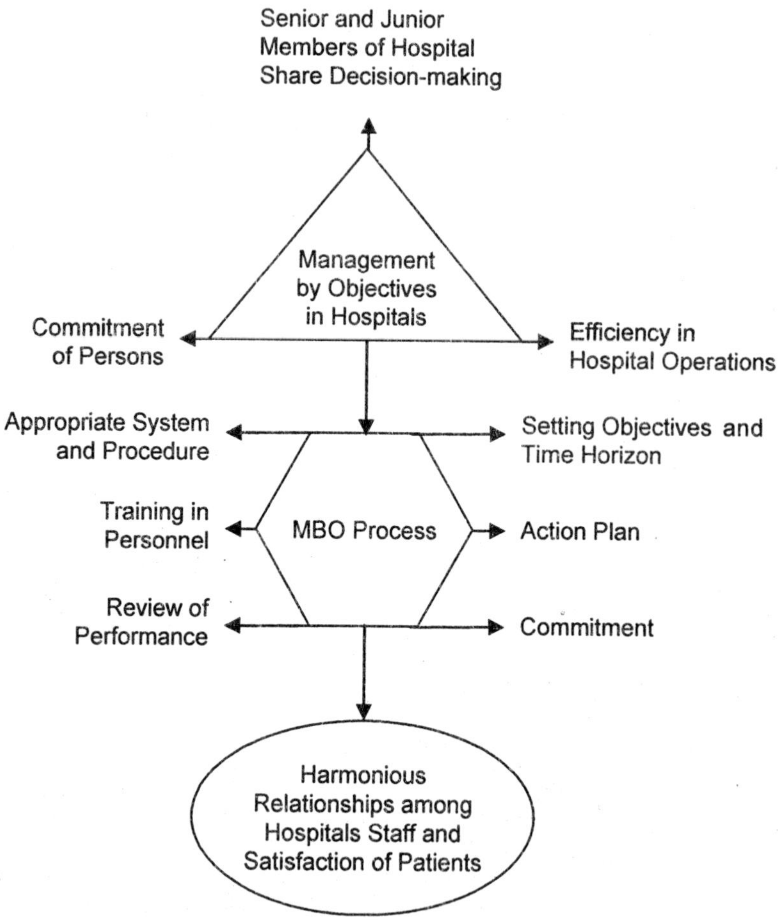

has provoked administrators to look over and beyond hospitals and other non-profit hospitals for getting familiar with new managerial ideas that could enable them to focus their attention on objectives and integrate efforts towards their attainment. A couple of decades ago few business enterprises in the world and only a microscopic minority of non-profit organisations were found to be applying MBO. Ever since the concept was developed in mid-fifties it has treaded a long distance and has inched from its initial, fledgling stage of improving the performance of the individual manager to organisational effectiveness. It has broken all geographical barriers and has been widely used not only in U.S.A., Canada, Japan but almost all over the globe. After having witnessed its success in business enterprises, the non-profit sector like hospitals has begun to adopt MBO at a rather startling pace.

Need for MBO in Hospitals

The need for setting objectives in hospitals hardly needs an emphasis. Actually, hospitals particularly in a developing country like India which is caught in a poverty syndrome of inefficiency is a very fertile area for its adoption. A broad survey of most of the hospitals in India shows that a majority of personnel working in hospitals are not clear about their duties and responsibilities resulting in poor performance. If hospitals are to be managed effectively and put on an even keel, these urgently need a system by which the objectives are properly set, prioritisation settled, responsibility for their achievement fixed, a thorough follow-up and a viable feedback system that has the blessings of the top man.[1]

Hospitals are today becoming inefficient causing inconvenience to patients and loss of prestige and reputation of hospitals both in private and Government sector. Even hundreds of cases are lying in courts for many issues of the hospital. In addition, complaints are being lodged by patients against hospitals. These and other problems can be lessened through MBO approach. Since the top leadership does not understand MBO approach, and even if understands it, does not follow resulting in many problems. MBO approach in hospitals can solve many of the existing and emerging problems. Before we discuss the steps to be undertaken for this approach to be used in hospitals, let us discuss the meaning of MBO.

Meaning

MBO is an approach which directs its main attention on objectives to improve administrative efficiency and effectiveness. Its emphasis is on results rather than activities.

Peter Drucker defines the Philosophy of MBO thus: "What the Business enterprise needs is a principle of management that will give full scope to individual strength and responsibility, and at the same time give common direction of vision and effort, establish teamwork and harmonize the goal of the individual with the common weal. . . . The only principle that can do this is management by objectives and self-control. It makes the common weal the aim of every manager. It substitutes control from outside by control from within. It motivates the manager to action, not because somebody tells him to do something or takes him into doing it, but because the objective needs of his task demand it He acts because somebody wants him to but because he himself decides that he has to-He acts, in other words, as a free man."

According to George Odiorne, "MBO (Management By Objectives) is a system wherein the superior and the subordinate managers of an organisation jointly define its common goals, define each individual's major areas of responsibility in terms of the results expected of him and use these measures as guides for operating the unit and assessing the contribution of each of its members."[2]

Prof. Reddin says that MBO is "the establishment of effectiveness areas and effectiveness standards for managerial positions and the periodic conversion of these into measurable time bound objectives linked vertically and horizontally with future planning."[3]

From these definitions it is clear that MBO is an approach which can help us in coinciding the objectives of the organisation and the individuals working in it and their ultimate achievement. It brings commitment on the part of personnel resulting in ultimate organisational efficiency.

Humble considers MBO as "a dynamic system which seeks to integrate the company's need to clarify and achieve its profit and growth goals with the manager's need to contribute and develop himself." In his view, MBO is a demanding and rewarding style of managing a business[4] Dale D. McConkey has defined it "as an approach to management planning and evaluation in which specific target for a year or some other length of time are established for each manager on the basis of result which each must achieve, if the overall objectives of the company are to be realized. At the end of the period, the actual results achieved are measured against the original goals, that is against the expected results which each manager knows, he is responsible for achieving."

In spite of these definitions, still there is no clarification about its meaning. Walter S. Wikstrom wrote, "Management by Objectives has become an all-purpose term, meaning almost anything one chooses to have it meaning."[5] More recently, Dale D. McConkey noted that no data on the number of organisations using MBO exist, primarily because of the "uncertainty concerning what MBO is."[6]

J. Philip has enlisted the following characteristics of MBO system:

- Some form of corporate or unit plan by which the objectives are laid down;
- Measurable and time-bound objectives for each managerial position;
- Objectives for each position are established by the job-holder and the boss together;
- Mutually agree job improvement plans to facilitate the accomplishments of objectives;
- Periodic reviews and updating, whereas necessary of the mutually agreed objectives by the boss and the subordinates together;
- Such mutually agreed objectives form the basis of performance evaluation;
- Sharp definition of responsibilities and authorities for positions, which brings in clarity in the organisations; and
- Aligning and linking of objectives up, down and across.

Ingredients of MBO

We mention here some essential ingredients required for the success of MBO:

(a) Active participation and involvement of the subordinates in Planning, implementation and evaluation.
(b) Emphasis on team spirit and team approach.
(c) Open Communication among the members of the Organisation irrespective of their status.
(d) Increased skill in inter-personal communication.
(e) Personal counseling and guidance.

MBO PROCESS

1. Setting Objectives

The first important thing in this direction is to determine key result areas expected from Hospital management. After establishing Key Result areas, the next task is to set objectives for all department participating in Hospital Management. The aim of setting objectives in specific terms at every echelon is to help employees in understanding as to what is expected to be done by them. This makes the individuals precise in their task. However, it must be kept in mind that objectives should be set jointly by superiors and the subordinates of Hospital. The superiors in Hospitals need to inject in them a spirit of raising their sights towards higher objectives through counseling and thus leading them from a diffidence to confidence.

Stephen J. Caroll, Jr. and Henry, H. Tosi Jr. in their book, Management by Objectives (1973, p. 72) have slightly spelled out the parameters of sound objectives. To quote them:

> In order to be sound, the objectives of each Hospital or a unit of an hospital must be: (1) clear, concise and unambiguous, (2) accurate in terms of the true end state or condition sought, (3) consistent with policies, procedures and plans as they apply to the unit, (4) within the competence of the man or represent a reasonable learning and development experience for him, and (5) interesting, motivating and or challenging whenever possible.

People work well together when they agree with one another. To fulfil the objectives of an hospitals those who work for the hospital should know what its objectives are. People who do not know what these objectives are may waste much of their efforts on activities that do not bring the objectives any nearer to achievement. People who are opposed to the objectives may obstruct the work of the hospitals. It is very difficult, if not, impossible, for real progress to be made without the active participation of all the members.

2. Action Planning

In order to translate the objectives into practice, there is a need to design the action planning which is of great significance in activities like

Hospital management as here action planning is of great significance. This would mean to decide about right strategies, allocation of finances and scheduling.

3. Commitment in the Ideology of the Programme

All the members of a hospitals must share the rationale and philosophy of the programme to be implemented, i.e. service to disease affected people. This would generate loyalty and commitment among them.

4. Review of Performance

One of the important ingredients of MBO is a periodic review of performance. Both the superiors and the subordinates meet periodically to review progress towards these objectives. These reviews help them in identifying the problems that exist and how these can be resolved. If need be, objectives may be revamped and revised for the ensuing review period. In fact, these reviews are "future-oriented" and focus is on corrective action and planning. This is the operation of the self-control in the MBO process.[7] To be fair and meaningful, such reviews should be based on measurable performance rather than on some subjective criteria such as attitude or ability.[8] There is a need of quarterly review. Robert McNamara has listed five positive results of quarterly review:

1. It forces a dialogue between the boss and the managers, improving teamwork even between executives who may not like each other.
2. It raises the superiors awareness of praiseworthy performers who could become lost in a big organisation and brings deadwood into the open for accountability.
3. Managers walk away feeling that they are their own boss with individualized goals—"in charge" and not a boss's flankly or gofer.
4. Managers become more productive as self-motivation increases.
5. "I've never found a better way to stimulate fresh approaches to problem-solving or to generation of new ideas."

Lacocca does admit that the system is not infallible. It works well in situations like—where (a) fixed goals are to be met; (b) owner complaints are to be satisfied; (c) costs are either to be reduced or kept from increasing above a certain percentage, etc. The review is a far less definable concept in public relations, labour relations, or advertising.[9]

5. Time Horizon

Adaptability to change differ from organisation to organisation. Therefore, every organisation must decide the appropriate time for the introduction of MBO so that it can produce result. before introduction of MBO in any organisation, a good organisational climate is a sine-qua-non for the success of MBO.

6. Requisite Training to Personnel

Since, it is very difficult to change the human mind, therefore, there is a constant need to educate the personnel about the benefits of MBO to the personnel and ultimately to the organisation. We must, therefore, organize formal courses for them so that they can learn the art and science of MBO and can make use of it in practice

7. Appropriate Systems and procedures

The existing organisations using traditional and meticulous procedures and methods need change to accommodate the fructification of the new technique of MBO. All the procedures need to be simplified and should be based on mutual trust and confidence rather than on legal framework.

MBO IN PRACTICE

A large number of organisations in developed and developing countries are making use of this concept. There has been both the experiences—successes and failures. Where MBO has not been success, the fault lies with wrong introduction. MBO in India was introduced in the early seventies on the British pattern. About 100 companies are making use of this technique. Hindustan Copper Limited, a Public Sector Undertaking has introduced it with a success. In the private sector, Madura Coats, Bharat Bijlee, etc. have introduced it with a success.

However, in Public Administration, it has not been introduced since there are many problems which need solution. We must try experiments in Universities, Hospitals and other sectors to make the Public Administration result-oriented.

U.S.A.—Hospitals (Experiments)

A study of MBO in hospitals conducted by Luthans and Sellenin[10] revealed that 41 per cent of the hospitals surveyed were using MBO system and another 33 per cent had plans to start it in the near future. Further great majority of the respondents indicated that MBO had contributed in improving performance particularly in the areas of planning co-ordination, control and communications.

It may be useful to apprise ourselves with the sweet and sour experiences of an administrator who had applied MBO in some non-profit hospitals. Though his experiences with MBO span only over a period of three years, yet his findings are quite revealing for any hospital which is keen and determined to launch MBO for increasing its efficiency and effectiveness. He is of the opinion that on the balancing scale, the benefit which an organisation would derive by use of MBO would always outweigh the quantum of expenditure in terms of time and money and effort.[11]

1. "Regardless of the effort put forth, enthusiasm and utilisation of MBO is cyclic.
2. Only about 60 per cent of those that started the programme are still successfully using the approach. However, in light of factors such as background, personal limitations and other organisational circumstances, this percentage seems acceptable to us.
3. The greatest enemy of a MBO programme in a non-profit organisation is apathy. With the recent advent of "global budgeting . . . perhaps realistic incentive programmes will be devised in a way that successful MBO performances can be rewarded in more tangible terms."
4. Many projects that "should be done" are done because of MBO. Procrastination generally is the result of lack of commitment.
5. The contribution to communications both horizontally and vertically has been unreasonable.
6. Contribution of MBO to our budgeting process has been equally rewarding.
7. Since MBO is an essential ingredient of writing and executing a long-range plan, the programme will no doubt continue to prove invaluable, as we are currently in the primary stages of formulating such a plan.
8. On balance, the benefits we have gained far outweigh expenditure of time and money. Management by objectives is an interesting theory and a worthwhile practice.

The Indian Experience

The experience of a hospital in the state of Punjab in this respect are quite encouraging. It is a positive pointer to the future. The findings of a study by Drs. S.K. Sachar and C.M. Singh on Cost Efficient Health Care. "The Oswal Experiment" are:

> "It has elicited a commitment for performance, generated a sense of involvement and belonging and above all has helped to create a congenial work environment and foster 'espirit de corps'.[12]

BENEFITS OF MBO (See Chart 16.2)

In many hospitals, that every thing is decided at the top and the people at the lower levels of hierarchy never gets the chance to articulate either their perceptions or their apprehensions before their superiors. Ways of improving the working of the system can be suggested most realistically by people working at lower levels. Obviously a top

CHART 16.2

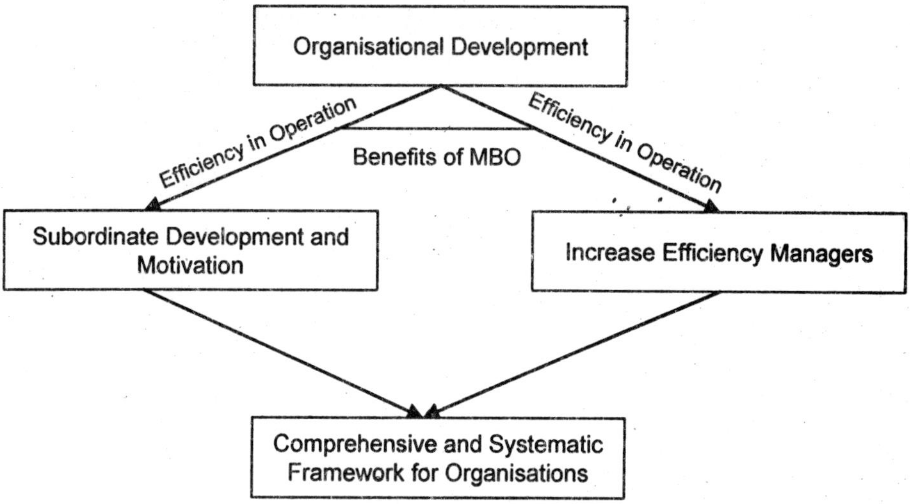

down organisation which thwarts self expression at these levels is bound to do badly because it fails to harness the knowledge, imagination and commitment of most of its personnel. It has been found that many a times, we come across subordinates whose comprehension, analytical ability and capacity to come up with solutions to new and complex problems was far superior than the higher ups. Thus, there is a need of MBO approach to pool knowledge, experience, ideas, and wisdom of all from top-down.

However, MBO plans work best where the persons involved in goal setting are able to have a clear perception and a correct understanding of co-relationship between organisation policies and their area of operations. It requires knowledge and harmony.

A. Organisational Development

Since MBO focuses on managerial efficiency, therefore, this sentiment spreads among all the members and thus each contribute to the development of the organisation. In this way, MBO, helps in ensuring that every employee's activity in the final analysis is aimed at attaining organisational goals. Besides, the gulf between the employees and the organisation narrows down leading to harmony and goodwill.

1. MBO improves effectiveness and increased profitability for the enterprise.
2. MBO ensures utilization of human resources.
3. MBO promote organisational changes to suit the present conditions.
4. It helps in improving structures, strategies and practices.
5. MBO makes planning more specific and purposeful

6. MBO promotes coordination and cooperation in the organisation.
7. MBO lays emphasis on delegation of authority.
8. MBO is not a complex system and is easily and clearly understood, and can be adopted and applied without much difficulty.
9. Voluntary commitments for performance by the employees in an organisation come forth as a result of MBO involvement.

B. Subordinate Development and Motivation

MBO gives greater role clarity and motivates them to hard work to achieve the objectives set by them. All persons in the organisation co-operate and enjoy the work. They take pride in the achievement of organisational goals. Subordinates become their own masters and thus enjoy autonomy and flexibility.

1. MBO enhances employee job satisfaction.
2. MBO ensures dignity to employees
3. It provides measurable objectives that the employee is expected to achieve.
4. MBO provides status and importance to subordinates.

C. Superiors remain relaxed and efficient

By introducing MBO not only the organisations benefit but individual managers too do gain to stand. Some of the possible benefits from the individual point of view are:

(a) There is a greater opportunity to make a personal contribution and to accept and carry out their responsibilities willingly and successfully.
(b) There is a less frustration as the individuals are aware of the Hospital objectives, what is expected of them (Time table of their goals) and what are the constraints on their authority?
(c) There is a better and more purposeful communication between him and his superior, peers and subordinates.
(d) There is a greater opportunity for personal growth.
(e) .It makes the evaluation process more equitable by focussing on specific achievements. It also lets subordinates know how well they are performing in the context of the organisational goals.
(f) It leads to more equitable material rewards and promotion plans as individual managers concentrate their efforts where they are most needed and likely to be rewarded. Moreover, individuals know that they will be evaluated, not on the basis of personal traits or superiors' bias but on how well they are hitting at the objectives they themselves have helped in conceiving.[13]

We may mention briefly the main advantages which can flow from the adoption of MBO approach in Organisations.

(a) Organisational efficiency.
(b) Determined and dedicated leadership.
(c) Better inter-personal relations and teamwork.
(d) Based on sound Organisational and Psychological Principles.
(e) Strengthens the performance appraisal system.
(f) Change in management styles.

Potentialities

To a reasonable extent, MBO has been successfully applied in all types of organisations—Business or non-business, the private and public sector, the government departments, trusts, large and small organisations in the developed and developing countries. Those include industrial organisations, educational and research institutions and various religious and hospital organisations.

However, it may be remembered that the MBO programme should not be introduced by any hospitals in a hurry. For ensuring its successful implementation, it must address itself a couple of questions and see that the answers are positive because only that will show its readiness for a launch. The questions are:[14]

1. Whether the hospitals has set clear goals, spotted out its priorities, set standards, determined performance measurement criteria and developed an "hospitals audit" of objectives to see its worth or not.
2. Whether MBO philosophy has permeated all the reaches in the hospitals hierarchy or not.[15]
3. Whether the organisation has taken all the necessary steps to have a close look at its hospitals structure, planning and control system and communication network, etc. or not.
4. Whether an organisation has a sound Management Information System (MIS) or not.[16]
5. Whether the organisation has examined its various policies particularly those pertaining to personnel such as reward system (aspects like relating the successful and timely completion of high-priority objectives) to gain maximum out of MBO or not. However, some people do question about the appropriateness of this linkage.
6. Whether all or majority of the organisations members do have faith in participate philosophy or not which is the Kernel of MBO.
7. Whether the MBO programme is fully and continuously bolstered by the top management or not as it is essential to keep the system alive and functioning.

8. Whether competent and trained managers, administrators and professionals are manning the key positions or not.
9. Whether the organisation has tailored the MBO programme to suit its ingenuity and environment or not.
10. Whether the hospitals has groomed itself to cope with the changes in internal and external environments, changes in technology, changes in value system and rising expectations and aspirations of the people who are entering into work and type of people of tomorrow. If this does not take place, there is always a danger of MBO becoming a more ritualistic form filling exercise.
11. Whether the top management has the patience, and stamina to wait and watch for three to four years needed for its success, what Koontz describes as the Principle of Commitment.
12. Whether the management is ready to commit resources in terms of time and energy. For example, some type of Performas etc. might have to be filled. A lot of paper work is involved.
13. And finally, whether the necessary 'portfolio of instruments' such as appraisal system, satisfaction questionnaire, and review of the system itself, etc. have been developed to improve it to render it responsive to the changing conditions of the work environment which it is being practised or not.[17]

CONCLUSION

MBO can be an excellent tool in improving Hospital reduction administrative efficiency in a conducive hospitals environment of transparency, accountability, responsiveness and good governance.

To conclude in the words of P.R. Ramaswamy,[18] In government, goals and targets are very important. These are assigned to departments and functionaries. Though they provide aim for actions and objectives for functions, very little enthusiasm and commitment is generated among the employees. For changing this, it is necessary to give employees a vision. It is a detailed and easily understandable picture of what the organisation is striving for. This vision has to be translated into meaningful functions/activities/tasks/sub-tasks and the targets have to be assigned in consultation with the employees. These targets have to be translated into inputs and outputs in quantitative terms so that the realism involved in the vision is appreciated. The present planning programming, budgeting and performance budgeting have to be knit together closely and their link to the vision of each organisation established.

J. Phillips rightly suggests that sufficient efforts must be made before introducing MBO in any hospitals. MBO should not be introduced in an organisation as a crash programme. Sufficient ground work should be done before embarking on the MBO programme. This is very essential to ensure that MBO does not crashland. Above all, top management interest, understanding and commitment to MBO should be ensured before the start up. Or else, it is bound to go up as one more of those interesting but unprofitable experiments that organisations go through only too often.[19]

It has been mentioned in our ancient scriptures as well. Rigveda says that as an administrator the kind was instructed to work for universal brotherhood, peace and development of mankind, following MBO like approach. To quote Rig Veda:

> Common be your Prayers
> Common be your End,
> Common be your purpose,
> Common be your Deliberations,
> Common be your desires,
> Unified be your Hearts,
> Unified be your intentions,
> Perfect be the Union amongst you.

Notes and References

1. Peter Drucker, Practice of Management, 1954, pp. 135-36.
2. George S. Odoirne: Management by Objectives, New York, Pitman, 1965, p. 55.
3. W.J. Reddin, Effective Management by Objectives, New York, McGraw Hill, 1970.
4. Humble, J.W.: Improving Management Performance, London, Management Publications, 1969, p. 5.
5. Walter S. Wikstrom, Managing by—and with Objectives (New York; National Industrial Conference Board, 1968).
6. Dale D. McConkey, "MBO—Twenty Years Later, Where Do We stand?" *Business Horizons*, August 1973, pp. 25-36.
7. B.L. Maheshwari, Management by Objectives, Tata McGraw Hill, New Delhi, p. 17.
8. Stoner and Wankel, *op. cit.*, p. 99.
9. Maynard M. Gordon, The Lacocca Management Technique, A Bantam Book, 1987, pp. 11-13.
10. Fed Ludhana and Jerry L. Sellenin, "MBO in Hospitals: A Step Towards Accountability", *Personnel Administrator*, No. 7 (Oct. 1976), pp. 42-45. Quoted in Stoner and Wanket, *op. cit.*, p. 98.
11. Prior to taking up this assignment as administrator of a large non-profit hospital in Ottawa. Garry D. Cardiff has played a significant role in installing MBO in another non-profit hospital. Dale D. McConkey, Applying MBO to non-profit organisation, Quoted in Diane Borst and Patrick J. Montana, *op. cit.*, pp. 150-51.
12. Proceedings of the Seventh Annual Conference — November 29 to December 1. 1986, held at Bombay on Cost Reduction in Hospitals and Health Care, Indian Society of Health Administration, Bangalore, p. 172.
13. J.W. Humble, Improving Management Performances—A Dynamic Approach to Management by Objectives (Mimeographed) See also Stoner and Wankel, *op. cit.*, p. 101.
14. The Complexion of Organisation 20 years hence would be quite different from

what it is today and Peter Drucker would like to describe as Information-based Organisation—"Organisations composed largely of specialists who direct and discipline their own performance through organisational feedback from colleagues, customers, and headquarters." According to him, we are entering a third period of change, first one taking place in the tag end of 19th century that of distinction between ownership and management and second one around 1925 which saw the concept of modern corporation. It is the managerial challenge of the future. Peter F. Drucker, the coming of New Organisation, HBR, Jan-Feb. 1988, pp. 45-53. Hospitals have already entered into the Zone of information-based organisations.

15. Based upon an Article, "MBO in Hospitals" by Dr. K.K. Mangla in Hospital Adm. and Management, Deep and Deep Publications, pp. 285-313.

16. However, it is high time that we review, if not revise our thinking in the matter. Even in countries like Japan where life-long employment and seniority-based reward system has been in vogue, the system is under pressure. The reliance on seniority as the prime, if not sole, criterion may satisfy a large number but it brings frustration to competent people and the consequences are Medicare and sub-medicare rise in hierarchy and what follows has been beautifully described in his. . . .

    Please see A.S. Gupta, Managing the Public Sector.

    Government culture plays havoc, *Times of India*, Sept., 30, 1988, p. 6.

    Also see, John A. Hall, Management by Objectives and its application to Branch Banking, *Journal of the Institute of Bankers*, London, April, 1970.

17. M. Mushker J., Management by Objectives in the Provision of Social Services, the *Indian Journal of Public Administration*, Vol. XXVI, July-Sept. 1980, No. 3, p. 678.

18. P.R. Ramaswamy, Implementing TQM in Government, In, *Management in Government*, January-March, 2000, p. 14.

19. J. Phillip, Management By Objectives, in *Management in Government*, eds. (B.C. Mathur, Diesht, C. Chandrasekharan), in *Management in Government*, New Delhi, 1979, GOI, Ministry of Information and Broadcasting, p. 272.

BOOKS BY THE SAME AUTHOR

1. International Administration: WHO South East-Asia Regional Office (New Delhi, 1977), Sterling Publishers
2. Principles, Problems and Prospects of Co-operative Administration (New Delhi, 1979), Sterling Publishers (Co-Author Dr. B.B. Goel)
3. Administration of Personnel in Co-operative (New Delhi, 1979), Sterling Publishers (Co-Author Dr. B.B. Goel)
4. Health Care Administration: Ecology, Principles and Modern Trends (New Delhi, 1980), Sterling Publishers
5. Health Care Administration: Policy-making and Planning (New Delhi, 1980), Sterling Publishers
6. Health Care Administration: Levels and Aspects (New Delhi, 1980), Sterling Publishers
7. International Civil Service: Principles, Problems and Prospects (New Delhi, 1984), Sterling Publishers
8. Public Health Administration (New Delhi, 1984), Sterling Publishers
9. Public Personnel Administration (New Delhi, 1984), Reprint 1987, Sterling Publishers
10. International Civil Services—Principles, Problems and Prospectives (New Delhi, 1984), Sterling Publishers.
11. Social Welfare Administration: Theory and Practice (Vols. I and II) (New Delhi, 1988), Deep & Deep Publications Pvt. Ltd.
12. Hospital Administration and Management (ed.) Co-Author Dr. R. Kumar in 3 volumes (New Delhi, 1989), Deep & Deep Publications Pvt. Ltd.
13. Policy and Administration: Family Planning & Beyond (New Delhi, 1990), Deep & Deep Publications Pvt. Ltd.
14. Modern Management Techniques (Revised and Reprinted) (New Delhi, 1990), Deep & Deep Publications Pvt. Ltd.
15. Development Planning and Administration (ed.) S. Bhatnagar (Co-editor) (New Delhi, 1992), Deep & Deep Publications Pvt. Ltd.
16. Financial Administration and Management (New Delhi, 1993), Sterling Publishers
17. Advanced Public Administration (New Delhi, 1993), Sterling Publishers

18. Personnel Administration and Management
(New Delhi, 1994), Deep & Deep Publications Pvt. Ltd.
19. Educational Policy and Administration
(New Delhi, 1994), Deep & Deep Publications Pvt. Ltd.
20. Slum Improvement Through Participatory Urban Based Community Structures
(New Delhi, 1999), Deep & Deep Publications Pvt. Ltd.
21. Distance Education in 21st Century
(New Delhi, 2000), Deep & Deep Publications Pvt. Ltd.
22. Health Care System and Management: Organization and Structure
(New Delhi, 2000), Deep & Deep Publications Pvt. Ltd.
23. Health Care System and Management: Policies and Programmes
(New Delhi, 2000), Deep & Deep Publications Pvt. Ltd.
24. Health Care System and Management: Management and Administration
(New Delhi, 2000), Deep & Deep Publications Pvt. Ltd.
25. Heath Care System and Management: Primary Health Care Management
(New Delhi, 2000), Deep & Deep Publications Pvt. Ltd.
26. Management Techniques: Principles and Practices
(New Delhi, 2001), Deep & Deep Publications Pvt. Ltd.
27. Encyclopaedia of Disaster Management in 3 Volumes
(New Delhi, 2001), Deep & Deep Publications Pvt. Ltd.
28. Management of Hospitals: Hospital Core Services
(New Delhi, 2002), Deep & Deep Publications Pvt. Ltd.
29. Management of Hospitals: Hospital Supportive Services
(New Delhi, 2002), Deep & Deep Publications Pvt. Ltd.
30. Management of Hospitals: Hospital Preventive and Promotive Services
(New Delhi, 2002), Deep & Deep Publications Pvt. Ltd.
31. Management of Hospitals: Hospital Managerial Services
(New Delhi, 2002), Deep & Deep Publications Pvt. Ltd.
32. Public Personal Administration
(New Delhi, 2002), Deep & Deep Publications Pvt. Ltd.
33. Public Financial Administration
(New Delhi, 2002), Deep & Deep Publications Pvt. Ltd.
34. Urban Development and Management
(New Delhi, 2002), Deep & Deep Publications Pvt. Ltd.
35. Public Administration: Theory and Practices
(New Delhi, 2003), Deep & Deep Publications Pvt. Ltd.
36. Advanced Public Administration (Revised and Enlarged Edition)
(New Delhi, 2003), Deep & Deep Publications Pvt. Ltd.

37. Panchayati Raj in India
(New Delhi, 2003), Deep & Deep Publications Pvt. Ltd.
38. Encyclopedia of Higher Education in 21st Century: Organisation and Structure
(New Delhi, 2004), Deep & Deep Publications Pvt. Ltd.
39. Encyclopaedia of Higher Education in 21st Century: Quality and Excellence
(New Delhi, 2004), Deep & Deep Publications Pvt. Ltd.
40. Encyclopedia of Higher Education in 21st Century, Extension Education Services
(New Delhi, 2004), Deep & Deep Publications Pvt. Ltd.
41. Stress Management and Education: An Indian Perspective
(New Delhi, 2004), Deep & Deep Publications Pvt. Ltd.
42. Human Values and Education:
(New Delhi, 2004), Deep & Deep Publications Pvt. Ltd.
43. Public Health Policy and Administration
(New Delhi, 2004), Deep & Deep Publications Pvt. Ltd.
44. Administration and Management of NGO's: Text and Case Studies
(New Delhi, 2004), Deep & Deep Publications Pvt. Ltd.
45. Nursing Services: Management and Administration
(New Delhi, 2005), Deep & Deep Publications Pvt. Ltd.
46. Population Policy and Family Welfare Administration
(New Delhi, 2005), Deep & Deep Publications Pvt. Ltd.
47. Human Resource Development in 21st Century
(New Delhi, 2005), Deep & Deep Publications Pvt. Ltd.
48. Encyclopaedia of Disaster Management (3 Volumes)
(New Delhi, 2006) Deep & Deep Publications Pvt. Ltd.
49. School Health Education
(New Delhi, 2007), Deep & Deep Publications Pvt. Ltd.
50. Health Education: Theory and Practices
(New Delhi, 2007), Deep & Deep Publications Pvt. Ltd.
51. Good Governance: An Integral Views
(New Delhi, 2007), Deep & Deep Publications Pvt. Ltd.
52. Right to Information and Good Governance
(New Delhi, 2007), Deep & Deep Publications Pvt. Ltd.
53. Disaster Management: Text and Case Studies
(New Delhi, 2007), Deep & Deep Publications Pvt. Ltd.
54. Hospital Administration: Theory and Practices
(New Delhi, 2007), Deep & Deep Publications Pvt. Ltd.
55. Environmental Health Values and Education,
(New Delhi, 2008), Deep & Deep Publications Pvt. Ltd.

56. Administrative and Management Thinkers: Revelvance in New Millennium
(New Delhi, 2008), Deep & Deep Publications Pvt. Ltd.
57. Principles and Practices of Human Values
(New Delhi, 2008), Deep & Deep Publications Pvt. Ltd.
58. Distance Education: Principles, Potentialities and Perspectives
(New Delhi, 2008), Deep & Deep Publications Pvt. Ltd.
59. Educational Administration and Management: An Integral View
(New Delhi, 2008), Deep & Deep Publications Pvt. Ltd.
60. Women Health Education
(New Delhi, 2008), Deep & Deep Publications Pvt. Ltd.
61. Health Care System and Hospital Administration
Vol. 1 (Organizational Structure)
(New Delhi, 2008), Deep & Deep Publications Pvt. Ltd.
62. Health Care System and Hospital Administration
Vol. 2 (Resources: Human, Finance and Material)
(New Delhi, 2008), Deep & Deep Publications Pvt. Ltd.
63. Health Care System and Hospital Administration
Vol. 3 (Policy-making and Programmes)
(New Delhi, 2008), Deep & Deep Publications Pvt. Ltd.
64. Health Care System and Hospital Administration
Vol. 4 (Emerging and Thrust Areas)
(New Delhi, 2008), Deep & Deep Publications Pvt. Ltd.
65. Health Care System and Hospital Administration
Vol. 5 (Primary/Rural Health Care)
(New Delhi, 2008), Deep & Deep Publications Pvt. Ltd.
66. Health Care System and Hospital Administration
Vol. 6 (Secondary and Tertiary Health Care)
(New Delhi, 2008), Deep & Deep Publications Pvt. Ltd.
67. Health Care System and Hospital Administration
Vol. 7 (Management Techniques and Good Governance)
(New Delhi, 2008), Deep & Deep Publications Pvt. Ltd.
68. Education of Lifestyle and Lifetime Diseases
(Deep & Deep Publications Pvt. Ltd.)
69. Health Education Administration—From International Level to Village Level
(Deep & Deep Publications Pvt. Ltd.)
70. Education for Healthy Urban Cities
(Deep & Deep Publications Pvt. Ltd.)
71. Rural Health Education
(Deep & Deep Publications Pvt. Ltd.)

Bibliography

Acton Society Trust, Hospitals and the State: Hospital Organisation and Administration under the National Health Service Series, London: Action Society Trust, 1956, 54p.

Acton Society Trust, Hospitals and the State: Hospital Organisation and Administration under the National Health Service, London: The Trust, 1959, iii, 80p.

Andhra Pradesh, Health and Local Administration Department Panchayats Executive Officers Regulations relating to Recruitment, etc., Hyderabad: The Author, 1956, l6p.

Bannington, B.G., English Public Health Administration, 2nd ed., London: P.S. King, 1929, 325p.

Berkov, Robert, The World Health Organisation: A Study in Decentralized International Administration, Geneva Droz, 1957, 173p.

Better Health by Community Projects Administration, Planning Commission, New Delhi: Community Projects, Planning Commission, n.d., 32p.

Blum, Henrik L., Public Administration: A Public Health Viewpoint, N.Y.: Macmillan, 1963, 532p.

Hugh Flanagan and Peter Spurgeon, Public Sector Managerial Effectiveness: Theory and Practice in the National Health Service, Buckingham: Open Univ. Press, 1996, 128p.

Freeman, Ruth B., Administration of Public Health Services and Edward M. Holmes, Philadelphia: Saunders, 1960, 507p.

Goddard, H.A., Principles of Administration Applied to Nursing Service by H.A. Goddard, Geneva: World Health Organisation, 1958, 106p.

Goel, Rajneesh, Community Health Care, New Delhi: Deep & Deep Publications Pvt. Ltd., 2004, 403p.

Goel, S.L., Health and Care Administration: Policy-making and Planning, Delhi: Sterling, 1980, 288p.

Goel, S.L, Health Care Administration: Ecology, Principles and Modern Trends, Delhi: Sterling, 1980, 233p.

Goel, S.L., Health Care Administration: Levels and Aspects, Delhi: Sterling, 1980, 245p.

Goel, S.L., Health Care System and Management, New Delhi: Deep & Deep Publications Pvt. Ltd., 2004, 4 Vols.

Goel, S.L., International Administration: WHO South-East Asia Regional Office, Delhi: Sterling, 1977, 344p.

Goel, S.L., Population Policy and Family Welfare: Reproductive and Child Health Administration, New Delhi: Deep & Deep Publications Pvt. Ltd., 2005, 526p.

Goel, S.L., Public Health Administration, Delhi: Sterling, 1984, 472p.

Goel, S.L, Public Health Policy and Administration, New Delhi: Deep & Deep Publications Pvt. Ltd., 2005, 651p.

Graduate Study in Public Administration: A Guide to Graduate Programs by Office of Education, Department of Health, Education and Welfare, Washington: United States Government Printing Office, 1961, 158+p.

Greenfield, Margert, State-Local Service for Mental Health, Bureau of Public Administration, Berkeley: The Bureau, 1955, 93p.

Guangde, Sun, Health Care Administration in China, Westport: Greenport, 1993, pp. 53-62.

Handbook on Human Services Administration, edited by Jack Rabin and Marcia B. Steinhauer, New York: Marcel Dekker, 1988, 604p.

Health Policy Research in South Asia: Building Capacity for Reform, edited by Abdo S. Yazbeck and David H. Peters, Washington, D.C.: World Bank, 2003, 428p.

Heaver, Richard, Managing Primary Health Care: Implications of the Health Transition, Washington, D.C.: World Bank, 1995, 41p.

Health Status of the Underprivileged, New Delhi: Centre for Urban Studies, Indian Institute of Public Administration, 1991, 225p.

Indian Institute of Public Administration, Centre for Urban Studies, Urban Health System, edited by P.K. Umashankar and Girish K. Misra, New Delhi: Reliance and IIPA, 1993, 259p.

Institute for Training in Municipal Administration, Administration of Community Health Services, Chicago: ICMA, 1961, 560p.

Johnston, Timothy, Investing in Health: Development Effectiveness in the Health, Nutrition, and Population Sector, Washington, D.C.: World Bank, 1999, 69p.

Khandewale, Shreekant V., Health Administration and the Weaker Sections in an Indian Metropolis, Delhi: Devika, 1996, 231p.

Klinoubol, Kriengkrai, Public Health Development and Administration: A Study of Developing Economy, Delhi: Deep & Deep Publications Pvt. Ltd., 1989. 436p.

Local Self-Government Administration in States of India, 1956, New Delhi: Ministry of Health, 1956, 149p.

Local Self-government Administration in States of India, 1962, Ministry of Health, Delhi: The Manager of Publications, 1962, 161+p.

Legislature Committee on Local Administration by Health, Education and Local Administration Department, Madras, Madras: Health, Education and Local Administration Department, 1958, 5 Parts.

Morden, Margaret Gorsuch, Cooperative Health Administration in Metropolitan, Los Angeles: The Bureau, 1949, 52p.

Panchayat Manual, Madras: Health, Education and Local Administration Department, 1956, 368+p.

Papers in Public Administration, No. 6, Ann Arbor: The Bureau, 1950, 85p.

Public Services M.B.A. Induction Module: India-U.K. context (August-September, 1999: Indian Institute of Public Administration, New Delhi), Gender-related Issues (course material), New Delhi: Indian Institute of Public Administration, 1999, vp.

Report of the Regional Training Seminar on Social Security Administration, New Delhi: Regional Office for Asia and Oceania, 1979, 75p.

Rowbottom, R., Hospital Organisation: A Progress Report on the Brunel Health Services Project, London: Heinemann, 1973, 3l4p.

Survey of Research in Public Administration, 1980-90, edited by V.A. Pai Panandiker, Delhi: Konark, 1997, 631p.

Tebow, Hilda P., Staff-Development as an Integral Part of Administration, Washington, D.C.: Department of Health, Education and Welfare, 1959, 33+p.

The Indo-US Symposium on Community Mental Health at National Institute of Mental Health and Neuro Sciences, Bangalore: National Institute of Mental Health and Neuro Sciences, 1992, 520p.

Weaver, Jerry L., Conflict and Control in Health Care Administration, Beverly Hills: n.p., 1975, 197p.

Welfare Administration and Social Welfare Around the World, by Department of Health, Education and Welfare, United States, Washington: Government Printing Office, 1963, 9p.

Wishwakarma, R.K., Health Status of the Underprivileged, New Delhi: Centre for Urban Studies, Indian Institute of Public Administration, 1993, 283p.

Index